SAFE CARE IN PAEDIATRICS

SAFE CARE IN PAEDIATRICS

Alf Nicholson, FRCPCH, FRCPI
Professor and Vice President for Academic Affairs/Head of School of Medicine
Royal College of Surgeons in Ireland (RCSI), Bahrain
Kingdom of Bahrain

John Murphy, DCH, FRCPI
Consultant Neonatologist, The National Maternity Hospital, Holles Street, Dublin
Children's Hospital Ireland (CHI) at Temple Street
Associate Professor of Neonatology, Royal College of Surgeons in Ireland (RCSI)
National Clinical Lead in Neonatology Ireland

Sarah Taaffe, MRCPCH, MRCGP, Dip. IBLM
Assistant Scheme Director in GP Education, Former Paediatric Training Lead
Irish College of General Practitioners, Ireland

Kevin Dunne, DCH, FRCPCH
Professor of Paediatrics and Child Health, Department of Paediatrics
Royal College of Surgeons in Ireland (RCSI), Bahrain
Kingdom of Bahrain

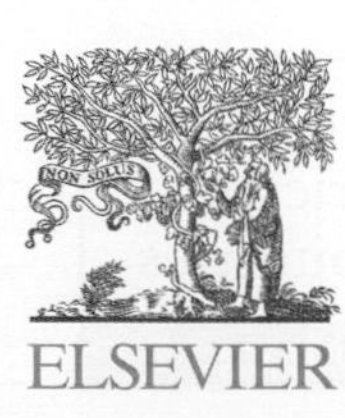

Notices

Practitioners and researchers must always rely on their own experience and knowledge in evaluating and using any information, methods, compounds or experiments described herein. Because of rapid advances in the medical sciences, in particular, independent verification of diagnoses and drug dosages should be made. To the fullest extent of the law, no responsibility is assumed by Elsevier, authors, editors or contributors for any injury and/or damage to persons or property as a matter of products liability, negligence or otherwise, or from any use or operation of any methods, products, instructions, or ideas contained in the material herein.

ISBN: 978-0-4431-0885-3

Content Strategist: Alexandra Mortimer
Content Project Manager: Ayan Dhar
Design: Miles Hitchen
Marketing Manager: Deborah Watkins

Printed in India

Last digit is the print number: 9 8 7 6 5 4 3 2 1

To all our families for their love and patience

—Alf, John, Sarah and Kevin

FOREWORD

It was with a genuine sense of anticipation that I read the latest paediatric textbook edited by Alf Nicholson, John Murphy, Sarah Taaffe and Kevin Dunne, titled *Safe Care in Paediatrics*.

With well over a hundred years of combined paediatric experience and expertise between them, I knew readers were in good hands. The content is not only enjoyable to read but also highly educational, relevant, informative and accessible.

I'd like to start at the end. The final chapter in this book delves refreshingly into the well-being and mental health of our colleagues – a topic that I suspect has rarely been examined in books like this, in years gone by. But with the peak of the COVID pandemic firmly in the rear-view mirror, we're now coming to grips with the alarming rates of burnout amongst healthcare staff. To see a full chapter dedicated to this important issue sends a powerful message. It is well known that there is a direct link between staff well-being and improved patient outcomes, and all of us have a role in creating a thriving work environment where staff feel secure, safe and valued.

Being involved in the care of sick children is a great privilege and with this comes great responsibility. Unfortunately, we won't always get everything right. Errors in healthcare occur every day and many are preventable through adequate systems of clinical governance. However, a no-blame culture is essential to promote not only the timely reporting of incidents but also importantly the opportunity to learn and implement strategies that reduce the likelihood of such incidents from occurring again. In reviewing significant incidents, it is common to examine the specific moments when an additional intervention, question or observation may have changed the clinical trajectory for a patient and led to an altogether different outcome. Often, these relate to human factors such as fatigue, cognitive bias or overload, and the critical importance of these in clinical incidents cannot be underestimated.

This book is unique in that it is written primarily through a safety lens with a clear focus on reducing avoidable harm. There is so much useful content crammed into these 20 short chapters that take readers on a journey from neonates through to adolescence, via subspecialties, and viewed through the different settings where paediatric care is delivered.

With a clear, predictable, and deliberate layout, individual chapters will quickly become familiar to readers. Chapters are short, are easy to read and provide readers with 'clinical pearls' and 'pitfalls to avoid' through a series of extremely well-illustrated 'clinical histories'. Although the clinical histories may be familiar to many in community and tertiary hospital settings, the level of detail provided is just right to ensure content is valuable to those working at the coalface, irrespective of where care is being provided or the level of experience of the provider. Whether you're a paediatric medical trainee, a community practice nurse, an allied health clinician, a hospital-based ward nurse, a paramedic or the most seasoned and experienced GP or specialist, there are nuggets of wisdom here for everyone.

The concept of teamwork, actively engaging with and listening to colleagues and parents, is an important theme throughout this book. It's understanding that 'none of us is as smart as all of us'. The 'three strikes and you are in' rule is as relevant today as it was when I started paediatric training. A key principle emphasised throughout is the importance of 'safety-netting'. Providing clear advice to parents regarding the expected clinical trajectory of an illness and resolution, what symptoms and signs to look out for when this does not occur and when to re-present for further review is not only good clinical practice but, when practiced repeatedly with discipline, will save lives.

A true strength of the book is its ability to relate to so many different professionals who work with children in both community and hospital settings. With this in mind, several chapters are particularly worth mentioning for their educational content. These include the chapters on newborn and 6-week examination, diagnosing cancer in childhood, child protection and safeguarding concerns and mental health issues in adolescence. I also found the chapter on ordering and interpreting tests in children highly valuable and informative, with extremely relevant advice on point-of-care and routine testing, allergy testing and ECG interpretation, all the way through to advanced genomic testing. Importantly, the focus throughout remains on avoiding pitfalls and potential mistakes when interpreting test results.

Given their combined experience, it must have been difficult for the editors to select 12 memorable diagnoses to present in the penultimate chapter. I personally challenged myself to see how early I could reach a diagnosis.

It was such a joy to read every individual chapter, not only by the editors themselves but also by the contributions from esteemed paediatric colleagues who have contributed so much to their individual fields, many of whom I have had the fortune of working with or knowing throughout my paediatric career. This book was always going to deliver in spades, and it does not disappoint.

By A/Prof Tom Connell,
Paediatrician and Chief Medical Officer,
Royal Children's Hospital Melbourne

PREFACE

The purpose of this textbook is to enable and support the reader in the medical care of children. The content covers hospital-based paediatrics, neonatology and general practice. The book has been written for all those charged with clinical decision-making in both the community and hospital, be they from a medical, nursing or healthcare and social care professional background.

We are particularly pleased that an experienced family doctor is part of our senior editorial team. We are especially keen that this book should resonate with both family doctors and trainees in both paediatrics and general practice.

Right at the core of acute paediatrics is a key conundrum. While the chance of a serious illness in infants, children or young people seen in family practice is low, the consequences of not recognising and treating serious illness are stark and can be devastating for both the family and the professionals involved.

Errors do happen relatively frequently in paediatrics and most are not associated with harm.

Now and then, sentinel events occur with serious consequences for a child and their family. The spirit of this book is to explore in detail pitfalls that, once we are aware of them, can perhaps be largely avoided.

Our aim is to promote safe care for newborns, children and adolescents. Using clinical case scenarios, we clearly identify symptoms and signs that should alert healthcare professionals and offer clear advice to show how mistakes can be avoided.

The book spans 20 chapters, with the opening 2 chapters shining a light on the science of safe care in children and innate parallels (and indeed differences) with the aviation industry. We concur with the view that errors in healthcare should be seen as precious learning opportunities that can and should be shared throughout the system. This shared learning aims to ensure that errors are not repeated. We explore the growing importance of artificial intelligence and are grateful for insightful editorial input from both Jamal Hashem and Zubin Daruwalla.

Topics in the early chapters include the recognition of the sick child and the approach to the child with a fever or a worrisome rash. These are major areas of concern in both primary care and the emergency department setting. We describe in detail rashes of concern and their potential clinical significance augmented by high-quality clinical images.

In the following chapters we use a symptom-based approach, taking the reader from a primary care setting all the way to a tertiary paediatric service. Each chapter has been edited by at least one subject matter expert, imparting their professional expertise to the reader.

We are truly indebted to our chapter editors for highlighting the key practical tips in management. In each chapter we cite typical clinical scenarios and describe clinical pearls and the pitfalls that should be avoided. We also describe challenges in the diagnosis of common cancers seen in children and adolescents where the mantra 'three strikes and you are in' is apt in that if a parent re-presents on three occasions with their child, then serious illness, including cancer, should be considered. We thank Drs Jennifer Kelly and Sarah Taaffe for offering a first-responder perspective in diagnosing cancer.

Adolescent mental health issues merit a detailed chapter in view of their frequency and we thank Professor Fiona McNicholas for her unique insights and Dr Anna Beug for reviewing the chapter.

We reflect on the importance of requesting and interpreting investigations: modern genomic tests as well as radiology are discussed with worked examples and an array of high-quality radiological images.

We appreciate that readers do like the ultra-rare 'once in a lifetime' diagnosis and we highlight 12 such cases in the penultimate chapter.

Finally, we look at the key area of promoting resilience and how to avoid so-called burnout in healthcare professionals dealing with children. This is a key area of concern for all professionals. Developing personal resilience, however, is only half the answer. Many of the factors that lead to burnout are organisational, and a systems approach to well-being is also crucial.

In this final chapter we are grateful to a number of contributors including Drs Reena Kotecha and Elaine Cooke, who kindly reviewed the chapter and offered helpful suggestions.

We are indebted to the skill and professionalism of the Elsevier publishing team led by Ms Alexandra Mortimer and Mr Ayan Dhar. We also thank Mr Fintan Foy, CEO, and Dr John Farrell, Chairperson of the Irish College of General Practitioners, for their collaborative effort in writing this book. Special thanks to Ms Bincy Mathew for her secretarial support through the many drafts. We thank Dr Bindhu Nair, Manager – Library & Learning Resource Centre RCSI Bahrain for her support in literature searches and retrieval.

Finally, we are grateful to Prof Tom Connell, Paediatrician and Chief Medical Officer at the Royal Children's Hospital in Melbourne, for kindly writing the foreword for this book.

We hope you enjoy and benefit from this book and that it serves as a companion book and helpful aid throughout your career.

Alf Nicholson
John Murphy
Sarah Taaffe
Kevin Dunne

CONTRIBUTORS

Carol Blackburn, RCPI, MB, BCh, BAO, BMedSci
Consultant in Paediatric Emergency Medicine
Department of Paediatric Emergency Medicine, Childrens Health Ireland (CHI) at Crumlin
Dublin, Ireland

Billy Bourke, MD, FRCPI
Consultant Paediatric Gastroenterologist/Associate Professor of Paediatrics
University College Dublin
National Childrens Research Centre, CHI at Crumlin Dublin, Ireland

Annemarie Broderick, FRCPI
Consultant Paediatric Gastroenterologist
CHI at Crumlin
Dublin, Ireland

Fiona Browne, MB, BCh, BAO, MSc, MRCPI
Consultant Dermatologist
CHI at Crumlin and Temple Street
Dublin, Ireland

Karina Butler, MB, BCh, BAO, MRCPI, FFPHMI (Hon.)
UCD Clinical Professor of Paediatrics
Paediatrician with a special interest in infectious diseases
CHI at Crumlin and Temple Street
Dublin, Ireland

Michael Capra, MBBCH, Dip. Obst., DCH, MMedSci (Clin Edu), FRCPI
Consultant Paediatric Oncologist, CHI at Crumlin
Dublin, Ireland

Ciaran Carthy
Airline Safety Auditor/Airline Captain (Retired)

Desmond Cox, FRCPI
Consultant Respiratory Paediatrician
CHI at Crumlin
Dublin, Ireland

Ellen Crushell, FRCPI, FRCPCH
Paediatrician with a special interest in metabolic disorders
CHI at Crumlin and Temple Street
Dublin, Ireland

Aisling Dunne, MB, BCh, BAO, MRCPI
Basic Specialist Paediatric Trainee
CHI at Temple Street
Dublin, Ireland

James Foley, MB, BCh, BAO, FRCEM, MSc, PgCert
Consultant in Emergency Medicine
Galway University Hospital
Galway, Republic of Ireland

Jamal Hashem, MBBCh, BAO, LRCPI (NUI), MRCSI, MSc (HCM)
Lecturer in Surgery and Academic Director of Artificial Intelligence
Royal College of Surgeons in Ireland (RCSI) Bahrain
Kingdom of Bahrain

Jonathan Hourihane, FRCPCH, FRCPI
Professor of Paediatrics and Child Health
Royal College of Surgeons in Ireland (RCSI)
Dublin, Ireland

Neale Kalis, MBChB, M Med (Stell Peads), FCP (SA Peads)
Consultant Paediatric Cardiologist, Mohammed bin Khalifa bin Salman Al Khalifa Specialist Cardiac Centre (MKCC), Kingdom of Bahrain and
Professor of Paediatrics, Royal College of Surgeons in Ireland (RCSI)
Bahrain, Kingdom of Bahrain

Sabine Maguire, MBE, MBBCh, MRCPI, FRCPCH
Honorary Research Fellow
Cardiff University
Cardiff, Wales, UK

Hani Malik, MB, BCh, BAO, ABFM, PGDip HPEd, MSc LIH, FHEA
Consultant Family Physician and Lecturer in Family Medicine
Royal College of Surgeons in Ireland (RCSI) Bahrain, Kingdom of Bahrain
Busaiteen, Bahrain

Niamh McGrath, MD, MRCPI
Paediatrician with a special interest in endocrinology
University College Hospital
Galway, Ireland

Fiona McNicholas, MB, MD, FRCPsych, Dip. Clin. Psychotherapy
Full Professor and Academic Lead in Child and Adolescent Psychiatry SMMS UCD
Consultant in Child and Adolescent Psychiatry
Department of Paediatric Liaison Psychiatry
Lucena Clinic, Rathgar, and CHI at Crumlin
Dublin, Ireland

Alan Mortell, MB, BCh, BAO, FRCSI, MD, FEBPS, FRCS (Paed. Surg.)
Associate Professor of Paediatric Surgery
Royal College of Surgeons in Ireland (RCSI)
Consultant Paediatric Surgeon
CHI at Crumlin and Temple Street
Dublin, Ireland

Ciaran O'Boyle, BSc, PhD, DipTheol, DipOrgLead
Professor of Psychology and Director of the Royal College of Surgeons in Ireland (RCSI)
Centre for Positive Health Science
Dublin, Ireland

James O'Byrne, PhD, MRCPI
Associate Professor in Genetics
Mater Hospital
Dublin, Ireland

Aengus O'Marcaigh, MD. FRCPI, FFPaed, FAAP
Consultant Paediatric Haematologist, CHI at Crumlin
Dublin, Ireland

Terence Prendiville, MD, FRCPI
Professor of Paediatric Cardiology, CHI at Crumlin
Dublin, Ireland

Michael Riordan, MD, FRCPCH
Paediatric Nephrologist
CHI at Crumlin and Temple Street
Dublin, Ireland

Amre Shahwan, MD, MRCPCH
Consultant Clinical Neurophysiologist and Epileptologist
Royal College of Surgeons in Ireland (RCSI)
CHI at Temple Street
Dublin, Ireland

Yusra Sheikh, MBChB, FFR RCSI, FRCR
Administrative Head of Radiology Department
CHI at Temple Street
Dublin, Ireland

CONTENTS

1

Towards Safer Care for Children

Alf Nicholson, Jamal Hashem

'We are what we repeatedly do. Excellence is not an act but a habit'.
—***Aristotle***

CHAPTER OUTLINE

SETTING THE SCENE

Successful medical care of children requires many things to go right, and that is exactly what happens in the vast majority of cases. Parents and families want healthcare professionals (nurses, allied health professionals, primary care doctors and paediatricians) they can trust and have confidence in. We need to be transparent with families and involve them in decisions relating to their children's health.

Significant progress has been reported in the UK in terms of child and adolescent health with improved glycaemic control in diabetes mellitus, reduced hospitalisations in both asthma and epilepsy and reduced teenage pregnancies. Child health inequalities and a rising prevalence of significant mental health and emotional disorders in adolescence are tougher nuts to crack.

As doctors, we tend to be perfectionists and may find it difficult to accept our own failures or admit we have made an error. Modern healthcare is complex. Success can only happen when we admit to our mistakes, learn from them and create a working environment and culture where it is 'safe' to fail. As expertly enunciated by Matthew Syed in his bestseller book titled *Black Box Thinking*,[1] the problem is not just the consequences of failure but also the attitude towards failure. For us in healthcare, it is about having the desire and tenacity to investigate the lessons that often exist when we fail but which we rarely exploit.

So often in healthcare, competence is equated with clinical perfection, and this perfection is in essence a grand illusion.[1] This contrasts quite starkly with the airline industry, where failure is seen as a precious learning opportunity for all pilots and airlines.[2] Quite often in healthcare, even if mistakes are detected, the learning opportunities do not flow through the system.

Doctors are sometimes oblivious to their mistakes because they have already reframed them. This means that doctors make the same mistakes over and over again while growing in the mistaken conviction that they are infallible.

As Eleanor Roosevelt said, '*Learn from the mistakes of others. You cannot live long enough to make them all yourself*'.

This book is all about exploring the potential pitfalls for the healthcare professional dealing with children to share the learning and avoid making the very same mistakes.

The key message is to think again when the child's clinical course is not in keeping with the initial diagnosis. This is termed cognitive dissonance. 'There is something different about this child's case' is often the first step on the pathway to the correct diagnosis. The confidence to escalate a case, where appropriate, is an important skill for every doctor dealing with children.

LIVING IN A DIGITAL WORLD

Future medical education will need to embrace advances in genomics, artificial intelligence (AI), robotics and online medicine.[3] A project termed the 100,000 Genomes Project[4] has already had an impact in enabling the practice of medicine to focus on being more predictive, preventive and personalised and to have both patient and family participation. Treatment of cystic fibrosis now focuses on which gene mutation is responsible.[5] The impact of robotics to date has been significant in surgical practice but a trained surgeon is still required to operate the robot.

While telemedicine, artificial intelligence (AI) and robotics will help in mitigating deficits in terms of the healthcare workforce, health professionals working in either family practice or in hospitals are very likely to continue to be the cornerstone of healthcare delivery. The role of doctors will inevitably change as AI is used to interpret electrocardiograms, skin lesions, radiology tests and pathology specimens with a fidelity approaching and, in time, superior to doctors. In truth, our brightest future is a symbiosis of doctors and AI working together, each augmenting the other.

AI has relevance to general practice as it may supplement or enhance diagnostic intelligence.[6,7] Several AI-based symptom checkers aim to increase the accuracy and reliability of advice and guidance to be given by a family doctor.[8] Unfortunately, symptom checkers are risk averse and they do tend to encourage users to seek advice from their family doctor when self-care would be both perfectly reasonable and safe.[7] We need to strike a balance between missing a serious illness in a child and completely overwhelming family practice surgeries or out-of-hours services.

A key element of any paediatric consultation is to monitor symptoms over time and certain new AI tools may help in this regard. Wearable biosensors may track important physiological data such as heart rate, respiratory rate, or temperature and offer helpful additional information and potentially simple, life-saving recommendations.

AI may have applications in the diagnosis of retinopathy of prematurity, where AI tools could help in the triage of retinal photographs.[9] Tools are in development that might help predict severe asthma or sepsis in children. There is an increasing utility for using AI as an aid to clinical judgement. In a family practice setting, AI appears to help most in deciding the most appropriate course of action to take (refer or not) rather than making a precise diagnosis.

> While it is highly unlikely that doctors will be completely replaced by technology, it is highly likely that any doctor who does not embrace technology will be replaced by one who does.

Therefore, AI will not replace diagnostic intelligence but has the potential to augment it.[7]

ELECTRONIC HEALTH RECORDS

Like them or loath them, electronic healthcare records (EHRs) are here to stay[10] (Fig. 1.1). EHRs obviate the need for bulky and chaotic charts, help to monitor progress in a child who is deteriorating and are always accessible.

EHRs are, as we have learned, vulnerable to cyberattacks.[11] It is true that EHRs may be plagued with excessive and often redundant information and may lack a clear structure. There is also the risk of taking 'cut and paste' shortcuts instead of entering a contemporary clinical assessment of the child's condition. EHRs need to be connected with family practice records in a seamless way, and this integration can be a challenge. EHRs are expensive to introduce and to maintain.

Remote access to EHRs enables doctors to access patient observations, radiology and laboratory results, clinic letters, emails and electronic prescriptions. Senior

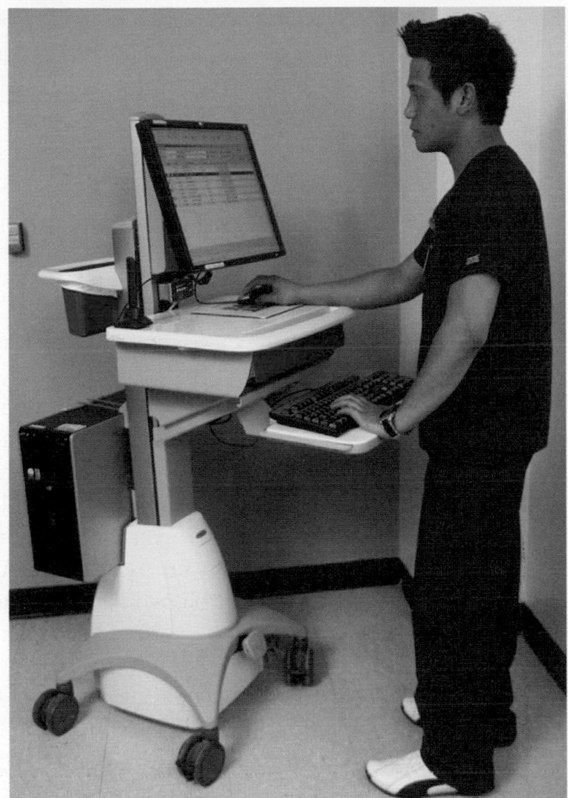

Fig. 1.1 The nursing assistant uses an electronic health record (electronic medical record). (Source: *Mosby's® Essentials for Nursing Assistants*. 7th ed. 2023.)

clinicians (who are often on call from home) may find remote access to the above data out of hours to give a very accurate reflection of the child's current status, and they may make changes to the child's treatment based on this remote access. This may serve to improve patient safety but may also promote 'micro-management', heightened anxiety and associated stress and burnout. In our view, it is hard to beat a further history and clinical examination of the child, and remote access to the EHR may take the on-site on-call team out of the key decision-making loop.

> Remote access may be very helpful for tertiary subspecialists to offer advice based on the latest trends in the child's condition and may help to justify formal transfer.

Medication errors are of particular concern as a new system is put in place. Other teething issues include delays in patient care and increased need for documentation with consequent delay in discharges.

CARE CLOSER TO HOME

Children and young people have fully embraced technology with over 90% possessing a mobile phone, and they are enthusiastic users of a variety of applications that improve their health. They now view technology to be part of everyday life. Technology may help to improve integration of care between the hospital and the community and is helpful in preventive care which is such a key part of child and adolescent health.

> Chronic illnesses such as diabetes, cystic fibrosis and sickle cell disease have been traditionally largely managed in a hospital setting, and new technologies enable more and more care to be delivered in a home or community setting which is far less expensive and favoured by families.

This care delivery model for chronic conditions helps reduce hospital attendance, allows the children to attend school more often and helps avoid days off work for parents. A 4-hour round trip for a 20-minute routine consultation does not make much sense and is not cost-efficient.

Telemedicine is helpful especially for families living in remote areas and may help reduce the need for hospital attendance and may provide timely advice to deal with symptom escalation enabling the child to remain at home.

The Digital Child Health Transformation Programme,[12] which commenced in the UK in 2021, will enable an online record of a child's health and development and enable goal setting for health and well-being of individual children. Technology will also help smoother transition to adult services for children with chronic conditions. For new technology, families and children need to be involved in every step of new innovations. All design should focus on being user-friendly.

SAFE PRACTICE FOR PRIMARY CARE PRACTITIONERS

One of the key challenges is supporting primary care doctors in this fast-changing and developing world of modern paediatrics. Most have received just 6 weeks of undergraduate training and thereafter 3 to 6 months in hospital-based paediatrics.

There is no doubt that the provision of healthcare in a primary care setting (largely in family practice) has become increasingly complex, and this relates to the pressures of short consultation times, the increasingly complex nature of children with chronic disease or multiple morbidities and the fragmented nature of service delivery between primary and secondary care.[13] An accurate estimation of the frequency of adverse events in primary care is very difficult, and the use of malpractice claims brought against family doctors is not a reliable proxy measure of adverse events in primary care.

Family doctors play a key role, and their workload is very high. The average time spent in a consultation (child or adult) is under 10 to 15 minutes. Children account for 25% of attendances in general practice. Overall, the number of children referred to the hospital services is just over 2% but comfort with children, limited training in paediatrics and a prior adverse clinical event involving a child may lead to a rise in referral rates. Among a high number of children seen with minor illness will be a small number of children with a serious underlying diagnosis and picking these out is very challenging (Fig. 1.2). In each chapter, we will focus with clinical scenarios on how the infant or child may present to their primary care doctor.

A detailed systematic review of malpractice claims in primary care was published in 2013. This showed that claims involving family doctors have greatly increased and, in Australia, they were the group with the highest number of malpractice claims.[13]

> Delay in diagnosis is the medical misadventure most often cited against family doctors.

This may include a failure to order a diagnostic test or to create a proper follow-up plan, failure to obtain an adequate history or perform a physical examination or the incorrect interpretation of a diagnostic test. [14]

For children under 24 months of age, dehydration, meningitis and developmental dysplasia of the hip were the conditions most involved in claims against family doctors.

For children from 2 to 12 years of age, pneumonia, malignancy and appendicitis were the claims most often cited against family doctors and, for adolescents, trauma, torsion of the testis and malignancy.

> Missed or delayed diagnosis of meningitis accounted for just 1 in 100 claims but accounted for 30% of overall settlements against GPs.[13]

Shortcuts in reasoning (or heuristics) are an important entity in faulty decision making. Family doctors may be tempted to go for the common diagnosis and may also maintain initial impressions despite the child not improving (termed 'anchoring heuristics'). In primary care there is often a lower prevalence of serious disease, and this further challenges the doctor to formulate an appropriate list of differential diagnoses, gather information to test these diagnostic possibilities and then go on to accept or reject these differential diagnoses.[13]

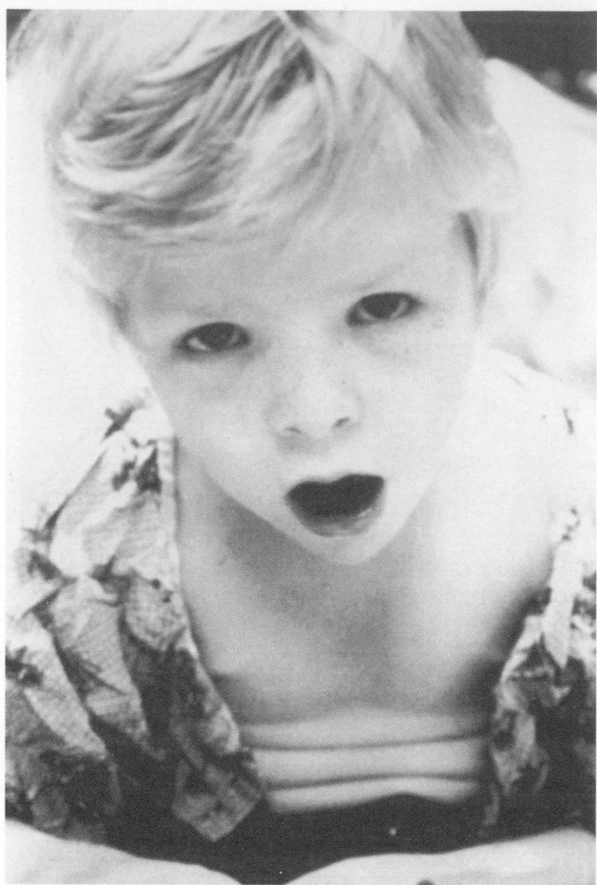

Fig. 1.2 Child with epiglottitis. Characteristic posture in a patient with epiglottitis. The child is leaning forward and drooling and the neck is hyperextended. (Source: from Sharma, Anjali, et al. In Kliegman RM, Lye PS, Bordini B, Toth H, & Basel D, (eds.). *Nelson Pediatric Symptom-based Diagnosis*. Elsevier; 39–60.e1.)

For any doctor, facing a malpractice claim has very serious implications. One clinical implication can be the subsequent practice of defensive medicine with resultant over-referral and over-investigation and a morbid fear of further litigation. Doctors facing litigation proceedings experience very high levels of psychological stress and may consider leaving medicine or early retirement.

INTEGRATING ACUTE SERVICES FOR CHILDREN

There are many examples of integrated care models and most involve a consultant paediatrician joining a primary care network with joint clinics, 'hot lines' and a very strong connectivity between those in the community and those working in a hospital. Key elements of success are open access to specialist advice, regular multidisciplinary meetings, and parental education. These models do reduce unnecessary urgent care activity. This helps to build strong professional relationships between those working in the community and those in hospital.

Therefore, in complex health systems, care of the highest quality depends on 'joined up' care that is focused on patient and family needs. Integration of care will improve health outcomes and child and family experiences. Communication deficits between healthcare professionals and poor communication with parents are frequently cited as key in medico-legal cases involving children.

> The key to a successful healthcare system for children and adolescents is bridging that gap between primary and secondary care.

The debate as to whether primary care paediatricians might offer a better health service for children in countries such as the UK and Ireland still rages on.[15–18] There is little evidence that primary care paediatricians alone would improve health outcomes and many feel that better training of family doctors and a more integrated model of care (as outlined above) would offer a better and more sustainable solution. We should adopt more flexible models with child health family practice hubs, additional advanced nurse practitioners with special skills in paediatrics in the community and, in the new world of artificial intelligence, the expansion of virtual opinions from paediatric specialists as required. Increasing access to diagnostics and extending family practice training in paediatrics would both help. A far greater integration of training curricula in paediatrics and general practice would be of benefit.

> Most (if not all) family doctors view looking after children as one of the core purposes and joys of being a family doctor.

PROMOTING DIAGNOSTIC EXCELLENCE IN HOSPITAL

Paediatricians have described how, in a hospital setting, they are aware of, on average, one or two diagnostic errors leading to harm per year which equates to 30 to 60 such errors over a 30-year career in paediatrics.

Making a diagnosis is, at times, a complex process where the child's symptoms evolve, multiple interactions with healthcare professionals occur and where new information may surface over time. Diagnostic errors may result from the inadequate gathering of data, inadequate processing of information or application of knowledge.[19]

Doctors should seek diagnostic feedback by keeping a record of patients where the diagnosis remains elusive, engaging in peer discussion around challenging cases and actively seeking feedback from colleagues.

The use of smartphone apps, social media and journal websites help to add concise summaries of a wide range of presentations and thereby increase the number of children 'seen' each day.

Always take a brief pause to reflect on whether an alternative diagnosis might be entertained.

Finally, try to foster critical thinking in everyday practice and always consider diagnoses as provisional and therefore subject to revision.[19] Always maintain a healthy scepticism, especially with children who come to see you already with a diagnostic label.

> Most often diagnostic error is a result of human rather than systems error.

Errors in clinical reasoning are more likely when heuristics are invoked. In essence heuristics are patterns of recognition or 'rules of thumb' and are very useful in situations where there are high volumes of patients. The key element of a clinical consultation is knowing when to move from heuristics to a more deliberate analytical approach, and occasionally we fail as paediatricians in that step. Most frontline paediatricians and family doctors rely on their intuition, but the clear lesson is that if the child is not improving or is indeed deteriorating, a more analytical approach is required to look for rarer diagnoses. Heuristic processes are especially prone to error when the presentation is atypical (such as fever only in Kawasaki disease or an atypical presentation of acute appendicitis).

> A team approach is essential in hospital practice on the basis of the principle 'none of us is as smart as all of us'.

Team Discussions, Communication and Medical Handover

A key strategy to reduce diagnostic error involves making diagnostic reasoning a team sport by engaging in interprofessional 'huddles' either after outpatient clinics or prior to or following inpatient rounds.

This team discussion during or after the ward round or at the end of the outpatient session allows for deeper analysis of the presenting symptoms and the potential to explore rarer diagnoses and a healthy scepticism in readily accepting the diagnosis. Team members from a variety of disciplines (such as the nursing team and health and social care professionals) add further depth to the discussion. Try to meet with and seek advice from key professionals such as those working in laboratory medicine, radiology and pathology. In these conversations, prior diagnostic evaluations are unpacked in detail and new and perhaps rarer diagnoses are entertained.

Handover is, without doubt, a critical item in a doctor's toolbox. Handover may be rushed and may have interruptions and distractions where vital pieces of information may be lost. This may lead to what is said not being heard or understood and what is understood may not be done. We certainly need to look at ways to improve medical handover.[20]

In summary we all use heuristics (in essence 'rules of thumb') to good effect in dealing with regular presentations of illness in children, and the real challenge as specialists is to know and sense when we should dispense with heuristics and take a deeper and more analytical approach. This skill is not easily attained and requires a team approach and an ever-curious mind with lots of humility.

> We should always try to pick out that single child from the ward round or clinic where the symptoms do not quite fit and use analytical reasoning, and this approach is the best way to reduce diagnostic errors.

Making a correct and timely diagnosis while using the fewest resources, managing uncertainty and improving patient experience all lead to diagnostic excellence[19] (Table 1.1).

TABLE 1.1 Improving Diagnostic Excellence in Clinicians
Seek and learn from feedback from a variety of sources
Be digitally aware and use e-resources
Address bias in clinical decision making
Work as a team of healthcare professionals and learn from each other
Practice reflective and critical thinking

Adapted from Singh H, Connor DW, Dhaliwal G. Five strategies for clinicians to advance diagnostic intelligence. *BMJ* 2022:376e068044/doi:101136/bmj-2021-068044.

MEDICATION SAFETY

Children are a high-risk population for medication errors due to weight-based dosing, dilution to administer small volumes, their inability to self-administer medication or to communicate reliably side effects and immature hepatic and renal systems of drug metabolism.[21]

> Medication errors can occur during any step of the medication process. These steps include prescribing, transcribing, dispensing, administration, and the monitoring of medications.

Computerised Prescription Order Entry

Most EHRs have computerised prescription order entry (CPOE) and the benefits of CPOE include elimination of illegible orders and reliable clinical decision support tools to help clinicians with medication orders. CPOE does reduce the risk of medication errors (Fig. 1.3).

Pharmacists

Pharmacists play a key role especially in an intensive care setting and their professional input has been found to reduce the frequency of medication errors. Attendance of pharmacists at ward rounds helps with complex patients, medication reconciliation and potential drug interactions.

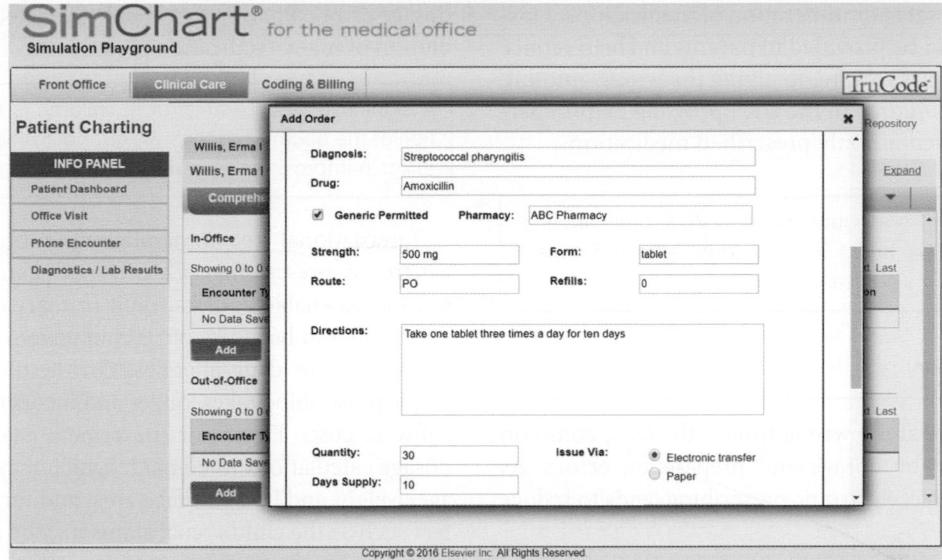

Fig. 1.3 With e-prescribing, providers can enter the prescription information into the electronic health record and send it to the pharmacy. The pharmacist can easily read the information, which reduces the chance of errors. (*Kinn's Medical Assisting Fundamentals: Administrative and Clinical Competencies With Anatomy & Physiology*. 2nd ed. 2022.)

Dispensing Medications

Mobile applications and workflow management systems are available to assist the process from medication ordering to dispensing, but constant updating is required.

Barcoding and Medication Administration

Barcoding administration systems will decrease administration errors. Barcodes confirm the identity of the child and the medication to be administered. These have been shown to be very effective in reducing administration errors by up to 50%. During medication rounds, distractions and interruptions need to be reduced, and one way is for the two nurses involved to each wear a plastic apron of a particular colour to signify they are on a medication round and should not be disturbed.

SMART Pumps

Safe medication administration through technologies (or SMART) pumps are infusion delivery systems that help to reduce reliance on memory when calculating infusion pump doses and rates of infusion. This technology has the potential to reduce medication errors including the overdosing of high-risk medications[21] (Fig. 1.4).

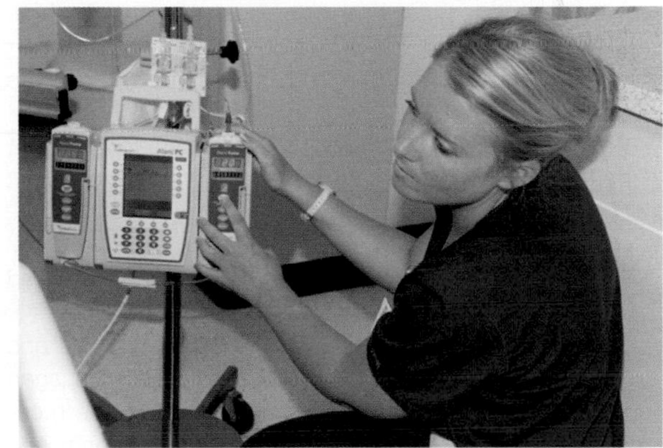

Fig. 1.4 Smart pumps offer integration between the pump and the electronic health record, including auto-pump programming. (*Leading and Managing in Nursing*. 8th ed. 2023.)

MEDICATION SAFETY IN THE COMMUNITY

Sadly, parents may be reluctant to use standard dosing instruments, preferring to revert to a 'teaspoon' or 'tablespoon', and this may lead to inaccuracies in administration. Initiatives to improve medication safety in the community include improvements in packaging, dose standardisation and education regarding the importance of safe administration of medications. Dosing tools should be provided to parents and help reduce medication errors relating to giving the wrong amount. *Medicines for Children* in the UK[22] provides helpful parent leaflets for commonly prescribed medications.

> Medication errors account for 10 to 20% of all adverse events in the UK and 1 in 15 children admitted experience a clinically significant prescribing error.[23]

THE IMPACT

Giving the dose at the wrong time is the most common error, followed by dosage and preparation errors. As mentioned above, electronic prescribing tends to reduce dosage errors. Pharmacists enable the detection and resolution of many medication errors.

> A significant source of error in children is the prescription of the doctor, and thus we all should invest time and effort in improving the quality of prescribing.

International recommendations now all support electronic prescribing (CPOE) and clinical decision support to enable doctors (both primary care and paediatricians) to be aware of risks of adverse effects, drug interactions or drug allergies. On the downside, electronic prescribing takes longer and incurs hardware and software costs. Electronic prescribing enables complex dosage calculations to be made which may be based on age, weight and body surface area, and further parameters such as the child's renal status may be added in.

KEY LEARNING POINTS

Patient safety is an integral part of quality care and should not be seen as a luxury. Parents of sick children (and indeed the children themselves) need to leave the consultation with a sense of resolution. Families need to feel that the focus has been on them, that their clinician has listened, paid attention and shown due concern.[24]

It does appear that AI has a big future in healthcare, but it does need human creativity to make it both relevant and practical.

Smartphone technology and algorithms may be especially useful to treat children living in remote, underserved regions with little paediatric expertise available.

Chronic illnesses such as diabetes, cystic fibrosis and sickle cell disease have been traditionally largely managed in a hospital setting, and new technologies enable more and more care to be delivered in a home or community setting which is far less expensive and favoured by families.

All new applications of technology need feedback and input from patients and families prior to widespread implementation. Families should be involved in each step of innovation to ensure that the product is fit for purpose.

Missed or delayed diagnosis of meningitis accounted for just 1 in 100 claims but accounted for 30% of overall settlements against family doctors.[13]

In primary care there is often a lower prevalence of serious disease, and this further challenges the family doctor to formulate an appropriate list of differential diagnoses, gather information to test these diagnostic possibilities and then go on to accept or reject these differential diagnoses.

For a primary care doctor or paediatrician, facing a malpractice claim has very serious implications. One clinical implication can be the subsequent practice of defensive medicine with resultant over-referral and over-investigation and a morbid fear of further litigation.[13]

Inter-professional communication and handover are key in reducing diagnostic error and in picking up clinical deterioration.

Medication safety has particular relevance to paediatrics.

New interventions that have become increasingly popular include computerised provider order entry (CPOE) with additional clinical decision support, barcoding technology, SMART pumps, and innovative workflow management systems.

Initiatives to improve medication safety in the community include improvements in packaging, dose standardisation and education regarding the importance of safe administration of medications.

REFERENCES

1. Syed M. *Black Box Thinking. Marginal gains and the secrets of high performance*. John Murray Publishers; 2020.
2. Kapur N, Parand A, Soukup T, Reader T, Sevdalis N. Aviation and healthcare: a comparative review with implications for patient safety. *JRSM Open*. 2015 Dec 2;7(1):2054270415616548. doi:10.1177/2054270415616548.
3. Stephenson T. RCGP William Pickles Lecture 2019: Training tomorrow's doctors, 1851–2051. *Br J Gen Pract*. 2019 Sep 26;69(687):515–516. doi:10.3399/bjgp19X705929.
4. 100,000 Genomes Project Pilot Investigators, Smedley D, Smith KR, et al. 100,000 Genomes Pilot on Rare-Disease Diagnosis in Health Care – Preliminary report. *N Engl J Med*. 2021;385(20):1868–1880. doi:10.1056/NEJMoa2035790.
5. Maule G, Arosio D, Cereseto A. Gene therapy for cystic fibrosis: progress and challenges of genome editing. *Int J Mol Sci*. 2020 May 30;21(11):3903. doi:10.3390/ijms21113903.
6. Li L. Artificial intelligence and diagnosis in general practice. *Br J Gen Pract*. 2019 Aug 29;69(686):430. doi:10.3399/bjgp19X705197.
7. Summerton N, Cansdale M. Artificial intelligence and diagnosis in general practice. *Br J Gen Pract*. 2019;69(684):324–325. doi:10.3399/bjgp19X704165.
8. Miller S, Gilbert S, Virani V, Wicks P. Patients' utilization and perception of an artificial intelligence-based symptom assessment and advice technology in a British primary care waiting room: exploratory pilot study. *JMIR Hum Factors*. 2020 Jul 10;7(3):e19713. doi:10.2196/19713.
9. Ting DSW, Pasquale LR, Peng L, et al. Artificial intelligence and deep learning in ophthalmology. *Br J Ophthalmol*. 2019;103(2):167–175. doi:10.1136/bjophthalmol-2018-313173.
10. Ranaweera M, Sharma V, Manna SS. NHS paediatric consultants' remote access to electronic health record: love it, loath it but won't get rid of it. *Arch Dis Child*. 2019;104(10):1019. doi:10.1136/archdischild-2019-317945.
11. Jercich K. HHS Cyber Arm Warns of EHR Vulnerabilities. 2022. Accessed at https://www.healthcareitnews.com/news/hhs-cyber-arm-warns-ehr-vulnerabilities
12. *Digital Child Health Transformation Programme*. NHS. Accessed at https://www.england.nhs.uk/digitaltechnology/child-health/#:~:text=The%20new%20Healthy%20Children%3A%20transforming,all%20children%20get%20the%20best
13. Wallace E, Lowry J, Smith SM, Fahey T. The epidemiology of malpractice claims in primary care: a systematic review. *BMJ Open*. 2013 Jul 18;3(7):e002929. doi:10.1136/bmjopen-2013-002929.
14. Gandhi TK, Kachalia A, Thomas EJ, et al. Missed and delayed diagnoses in the ambulatory setting: a study of closed malpractice claims. *Ann Intern Med*. 2006;145(7):488–496. doi:10.7326/0003-4819-145-7-200610030-00006.
15. Newson TP. Would primary care paediatricians improve UK child health outcomes? Yes. *Br J Gen Pract*. 2020 Mar 26;70(693):195–196. doi:10.3399/bjgp20X709229.
16. Ridd MJ, Thompson MJ. Would primary care paediatricians improve UK child health outcomes? No. *Br J Gen Pract*. 2020 Mar 26;70(693):196–197. doi:10.3399/bjgp20X709289.
17. Patel S, Hodgkinson T, Fowler R, Pryde K, Ward R. Integrating acute services for children and young people across primary and secondary care. *Br J Gen Pract*. 2020 Mar 26;70(693):158–159. doi:10.3399/bjgp20X708917.
18. Viner RM, Hargreaves DS. A forward view for child health: integrating across the system to improve health and reduce hospital attendances for children and young people. *Arch Dis Child*. 2018;103(2):117–118. doi:10.1136/archdischild-2017-314032.
19. Singh H, Connor DW, Dhaliwal G. Five strategies for clinicians to advance diagnostic intelligence. *BMJ*. 2022:376e068044. doi:10.1136/bmj-2021-068044.
20. Morgan M. Matt Morgan: the medical handover is broken. *BMJ*. 2022 Aug 30;378:o2091. doi:10.1136/bmj.o2091.
21. Kahn S, Abramson EL. What is new in paediatric medication safety? *Arch Dis Child*. 2019;104(6):596–599. doi:10.1136/archdischild-2018-315175.
22. *Medicines for Children UK*. Accessed at https://www.medicinesforchildren.org.uk/
23. Sutherland A, Phipps DL, Tomlin S, Ashcroft DM. Mapping the prevalence and nature of drug related problems among hospitalised children in the United Kingdom: a systematic review. *BMC Pediatr*. 2019;19(1):486. doi:10.1186/s12887-019-1875-y. Published 2019 Dec 11.
24. Kneebone R. Dissecting the consultation. *Lancet*. 2019;393(10183):1795. doi:10.1016/S0140-6736(19)30898-0.

ADDITIONAL READING

Bordini BJ, Stephany A, Kliegman R. Overcoming diagnostic errors in medical practice. *J Pediatr*. 2017;185:19–25. e1. doi:10.1016/j.jpeds.2017.02.065.

Cheung R, Shah R, McKeown R, Viner RM. State of child health: how is the UK doing? *Arch Dis Child*. 2021;106(4):313–314. doi:10.1136/archdischild-2020-319367.

Clark H, Coll-Seck AM, Banerjee A, et al. A future for the world's children? A WHO-UNICEF-Lancet Commission [published correction appears in Lancet. 2020 May 23;395(10237):1612]. *Lancet*. 2020;395(10224):605–658. doi:10.1016/S0140-6736(19)32540-1.

Clarke SL, Parmesar K, Saleem MA, Ramanan AV. Future of machine learning in paediatrics. *Arch Dis Child*. 2022;107(3):223–228. doi:10.1136/archdischild-2020-32102.

Dambha-Miller H, Everitt H, Little P. Clinical scores in primary care. *Br J Gen Pract*. 2020 Mar 26;70(693):163. doi:10.3399/bjgp20X708941.

Dimitri P. Child health technology: shaping the future of paediatrics and child health and improving NHS productivity. *Arch Dis Child*. 2019;104(2):184–188. doi:10.1136/archdischild-2017-314309.

Hill ID. Using QI to break bad habits. *J Pediatr*. 2020;225:1. Accessed at. https://www.jpeds.com/article/S0022-3476(20)31001-5/fulltext.

Holmes SM, Hansen H, Jenks A, et al. Misdiagnosis, mistreatment, and harm – When medical care ignores social forces. *N Engl J Med*. 2020;382(12):1083–1086. doi:10.1056/NEJMp1916269.

Jones D, Dunn L, Watt I, Macleod U. Safety netting for primary care: evidence from a literature review. *Br J Gen Pract*. 2019;69(678):e70–e79. doi:10.3399/bjgp18X700193.

Kickbusch I, Piselli D, Agrawal A, et al. The Lancet and Financial Times Commission on governing health futures 2030: growing up in a digital world. *Lancet*. 2021;398(10312):1727–1776. doi:10.1016/S0140-6736(21)01824-9.

Kneebone RL. Performing magic, performing medicine. *Lancet*. 2017;389:148–149. doi:10.1016/S0140-6736(17)30011-9.

Kneebone R, Houstoun W, Houghton N. Medicine, magic, and online performance. *Lancet*. 2021;398(10314):1868–1869. doi:10.1016/S0140-6736(21)02485-5.

Koller D, Rummens A, Le Pouesard M, et al. Patient disclosure of medical errors in paediatrics: a systematic literature review. *Paediatr Child Health*. 2016;21(4):e32–e38. doi:10.1093/pch/21.4.e32.

Leigh S, Mehta B, Dummer L, et al. Management of non-urgent paediatric emergency department attendances by GPs: a retrospective observational study. *Br J Gen Pract*. 2020 Dec 28;71(702):e22–e30. doi:10.3399/bjgp20X713885.

Marchalik D, Melnick E. Physicians in the digital age. *Lancet*. 2022;399(10321):231. doi:10.1016/S0140-6736(22)00021-6.

McAuliffe E, Hamza M, McDonnell T, et al. Children's unscheduled primary and emergency care in Ireland: a multimethod approach to understanding decision making, trends, outcomes and parental perspectives (CUPID): project protocol. *BMJ Open*. 2020 Aug 13;10(8):e036729. doi:10.1136/bmjopen-2019-036729.

Montejo M, Paniagua N, Saiz-Hernando C, Martinez-Indart L, Mintegi S, Benito J. Initiatives to reduce treatments in bronchiolitis in the emergency department and primary care. *Arch Dis Child*. 2021;106(3):294–300. doi:10.1136/archdischild-2019-318085.

Neighbour R. Safety netting: now doctors need it too. *Br J Gen Pract*. 2018;68(670):214–215. doi:10.3399/bjgp18X695849.

Neighbour R. *The Inner Consultation*. Kluwer Academic Publishers; 1987.

Ong C, Kachalia A. Safe harbors: liability reform for patients and physicians. *Bull Am Coll Surg*. 2013;98(3):41–44.

Perrem LM, Fanshawe TR, Sharif F, Plüddemann A, O'Neill MB. A national physician survey of diagnostic error in paediatrics. *Eur J Pediatr*. 2016;175(10):1387–1392. doi:10.1007/s00431-016-2772-0.

Shah A. Using data for improvement. *BMJ*. 2019 Feb 15;364:l189. doi:10.1136/bmj.l189.

Størdal K, Wyder C, Trobisch A, Grossman Z, Hadjipanayis A. Overtesting and overtreatment-statement from the European Academy of Paediatrics (EAP). *Eur J Pediatr*. 2019;178(12):1923–1927. doi:10.1007/s00431-019-03461-1.

Summerton N, Cansdale M. Artificial intelligence and diagnosis in general practice. *Br J Gen Pract*. 2019;69(684):324–325. doi:10.3399/bjgp19X704165.

Tou S, Wolthuis A, Gallagher AG. What surgeons can learn from other professionals – And not just from the pilots! *Colorectal Dis*. 2021;23(12):3059–3060. doi:10.1111/codi.15998.

The Future of Child Health Services: New Models of Care (2016). Nuffield Trust. 2016. Accessed at https://www.nuffieldtrust.org.uk/research/the-future-of-child-health-services-new-models-of-care

The Lancet. Patient safety is not a luxury. 2016;387(10024):1133. doi:10.1016/S0140-6736(16)30003-4.

The Lancet. Patient safety: too little, but not too late. *Lancet*. 2019;394(10202):895. doi:10.1016/S0140-6736(19)32080-X.

The Lancet. Can digital technologies improve health? *Lancet*. 2021;398(10312):1663. doi:10.1016/S0140-6736(21)02219-4. health and wellbeing in early childhood (2018). www.nuffieldtrust.org.uk.

The Nuffield Trust. International comparisons of health and wellbeing in early childhood. 2018. Accessed at https://www.nuffieldtrust.org.uk/research/international-comparisons-of-health-and-wellbeing-in-early-childhood.

2

Responding to Errors

Ciaran Carthy, Alf Nicholson

'To err is human, to cover up is unforgivable and to fail to learn is inexcusable'.
— Sir Liam Donaldson (2004)

CHAPTER OUTLINE

One of the great challenges in modern healthcare is to reduce preventable harm in both community and hospital settings. There has been an increasing recognition that doctors and other healthcare professionals simply cannot get it right all the time.

Diagnostic error includes unintentional diagnostic delays and missed or wrong diagnoses. Diagnostic error is indeed a 'blind spot' as such errors are rarely reported. Learning from diagnostic errors occurs infrequently in medicine.

Medicine has gained ideas from other high-risk industries, and we are now aware of human fallibility in flying airplanes, operating nuclear power stations or aircraft carriers. The airline industry acknowledges that human error can never be eliminated. In consequence, the primary focus in aviation is the mitigation of human error to be as low as reasonably practicable (termed the ALARP model).[1]

THE SCIENCE OF SAFER CARE FOR CHILDREN

We all know that humans are fallible, and therefore we need to focus on creating conditions under which professionals work to build defences and to mitigate errors.

> Three key elements in establishing a safe culture are reporting, flexibility and learning.

What is required is a structured investigation of events leading to an error or potential error, consistent and repeated technical and non-technical skills training, the promotion of resilience with adequate debriefing after events and team training in simulated environments. In a simulated environment, junior members should be encouraged to respectfully challenge more senior members when concerned about safety.

CULTURE OF RECORDING

We need to develop a culture of recording whereby data about adverse events is collected, analysed and disseminated.

> Frontline staff should be encouraged to report errors or adverse events without fear of sanction.[2]

Both families and staff should be able to communicate concerns easily and confidentially and receive timely and helpful feedback.

JUST CULTURE

We need to promote a just culture whereby the approach is firstly non-punitive and where human fallibility is acknowledged. However, there may be a small number of professionals who intentionally fail to adhere to policies and procedures and who must be held accountable for their actions.[2]

> In aviation, safety investigations and recommendations are not concerned with apportioning blame or liability. Their sole purpose is the prevention of future incidents and accidents.

FLEXIBILITY

Healthcare is constantly required to adapt to changing demands such as those placed on the system by the recent pandemic. Flexibility relies on teamwork, shared values, standard operating procedures, investment in training and prospective risk assessment.

A CULTURE OF LEARNING

This culture enables professionals to practice evidence-based medicine and to learn from both their mistakes and the mistakes of others. The use of root cause analysis helps to share the learning right throughout the system where mistakes are never hidden and where errors are disclosed to families with honesty and compassion.

KEY STRATEGIES IN PROMOTING SAFE CARE

The *Institute of Medicine Report*[3] from over 20 years ago highlights the key principles to promote safer care. Recognition of the deteriorating child is greatly helped by seeking family involvement and listening to parental concerns. In this regard, be aware of ethnic, cultural and language issues in addition to health literacy levels.

Leadership

We need to support and encourage senior clinicians to be involved in quality improvement initiatives.

> A key element of promoting a culture of safety is the engagement of clinicians at every level and the identification of 'champions' who promote and encourage a safe culture.

Information Technology

A key role of Information technology (IT) is in medication safety to enable decision support tools in terms of safe prescribing. The electronic health record (EHR) can track patient flow, notify abnormal results and help identify changes in clinical status. Other key issues are the integration of new software into existing systems and linking software to outside providers such as other paediatric departments or general practitioner surgeries. Clinicians may also experience alarm fatigue, be overwhelmed by excessive data and be tempted to copy and paste without editing. Transition of care back to a regional unit or to family practice can be challenging if EHRs are used. This may cause failures in the reconciliation of medications, duplications in investigations and a failure to respond to test results.

Quality Improvement in Action

Quality improvement (QI) initiatives in healthcare rely on the Deming principles using the Plan-Do-Study-Act model (Fig. 2.1). QI initiatives help to identify areas of non-compliance with current best practices or shortfalls in service delivery.[4] QI can also identify risks associated with change and to assess the readiness of a service to change. It is quite challenging to complete meaningful QI projects within a short space of time bearing in mind that most senior house officer rotations are for 6 months.

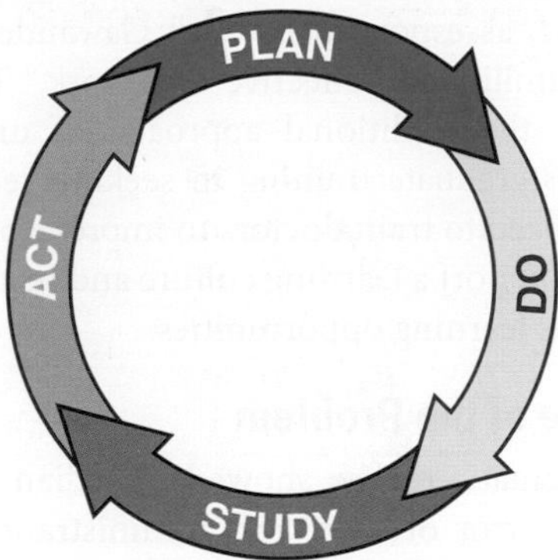

Fig. 2.1 The Plan-Do-Study-Act (PDSA) model of continuous quality improvement. The concept of the PDSA cycle was originally developed by Walter Shewhart, the pioneering statistician who developed statistical process control in the Bell Laboratories in the United States during the 1930s. It is often referred to as the 'Shewhart Cycle'. It was adopted in the 1950s by W. Edwards Deming and is often referred to as the 'Deming Wheel'. (Source: *Public Health Nursing: Population-Centered Health Care in the Community*. Tenth commemorative edition.)

Interprofessional involvement in Quality Improvement involving management, administrative and clinical staff is key in terms of likely impact.

Those embarking on a QI project should be supported by a named QI coach.

In writing up a QI project, the suggested outline should include, firstly, the project aim and the planned changes to be tested. Predictions should be included and, upon completion, an analysis of data, summary of results and a run chart should all clearly outline the outcome. Finally, describe the significance of the QI project both locally and nationally and reflect on the lessons learned overall.

Trainees are encouraged to present their work to their trainers, peers and the clinical team. Thereafter, presentation outside the hospital at a regional or national meeting and subsequent publication in a peer-reviewed journal should occur.

The 'Swiss Cheese' Model of Medical Error

This model was introduced by James Reason[5] as a means of understanding systemic error. It shifts attention away from the individual and places a greater emphasis on wider interlinked systems[6] (Fig. 2.2). It enables a root cause analysis of all the contributing factors to a poor outcome. Adverse events are contributed to by the complex nature of modern medical practice, human fallibility and the inherent uncertainty due to gaps in current medical knowledge. Traditional medical training has in the past focused on improving knowledge, whereas current thinking suggests the best approach is to understand human fallibility within the context of the complexity of modern healthcare.

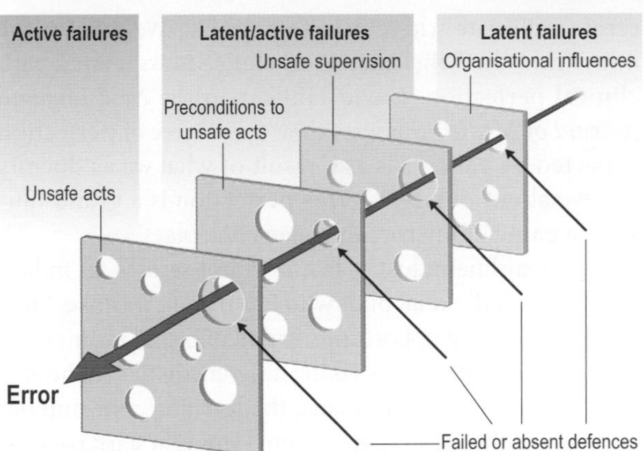

Fig. 2.2 The Swiss cheese model of human error. Each of the cheese slices acts as a barrier or block to an error occurring; the final chance to stop the error is elimination of the unsafe act itself. (Source: *Gray's Surgical Anatomy*. 2020.)

Adverse outcomes should really be a starting point for learning rather than a trigger for denial, shame and allocation of blame

Responding to Errors

In the airline industry, pilots, crew, maintenance personnel and air traffic controllers are encouraged and expected to report near misses and are commended when they do so.

In healthcare, by contrast, so-called 'whistle-blowers' may be given a very difficult time. In fact, the term 'whistle-blower' is not used in aviation. Doctors have in the past received very little training in understanding, detecting, preventing and responding to errors and thus may react poorly when an error occurs. It is preferable that if the doctor's performance is explored in a safe, caring and non-judgemental environment, a complaint or adverse event can be reframed as an opportunity towards improved practice and to provide support to the child and family who may have suffered harm.

There is no doubt that a progressive attitude to failure is the cornerstone of success in any organisation. Success requires us to learn from our mistakes and to create a climate where it is 'safe' to fail. We must move away from the belief that competence is associated with clinical perfection. David Hilfiker in the *New England Journal of Medicine* asserts that 'the degree of perfection expected by patients is as a result of what we as doctors believe about ourselves. This perfection is a grand illusion, a game of mirrors that everyone plays'.[7]

In the airline industry, failure is not seen as an indictment of an individual pilot who has made a mistake, but a precious learning opportunity for all pilots, all airlines and all regulators. The other striking difference is that, in healthcare, when mistakes are made, the learning opportunities do not flow throughout the system. This is in stark contrast to aviation, where data regarding errors is readily absorbed and shared by airlines across the world. As put by Professor James Reason 'healthcare is highly error-provoking and yet those who work in healthcare stigmatise fallibility'.[8]

So, what we need to learn from mistakes is, first and foremost, a system that harnesses errors as a means of driving progress and, of equal importance, a culture that allows such a system to flourish.

Many of us struggle to admit our personal failures and we tend to use cognitive dissonance to reframe, spin and even edit out our mistakes. In essence, we need to develop a Growth Mindset and thereby learn from our mistakes.

What is necessary is a cultural transformation to systematically capture near misses, to identify harm across a variety of care settings globally, to learn from each other and to empower patients and families to help us seek out and then aim to avoid preventable harm. So, rather than sink into despair, we need to look to other industries to see how they attempt to mitigate error and harm and a good place to start is the aviation industry. Clearly, looking after sick children and flying a passenger aircraft are very different human endeavours. Equally clear is the fact that, in both, there is little or no margin for error.

REDUCING HARM AND AVOIDING ERRORS IN HEALTHCARE

As healthcare has become increasingly complex, sadly there are multiple opportunities to cause unintended harm. Errors in paediatrics can range from the use of temporary names in the newborn nursery to diagnostic errors and prescribing errors in either family practice or in the hospital.

> Error traps are omnipresent within paediatrics.

We need, as espoused by Atul Gawande, a culture of trust, humility and effective teamwork.[9] There is no doubt that the traditional approach of undergraduate and postgraduate training in seeking certainty has failed. We need to train doctors to improve professional resilience, support a learning culture and regard adverse outcomes as learning opportunities.

The Scale of the Problem

A UK systematic review showed a median prevalence prescribing error of 6.5% and administration error of 11.1%.[10] Serious medication errors are most prevalent in critical care settings. Dose calculation errors are very common. The Vermont Oxford Network looks at outcomes of neonatal intensive care amongst very low birth weight infants and has reported that just under half of errors seen involve medication.[11]

> In hospital, the most frequently seen problem is medication error.

Lack of experience of staff in dealing with children allied to inexperience in performing technical procedures and in the calculation of medication doses in children is a key area of concern in the emergency department. Poor communication between pre-hospital and hospital staff, poor or no handover between shifts and poor communication between healthcare professionals and families can all contribute to errors. The nature of Paediatric Emergency Department attendances includes many children with undifferentiated illnesses which may lead to diagnostic errors, and this may be compounded when these presentations are out of hours when there may be sparse senior decision maker support.[12]

Errors in Primary Care

In primary care, the largest source of error (over 85%) again relates to medication.[13] Other errors seen frequently include incorrectly entered or misfiled patient information, delays in requesting laboratory tests, errors relating to vaccination or delays in referral to a specialist. Errors in diagnostic decision making may be due to inexperience, fatigue or lack of training. Primary care doctors manage both highly complex children across many specialties and a very large number of children with minor illness. They make countless clinical decisions every day and have significant workload pressures. Human factor awareness should be part of the annual appraisal of both primary care and specialist paediatric trainees.

Key Goals of Patient Safety Efforts

In a hospital setting, this involves a reduction in nosocomial infection, central line infections, surgical site infections and improvements in the recognition of the deteriorating child. The Paediatric Early Warning System is widely in use to pick up clinical deterioration but must be seen as more than just a score with interprofessional communication and response to family concerns key additional elements.[14]

We need to reduce stress and fatigue amongst trainees and efforts to reduce workplace stress are important.

> The safe and successful delivery of a service relies on a supportive organisational culture and helps promote staff well-being, morale and motivation.[15]

Supporting Trainees

The tragic story of Dr Bawa-Garba involved a young registrar who recently returned from maternity leave, who was required to cover six wards and to supervise multiple staff while her consultant was off-site.[16] In most people's eyes, this young doctor was scapegoated for the tragic death of a young child. Young trainees should always feel safe and valued. Overwhelming patient numbers and a lack of supervisory support exerts intolerable pressure on trainees.[16] Happily, in August 2018, a legal appeal supported by trainees in the UK and beyond against the decision to strike her from the medical register was upheld.[17] Health services and hospitals should be designed and administered with a compassionate and supportive approach that nurtures and values the valiant efforts of healthcare and other professionals within the system.

Long working hours are commonplace in medical training. A systematic review of the impact of restricting hours of work for trainees and safer care concluded, somewhat surprisingly, that the reduction of working hours for trainees had no impact on patient care or trainee wellness but did have a negative impact on trainee education.[18] So, a sole focus on duty hours alone will not improve either patient care or trainee wellness. In terms of night shifts, one study in the systematic review reported a favourable outcome for trainee wellness if 4 hours of protected time for sleep are built into the roster.

Shift work with night shifts showed interesting results and unfavourable outcomes with decreased sleep during off-duty, increased fatigue and greater stress compared to traditional on-call.

> Educational outcomes were adversely affected following night shifts with decreased attendance at teaching sessions, less time spent with attending physicians and less time and energy for independent reading.

Thus, recent literature points to less than favourable outcomes with restrictions in duty hours with the greatest impact on trainee education.[19,20] Night duty is especially unpopular.

Reduced time with consultants and reduced educational opportunities are significant negative outcomes of reduced working hours. Enhancing supervision by senior decision makers is the key intervention to improve patient safety in acute care settings and reductions of duty hours without increased supervision have a modest impact. Improved handover and night-time huddles are effective in reducing medical errors.

Staff who are awake longer than 10 hours may have increased error rates and judgement lapses, and it is recognised that people are notoriously poor judges of their own level of fatigue.

Second Opinions

Second opinions allow the assessment of a working diagnosis or treatment by a second independent physician. Second opinions may be sought by the physician alone or at the request of the family of the child.

> Up to 1 in 6 second opinions may lead to a change in diagnosis.

Parents may seek second opinions based on communication difficulties, differences in values or beliefs, comments on social media or a breakdown in trust between the family and the team.

The child's welfare is always paramount and the provider of the second opinion should have access to clinical notes, investigations and original images prior to seeing the child.[21] The child should be examined and the opinion of the doctor providing the second opinion should reflect the clinical facts. In cases where the first and second opinions differ, a mechanism to resolve these differences should be set out.[21] This may involve meetings of the multidisciplinary team, the involvement of the family and occasionally mediation.

Where mutual trust and respect between the attending team and the family has broken down, the doctor giving the second opinion may be required to take over care of the child. This requires prior consent of all parties (not least the child if competent) prior to transfer of care.[21]

Therefore, second opinions are increasingly being sought by families, and this may relate to the increased globalisation of healthcare, so-called health tourism and where innovative but perhaps unproven treatments are being sought. In general, outcome data on second opinion are divergent and scarce.[22]

THE AVIATION MODEL

> The most noteworthy achievement in international commercial aviation over the past 60 years has been in the area of improved safety management.

When quantifying this improvement, the safety statistics should be considered against the backdrop of the increasing size and complexity of the industry.

Improvement and innovation in airport facilities and layout, aircraft design, component reliability, navigation and air traffic management have all continued over the past 60 years.

> The most significant change in aviation, however, has been in efforts to mitigate human error.

Though difficult to quantify, it is believed that this safety management strategy has done more to reduce near-misses, incidents, accidents and fatalities than any other in the history of commercial aviation (see Fig. 2.3).

In stark contrast, in healthcare, it is estimated that there are 200,000 preventable medical deaths every year in the United States alone.[23] This equates to almost three fatal airline crashes per day.[15] As the renowned airline pilot Chesley Sullenberger (or *Sully*) noted, if such a level of fatalities were to happen in aviation, airlines would stop flying, airports would close and there would be congressional hearings and a presidential commission. No one would be allowed to fly until the problem had been solved.[15]

KEY FACTORS IN THE AVIATION INDUSTRY

Checklists

Checklists have been introduced to help pilots avoid the omission of one or more of a number of steps in a procedure, usually due to distraction or fatigue or the repetitive nature of the task.

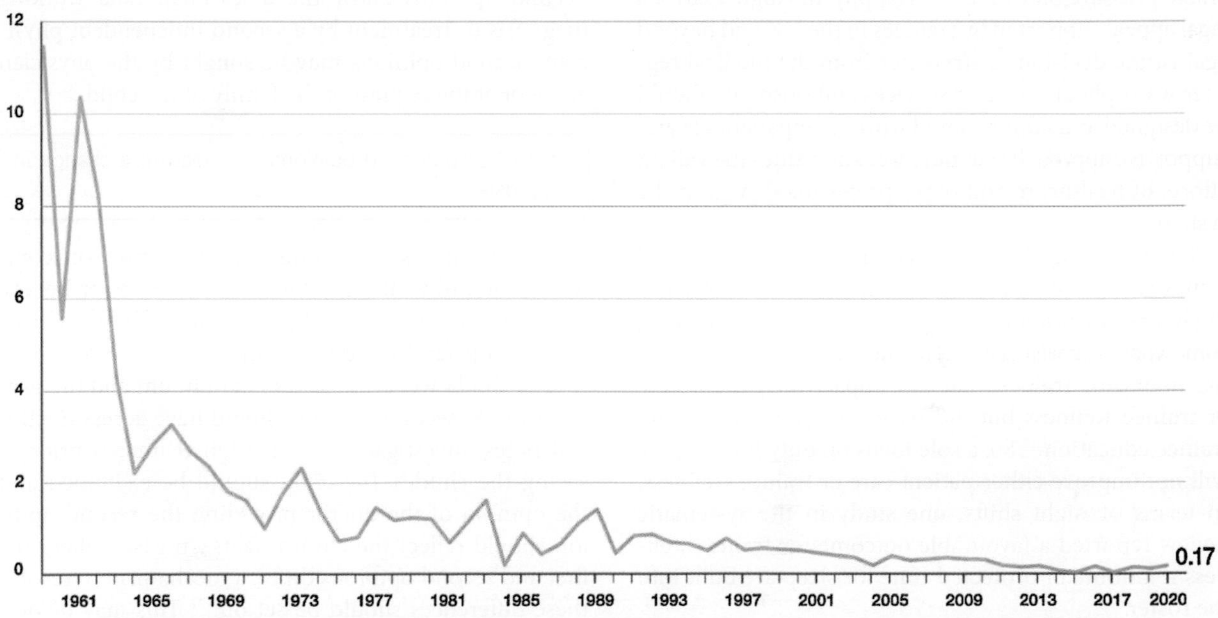

Fig. 2.3 Yearly fatal accident rate per million flights. In 2019, 4.5 billion passengers flew on 38.3 million commercial flights. There were 6 fatal accidents with 239 fatalities. (With kind permission from Airbus Head of Safety Promotion, accidentstats.airbus.com.)[31]

There are three types of checklists with one for simple, routine operations, a second for more complex operations and a third for emergency procedures.[15]

Normal checklists guide a crew through a sequence of actions related to a particular phase of flight. A good example is the 'Before Take-off Checklist'. It is precisely because the procedure is so familiar and repetitive that aviation sees the need to have a checklist, to ensure that one pilot performs the action item which is then verified by the other pilot.

Non-normal checklists are designed to assist pilots in abnormal and emergency scenarios where attempting to manage from memory would likely compound the situation.

Lastly, and to cover emergency situations where there is simply no time to access and execute a paper or electronic checklist there are 'Memory' or 'Recall' checklists. Clearly, in these scenarios, a timeout, huddle, groupthink, electronic or paper checklist is not appropriate. The correct actions must be executed in the correct sequence and without delay. Engine failure during take-off, explosive decompression and brake failure during landing are three examples of situations where immediate and swift action is necessary. In each of these situations the dynamic stage of the flight means that time is critical, there is no margin for error and stress levels are significantly increased.

These scenarios are akin to the acutely collapsed child in an emergency department where rapid sequenced responses as per Advanced Paediatric Life Support (APLS) are required. It is for this reason that 'Memory' checklists are the most trained and rehearsed in a pilot's initial and recurrent training program in the hope of ensuring immediate recall when needed.

Training

Initial pilot training is over 3 years and training to be a captain takes on average a further 10 years. Pilots are trained in the classroom, in a simulator and in an aircraft.

> Pilots are obliged, using a simulator, to undergo proficiency checks every 6 months.

During pilot training, there is a clear focus on the essential soft skills of leadership and teamwork, threat and error management, situational awareness, decision-making, workload management, briefing and debriefing, stress reduction and coping with fatigue. In surgery and anaesthesia, these soft skills are also assessed in some training programmes.[24,25]

CREW RESOURCE MANAGEMENT

Crew Resource Management (CRM) is the name adopted by the airline industry as the most appropriate title for its human factors programme.[26] CRM ensures that today's airline pilots regard their fellow crew members, air traffic control, autopilot and autothrust, checklists and Standard Operating Procedures (SOPs) as valuable resources.

The 'Two-Challenge' Rule

The most junior, timid, deferential crew member is empowered to speak up and, when necessary, challenge even the most senior, assertive and intimidating captain. In training, new recruits are taught to verbalise safety concerns and seniors are taught to encourage and listen to those concerns.

If one pilot has concerns about the performance of his/her colleague in flight, he or she *must* challenge the colleague by calling 'Speed' (if above or below target speed) or 'Altitude' (if above or below assigned altitude) or 'Heading' (if left or right of required direction). If a verbal response and physical correction of the deviation do not occur, the concerned pilot must challenge a second time, but with more assertion, and take over control of the aircraft (regardless of rank or experience). The 'two-challenge' rule is now being incorporated into resident training programmes.[27]

> Even if there are clear differences in the level of skill and experience between the pilot and co-pilot, safety is always the number one priority ahead of rank or title.

CRM enables respect for individual team roles. Direct eye contact, addressing others by their first name and always putting safety before self-esteem are key elements of CRM.

The 'Sterile Cockpit' in Aviation

While take-off, initial climb, final approach and landing phases account for just 4% of a typical flight, approximately half of onboard fatalities and two-thirds of fatal aircraft accidents occur during this time. Activities such as eating meals, friendly nonessential conversations both within the cockpit and between the cabin and cockpit crews and reading publications are not permitted during these times. These are also the most dynamic and complex stages of flight. The consequences of unnecessary distractions can be catastrophic at these times.

> A 'sterile cockpit' is in essence an environment free of unnecessary distractions and can be applied to certain situations such as drug ward rounds in a hospital setting.

Healthcare can be full of distractions and interruptions for bleep-carrying trainee doctors. Distracting events involving the anaesthetist are common and have been studied.[28]

PERFORMANCE ANALYSIS

All adverse events or near misses in aviation are investigated with thoroughness, and these include both the equipment and the individuals involved. Each investigation ends with a report and analysis of the sequence of events and finishes with conclusions and safety recommendations. An independent agency conducts the investigation in aviation, and a similar independent agency is required in healthcare.

> Reporting of incidents in aviation is blame-free, and near misses are also reported in detail.

In the airline industry, a major incident involving one airline is followed by shared learning by many airlines with these lessons becoming part of training with an emphasis on the design of equipment and training recommendations. The reporting of adverse events in aviation is immune from disciplinary action except if gross or wilful negligence is evident, in which case appropriate action is taken.

Cockpit Voice Recorders (CVRs) and Flight Data Recorders (FDRs) are the 'Black boxes' which must be fitted and serviceable on all commercial aircraft. The recorded data from these devices is invaluable in terms of assessing near misses and sentinel events.

COMPARISONS AND INNATE DIFFERENCES

Modern aviation is an inherently safe activity. In commercial aviation, the focus on safety is relentless, and it is central to both staff training and values. Staff who report concerns are protected due to an open and learning culture.[29] The airline industry has a blame-free culture in terms of safety incident reporting, whereas in healthcare it is still regarded as the priority for some, but sadly not the obligation of all.[15]

Commercial airlines tend not to schedule flights on routes that are nonprofitable or if adverse weather conditions, whereas acute healthcare must deal with all comers. By contrast, in healthcare, there is a relentless demand regardless of rota gaps, staff exhaustion, bed shortages or deficits in community support services.

IMPLICATIONS FOR HEALTHCARE

First and foremost, we need to embrace human factors training and focus on staff training and well-being as part of all work plans from the bedside to the boardroom. Continuing professional development should focus on patient safety and staff well-being.

KEY LEARNING POINTS

Medicine

Postgraduate training should stress the importance of communication within and between teams and with referring family doctors.

Attempt to share best practices in relation to patient safety initiatives and create a safety culture both in hospital and the community.

Maintain a focus on primary care and develop safety metrics that apply to family practice.

National paediatric error reporting systems should be developed, thereby enabling interprofessional learning because of reported errors.

Share materials and up-to-date information with families to improve their understanding of their child's condition.

Interventions that are proven to work include vigilant hand washing, timeouts before procedures, reconciliation of medications and child identification processes.[30]

Medical applications of checklists have been largely confined to the fields of surgery and infection control.

We should encourage leadership in patient safety initiatives at the local and national levels.

Always seek a second opinion if you are at a loss and the child is not getting better.

Aviation

The major achievement in international commercial aviation over the past 20 or 30 years relates to improved safety. Despite a doubling of worldwide flight hours over the past 20 years, the number of fatalities has fallen from approximately 450 to less than 250 per year.

Simulation training for pilots incorporates both technical and nontechnical skills. Pilots are required to undergo proficiency checks every 6 months in a simulator, during which both technical and nontechnical skills are evaluated.

Crew Resource Management (CRM) looks at how individual members of a team interact and the factors that influence their performance. The key features of CRM are cooperation, leadership, communication, workload management, enhanced situational awareness and decision making.

All adverse events or near misses in aviation are investigated with thoroughness, and these investigations include both the equipment, the environment and the individuals involved. Each investigation concludes with a report and analysis of the sequence of events and finishes with conclusions and safety recommendations.

Vive la Difference

An independent agency is responsible for conducting the investigation in aviation, and a similar independent agency is required in healthcare.

Black box recordings piece together both flight data and cockpit conversations and are carried on all commercial aircraft. They prove to be invaluable in terms of assessing near misses and sentinel events. No such 'black boxes' exist in healthcare.

Aviation has a far more mature and just culture in terms of the reporting of safety incidents, making it an inherently safe activity.

Staff who specialise in human factors and related psychological aspects of patient safety and staff well-being are required in healthcare.

REFERENCES

1. Melchers RE. On the ALARP approach to risk management. *Reliability Engineering & System Safety*. February 2001;71(2):201–208. doi:10.1016/S0951-8320(00)00096-X.
2. Mueller BU, Neuspiel DR, Fisher ERS. Council on Quality Improvement and Patient Safety, Committee on Hospital Care. Principles of Pediatric Patient Safety: Reducing Harm Due to Medical Care. *Pediatrics*. 2019;143(2):e20183649. doi:10.1542/peds.2018-3649.
3. Institute of Medicine (US) Committee on Quality of Health Care in America. In: Kohn LT, Corrigan JM, Donaldson MS, eds. *To Err is Human: Building a Safer Health System*. Washington (DC): National Academies Press (US); 2000.
4. Murphy JFA. Quality Improvement Projects for Doctors in Training. *Ir Med J*. 2022;115(3):556. Published 2022 Mar 16.
5. Reason J. Human error: models and management. *BMJ*. 2000;320(7237):768–770. doi:10.1136/bmj.320.7237.768.
6. Wiegmann DA, Wood LJ, Cohen TN, Shappell SA. Understanding the "Swiss Cheese Model" and Its Application to Patient Safety. *J Patient Saf*. 2022;18(2):119–123. doi:10.1097/PTS.0000000000000810.
7. Hilfiker D. Facing our mistakes. *N Engl J Med*. 1984;310(2):118–122. doi:10.1056/NEJM198401123100211.
8. Reason J. James Reason: patient safety, human error, and Swiss cheese. Interview by Karolina Peltomaa and Duncan Neuhauser. *Qual Manag Health Care*. 2012;21(1):59–63. doi:10.1097/QMH.0b013e3182418294.
9. Gawande A. *The Checklist Manifesto: How to Get Things Right*. Picador; First edition; January 4, 2011.
10. Sutherland A, Phipps DL, Tomlin S, et al. Mapping the prevalence and nature of drug related problems among hospitalised children in the United Kingdom: a systematic review. *BMC Pediatr*. 2019;19:486. doi:10.1186/s12887-019-1875-y.
11. Gray JE, Goldmann DA. Medication errors in the neonatal intensive care unit: special patients, unique issues. *Arch Dis Child Fetal Neonatal Ed*. 2004;89(6):F472–F473. doi:10.1136/adc.2003.046060.
12. Yoong SYC, Ang PH, Chong SL, et al. Common diagnoses among pediatric attendances at emergency departments. *BMC Pediatr*. 2021;21:172. doi:10.1186/s12887-021-02646-8.
13. Säfholm S, Bondesson Å, Modig S. Medication errors in primary health care records; a cross-sectional study in Southern Sweden. *BMC Fam Pract*. 2019;20(1):110. doi:10.1186/s12875-019-1001-0 Published 2019 Jul 31.
14. Chapman SM, Maconochie IK. Early warning scores in paediatrics: an overview. *Arch Dis Child*. 2019;104(4):395–399. doi:10.1136/archdischild-2018-314807.
15. Kapur N, Parand A, Soukup T, Reader T, Sevdalis N. Aviation and healthcare: a comparative review with implications for patient safety. *JRSM Open*. 2015;7(1):2054270415616548. doi:10.1177/2054270415616548. Published 2015 Dec 2.

16. Preisz A. Dr Bawa-Garba: The Virtue of Ethics and the Ethics of Virtue. *J Paediatr Child Health*. 2018;54(11):1283. doi:10.1111/jpc.14211.
17. Dyer C. Hadiza Bawa-Garba wins right to practise again. *BMJ*. 2018;362:k3510. doi:10.1136/bmj.k3510. Published 2018 Aug 14.
18. Morrow, G. and Burford, B. and Carter, M. and Illing, J. (2012) 'The impact of the Working Time Regulations on medical education and training: Literature review. Report for the General Medical Council'. Project Report. Durham University, Centre for Medical Education Research, Durham. Accessed at https://www.gmc-uk.org/-/media/gmc-site-images/about/theimpactoftheworkingtimeregulationsonmedicaleducationandtrainingliteraturereviewpdf51155615.pdf?la=en&hash=09E695D73667623B98E7ED6F5ADEFA1914A57073
19. Canter R. Impact of reduced working time on surgical training in the United Kingdom and Ireland. *Surgeon*. 2011;9(Suppl 1):S6–S7. doi:10.1016/j.surge.2010.11.020.
20. Peets A, Ayas NT. Restricting resident work hours: the good, the bad, and the ugly. *Crit Care Med*. 2012;40(3):960–966. doi:10.1097/CCM.0b013e3182413bc5.
21. Larcher V, Brierley J. Second medical opinions in paediatric practice; proposals for a framework for best practice. *Arch Dis Child*. 2020;105(3):213–215. doi:10.1136/archdischild-2019-317223.
22. Ruetters D, Keinki C, Schroth S, Liebl P, Huebner J. Is there evidence for a better health care for cancer patients after a second opinion? A systematic review. *J Cancer Res Clin Oncol*. 2016;142(7):1521–1528. doi:10.1007/s00432-015-2099-7.
23. Anderson JG, Abrahamson K. Your health care may kill you: medical errors. *Stud Health Technol Inform*. 2017;234:13–17.
24. Gerstle CR. Parallels in safety between aviation and healthcare. *J Pediatr Surg*. 2018;53(5):875–878. doi:10.1016/j.jpedsurg.2018.02.002.
25. Hardie JA, Oeppen RS, Shaw G, Holden C, Tayler N, Brennan PA. You have control: aviation communication application for safety-critical times in surgery. *Br J Oral Maxillofac Surg*. 2020;58(9):1073–1077. doi:10.1016/j.bjoms.2020.08.104.
26. Helmreich RL, Merritt AC, Wilhelm JA. The evolution of Crew Resource Management training in commercial aviation. *Int J Aviat Psychol*. 1999;9(1):19–32. doi:10.1207/s15327108ijap0901_.
27. Pian-Smith MC, Simon R, Minehart RD, et al. Teaching residents the two-challenge rule: a simulation-based approach to improve education and patient safety. *Simul Healthc*. 2009;4(2):84–91. doi:10.1097/SIH.0b013e31818cffd3.
28. Jothiraj H, Howland-Harris J, Evley R, Moppett IK. Distractions and the anaesthetist: a qualitative study of context and direction of distraction. *Br J Anaesth*. 2013;111(3):477–482. doi:10.1093/bja/aet108.
29. Oliver D. David Oliver: Are comparisons between acute healthcare and the aviation industry invidious? *BMJ*. 2018;361:k2203. doi:10.1136/bmj.k220. Published 2018 May 22.
30. Mueller BU, Neuspiel DR, Fisher ERS. Council on Quality Improvement and Patient Safety, Committee on Hospital Care. Principles of Pediatric Patient Safety: Reducing Harm Due to Medical Care. *Pediatrics*. 2019;143(2):e20183649. doi:10.1542/peds.2018-3649.
31. Airbus. A statistical Analysis of Commercial Aviation Accidents 1958–2021. With kind permission from Airbus Head of Safety Promotion. Accessed at Airbus accident-stats.airbus.com

ADDITIONAL READING

Abbasi K. First do no harm: the impossible oath. *BMJ: British Medical Journal (Online)*. Jul 19, 2019;366. doi:10.1136/bmj.l4734.

Bordini BJ, Stephany A, Kliegman R. Overcoming Diagnostic Errors in Medical Practice. *J Pediatr*. 2017;185:19–25.e1. doi:10.1016/j.jpeds.2017.02.065.

Davey P, Thakore S, Tully V. How to embed quality improvement into medical training. *BMJ*. 2022:376e055084. doi:10.1136/bmj2020:055084.

Hoban B. Learning to live with cognitive bias. *British Journal of General Practice*. 2022 Sep 1;72(722):433. doi:10.3399/bjgp22X720581 doi.

ICAO 2020 Annual Safety Report- Executive Summary. Accessed at https://www.icao.int/RASGPA/RASGPADocuments/ASR2020.pdf

ICAO Safety Indicators Study Group (SISG). *Annex 13 — Aircraft Accident and Incident Investigation*. 12th Edition; July 2020. Available at. https://store.icao.int/en/annexes/annex-13.

Nauta M, Grayeff S, Ponnusamy M, De Martino R, Yoong W. Human factors in general practice: what it means for practice, training, and CPD. *Br J Gen Pract*. 2019;69(689):592–593. doi:10.3399/bjgp19X706697. Published 2019 Nov 28.

Syed M. *Black Box Thinking*. London: John Murray Publishers; 2020.

Towell E. To Err is Human, to Cover up is Unforgivable. *The Bulletin of the Royal College of Surgeons of England*. 2010;92(7):232–233. Accessed at. https://publishing.rcseng.ac.uk/action/showCitFormats?doi=10.1308%2F147363510X514596.

Wilson H, Cunningham W. Being a doctor. Understanding medical practice. *Adverse Outcomes and Patient Safety*. Otago University Press; 2013:201–226.

3

Recognising the Sick Child

Carol Blackburn, Karina Butler

CHAPTER OUTLINE

Right at the core of acute paediatrics is a key conundrum – while the chances of a serious illness in infants and children presenting to primary care are very low the consequences of not recognising and treating serious illness are stark and can be devastating. Often, the clinical decision to allow home, refer to hospital or observe in hospital and treat is based on the application of experience supported by knowledge. This is a big ask of a family doctor with just three to 6 months of experience in paediatrics who may have never encountered a seriously ill child during their training.

Both in primary care and in hospital, prompt recognition is essential to optimise outcomes. In this regard, the parental level of concern is a key factor as are regular observation of vital signs, identifying and responding to concerns of the nursing staff and excellent communication. High uptake of immunisations has led to a striking fall in invasive meningococcal and pneumococcal disease (both thankfully now rare) but cases still occur. Early recognition confers better outcomes.

AN ACCURATE HISTORY AND EXAMINATION

History

An accurate history is essential. One needs to seek the key concerns and explore parental instinct in particular. A mother who returns to the family practice or to the emergency department with her young infant for a second or third time is clearly concerned, and a fresh view and, in the emergency department setting, review by a more senior clinician should take place. A young child that can smile or who appears to respond with interest to your presence and to the parents is unlikely to have sepsis or be seriously ill. On the other hand, a pale and unresponsive infant or child should raise significant concerns and prompt action.

Drowsiness, somnolence, reduced tone and being non-reactive are all worrying symptoms. Also of concern is a change in crying pattern with moaning being a notable feature.

Examination

Interpretation of physiological values such as temperature, respiratory rate and heart rate can be challenging in paediatrics. There are published validated, normal ranges for these variables which vary with age, but interpretation can still be problematic as heart rate can be affected by pain, fever and fear at any age; for example, the febrile infant with a sore ear who is due a feed might have a very elevated heart rate. Considering the trend of physiological values can be helpful; however, this is nigh on impossible in a general practice setting. A poor response to antipyretics does not predict the presence of sepsis, nor can it be ignored. Therefore, a rising heart rate well above the norm or a persistent tachycardia are both causes for concern but must be seen in context of other variables such as pain (often earache or nonspecific) and the responsiveness of the infant or child.

> It should always be remembered that an isolated tachycardia can be an early indicator of sepsis.

Clinical assessment should rely not just on physiological variables; a key element is observation of the infant or child undressed, checking for rashes, cold peripheries, central cyanosis and the responsiveness of the infant or child.

> A very simple clinical sign readily assessed by any clinician is the measurement of the capillary refill time (CRT). CRT is a proxy measure of skin perfusion

CRT should preferably be checked centrally on the sternal area but may be checked at the fingertip. Using an index finger, press the skin overlying the sternum or fingertip for 5 seconds using moderate pressure. Using a watch or phone, count the seconds it takes for the blanched skin to regain its original colour (Fig. 3.1). A normal CRT is 2 seconds or less.[1]

The finding of a *CRT of 3 seconds* or more should be considered a 'red flag' indicating that the infant or child is at higher risk of sepsis. CRT can be affected by the duration of pressure and the ambient temperature of the room with a longer duration of pressure and lower room temperature resulting in a prolongation of the CRT.[1]

The presence of focal neurological symptoms, such as a loss of power, is very concerning as is the presence of seizures.

SAFETY NETTING FOR FAMILY DOCTORS

Safety netting is particularly important in managing children presenting to family doctors, as many have nonspecific early symptoms with a small proportion having serious illness.[2] Diagnostic uncertainty should be communicated to the family and advice offered on worrisome or 'red flag' symptoms. The expected duration of the illness should be explained and parents advised where, how and when to seek further advice.

> Diagnostic uncertainty exists in the majority of consultations and this uncertainty should first be recognised and then communicated to the family.

Communicating Uncertainty

This is extremely important, as communicating uncertainty to the family is a key element of safety netting for family doctors. If the diagnosis is uncertain, this lack of certainty should be communicated to the family so that they feel empowered to re-attend if needed.

Advise parents about worrisome 'red flag' symptoms. It is important to highlight worrisome symptoms that

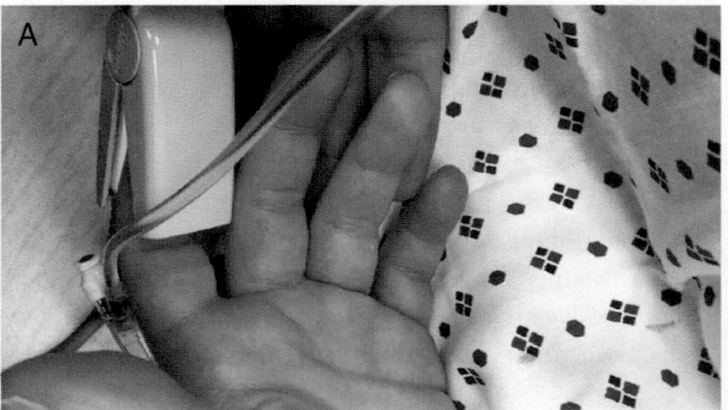

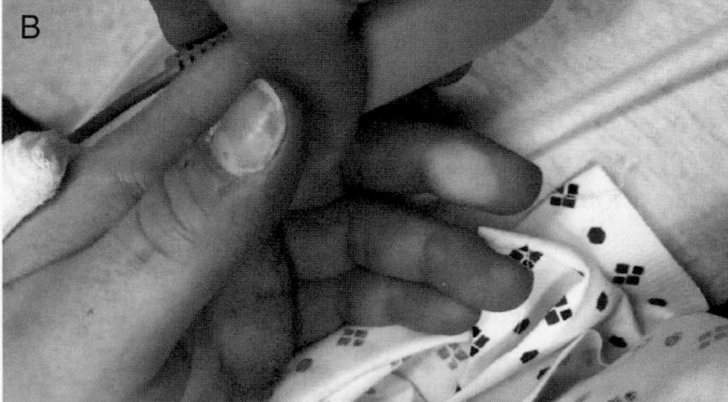

Fig. 3.1 (A) Normal capillary refill time of less than 3 seconds. (B) Abnormal capillary refill time of greater than 5 seconds. (Source: EMC, ISSN: 0733-8627, 2017.)

the parents should look out for including specific advice about the symptoms and signs that might indicate sepsis or meningitis.

> Non-resolution or progression of symptoms warrants a review and potentially referral to hospital, and this needs to be communicated to the family.

Highlight the Expected Course of the Illness Over Time

For instance, a viral illness and associated fever should resolve in 3 to 4 days. An acute cough relating to a respiratory tract infection may last up to 21 days. Parents should be made aware of the likely time course they might expect prior to recovery. This advice is equally applicable to trainees in the emergency department.

Seeking Further Advice

Parents, once they know the likely time course and potential red flag symptoms, also require information on how and where to seek further medical help.

> Families should feel empowered to return if symptoms persist or worsen.

Offer clear advice about re-contacting their family doctor in specific situations – for example, if progressive lethargy or a nonblanching rash occur in a child with fever. Some family doctors prefer to arrange a planned follow-up visit.

As a family doctor, you should ensure that parents understand the advice given and offer written instructions as required. Parental information leaflets on many common childhood illnesses are readily available. It is also important to document in the medical record that safety netting advice has been given.

Heuristics or 'Rules of Thumb'

Heuristics in essence is applying one's experience to solve a clinical problem and can be seen as both a blessing and a curse. We have all seen the wise and experienced paediatrician effortlessly pick out that single child from a lengthy ward round to focus attention on. Heuristics bypass a detailed problem-solving approach and allow for rapid and mostly correct decision-making. They can create several biases. These include confirmation bias where one looks for evidence to support a preconceived opinion, acceptance of a prior diagnosis without sufficient scepticism, bias due to over-confidence (a fatal flaw), jumping rapidly to a conclusion and the dreaded 'Eureka' moment that stops all further diagnostic enquiry.

The key skill for the clinician to develop, whether in primary care or paediatrics, is an awareness of the distinction between instinctive and analytical cognition. Both are required to safely manage sick children and the skill is knowing when to jump from instinctive to a more analytical approach. Too much of the latter and the surgery or emergency department grinds to a halt and too little carries the risk of missing an underlying rare or serious illness. *This is the absolute core of clinical paediatrics.*

Reflex decisions, grounded in a robust knowledge of paediatrics, enable many children to be treated relatively quickly. This approach will not work when the clinician is faced with a complex diagnosis or a diagnosis that is infrequently encountered.[3] Evidence-based clinical guidelines are helpful in this regard but where they are not available, a structured approach with a broad differential is the best route.

Parents, of course, are looking to professionals for a diagnosis and appropriate prompt treatment for their child. They wish to have the symptoms (such as pain) treated and seek certainty that the illness will resolve and that their child will make a full recovery.

> Parents are incredibly important partners when they present with their acutely ill child, not just in terms of the history but also in terms of their instincts of illness progression or resolution.
> Most have a 'sixth sense' that accurately reflects whether the child is getting better or worse.

The clinician must deal with an element of uncertainty and an overall low probability of serious illness. This is a delicate balance. One needs to avoid over-investigation and treatment yet remain able to recognise the rare instance of a child with a serious illness. Observation in hospital in a dedicated area in the emergency department over a defined period of several hours is incredibly helpful in informing decisions about investigation and treatment, but this option is not available to family doctors.

Clinical Decision Tools

The clinical decision tools most often used in primary care include the NICE Traffic Light system for managing the febrile child.[4,5] This tool is most useful at either end of the spectrum of presentation. The infant or young child who is feverish, responsive and smiling is very unlikely to have serious bacterial sepsis. The grey, pale, obtunded infant with poor peripheral perfusion, in contrast, is clearly a major concern and requires prompt hospital referral. The 'Amber' group is nowhere as clear-cut and open to interpretation.

> The problem is that every benign diagnosis has an evil twin, and it may be very difficult to tell them apart, especially in family practice.[2]

Recent observations have cast doubts about the use of the Traffic Light system in family practice.[4,5] Further research is needed to validate triage tools for use in this setting.

Safe System Framework in Hospital

The UK Royal College of Paediatrics and Child Health have highlighted *six key elements* that help to underpin a 'safe system' framework for children in hospital.[6] These include:

Safety Culture

A corporate commitment to patient safety, viewing safety as a priority and executive accountability in both the monitoring and measurement of patient safety.

Strong Partnership With Families

This is central to all efforts to improve the safety of infants and children in hospital.

Picking up the Deteriorating Child

This is central to the system and employs Paediatric Early Warning Scores (PEWS) to spot physiological deviations prior to overt deterioration.

Response to Deterioration

Ensuring a timely and accurate response is essential. This involves listening to parental concerns, excellent communication with other healthcare professionals, especially nurses, and ensuring concerns are acted upon.

A Learning Culture

Evaluate incidents to learn from them in a no-blame culture as seen in aviation.

Education and Training

Consistent training of existing and new staff in improvement science, PEWS and situational awareness.

Senior Decision-Makers

> Senior decision-makers are the safety net for the system and generally ensure a safe and accurate clinical assessment.

Clinicians with the necessary experience rarely rely solely on guidelines or tests to make diagnoses. Gut feeling is somewhat ill-defined but can be viewed as the intuitive feeling, often informed by experience, that something is not quite right even though the clinician is unsure why. Senior decision-makers should, as trainers, discuss why certain decisions were made and not just what decision was made. For paediatricians in training, the volume of cases seen and discussed adds to the level of clinical experience and enables them to make robust clinical decisions. There really is no substitute for seeing and treating as many children as possible while in training.

For the experienced primary care doctor, intuition still has a major role to play in clinical practice. This applies to the experienced family doctor who has seen many children with viral illnesses and who then recognises when a child is different and thereby refers to hospital. For a hospital senior decision-maker, the application of intuition occurs when a child presents to hospital with a certain diagnosis but does not follow the expected route to recovery and therefore a rare diagnosis or serious underlying illness becomes suspected. Intuition is a key skill in both situations in addition to published evidence, available guidelines and clinical pathway tools in order to make the best decisions in any given clinical scenario.[3]

PAEDIATRIC EARLY WARNING SCORES

Paediatric early warning scores (PEWS) have been in existence for over 15 years, and, in essence, help determine physiological parameters that identify infants and children at risk of clinical deterioration. In effect, PEWS scores convert clinical observations into a score and incorporate the concerns of nurses or family at the bedside, and this information helps clinicians recognise and rescue a sick child ideally before they deteriorate.

> The total PEWS score should never undermine or replace clinical judgement.

In hospitals where PEWS scores are in use, they may be applied to infants and children admitted to short-stay observation units in emergency departments or admitted to hospital. Clinical deterioration of infants and children in hospital is quite often preceded by a period of physiological instability. These periods can be detected through the serial monitoring of vital sign observation trends and other clinical signs at the bedside.[7] When recognised, this enables active intervention to avoid adverse events such as cardiac arrest, admission to paediatric intensive care or even death.

> Score-based PEWS should be accompanied by a defined escalation pathway that indicates the action to be taken.[6]

National PEWS programmes have been adopted in both Scotland and Ireland, but it has not been proven that they improve patient outcomes. PEWS scores have also been developed for specific patients (e.g. those with burns, congenital heart disease and those who are recipients of a bone marrow transplant), but it is as yet unclear if this improves prognosis.

PEWS on its own is unlikely to be effective and needs to be part of a system-wide approach to improve individual and team situational awareness. No PEWS will capture all children who are at risk of deterioration.

Standardised age-specific observation charts help prompt good decisions as does situational awareness in frontline healthcare staff. For healthcare professionals, one benefit of PEWS is a clear escalation pathway triggered by threshold scores. Finally, in the detection of the deteriorating child, clinical acumen remains important. Always consider that the patient's family are best placed to recognise when children are 'not right' or 'not themselves'.

THE SEPSIS 6 ALGORITHM

The mortality from severe sepsis with shock in infants and children in the developed world is 10% to 17%. We know that prompt (within one hour) initiation of antibiotics and intravenous fluids can significantly reduce both morbidity and mortality.[8] Thus, the recognition of sepsis is essential, but sadly, every year we continue to see examples highlighting the tragic consequences when sepsis is not recognised.

Formal teaching sessions delivered to trainees on the recognition and management of sepsis and septic shock and its time-critical nature have been shown to raise awareness and to improve trainee confidence in managing sepsis. Helpful resources include sepsis guidelines from the American College of Critical Care Medicine[9] and role play using the Sepsis 6 algorithm.

The paediatric **Sepsis 6 algorithm** involves the so-called 'Take 3, Give 3' approach that, in essence, is to take blood cultures, a serum lactate and monitor urinary output, and to give oxygen, prompt antibiotics and intravenous fluids.[10]

EVERYONE'S FEAR – MENINGITIS OR ENCEPHALITIS

> While the epidemiology of meningitis has changed substantially since the introduction of conjugate vaccines, acute bacterial meningitis continues to be the diagnosis that all family doctors fear missing the most and the condition where the highest litigation payouts occur.

Sadly, there is a sense of 'out of sight and thus out of mind' in that the prevalence of meningitis has declined markedly over the past 15 years, and family doctors are less likely to see a case during their time in Paediatrics or in practice, and this may make it more challenging to recognise. The three classical signs of meningism are neck stiffness (sometimes referred to as nuchal rigidity), Kernig's and Brudzinski's signs. These signs are not reliable in infants under 12 months of age.

Clinical Symptoms and Signs of Meningitis

> Classical symptoms and signs of meningitis are often absent in infancy.

In infants, symptoms and signs such as fever, vomiting, irritability and upper respiratory tract symptoms may predominate. A full or bulging fontanelle can sometimes be seen. (Fig. 3.2) In older children, nuchal rigidity and a positive Kernig's or Brudzinski's sign are clinical signs still relevant in modern paediatric practice. Of these, the Kernig's and Brudzinski's signs have a higher predictive value in the diagnosis of meningitis, and their presence confers a significant enough risk of meningitis to justify further investigations.[11]

Neck Stiffness

Firstly, ask the child to actively flex and extend the neck and see if there is any pain or limitation of movement.

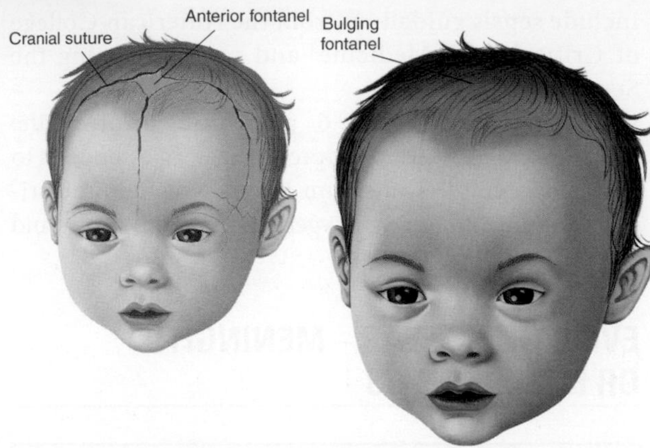

Fig. 3.2 Bulging fontanelle in bacterial meningitis.

Then the doctor should flex the child's neck and assess whether passive flexion is resisted. Meningism with neck stiffness can also be seen with acute follicular tonsillitis, acute otitis media, painful cervical lymphadenitis and cervical discitis.

> You should examine every febrile child for signs of illness, rash and neck stiffness.
>
> Your clinical note will then show that the diagnosis of meningitis was looked for even if no signs at that time.

Kernig's and Brudzinski's Signs (Fig. 3.3)

Position the child with their hips flexed to 90 degrees. Kernig's sign is positive if the child experiences pain, discomfort and limitation of extension on passive extension of the knee.

Ask the child to lie supine and passively flex the child's neck. Brudzinski's sign is positive if this passive flexion of the neck leads to a reflex flexion of the hip and knee.

Bacterial and Viral Meningitis

Over the past three decades, the successful introduction of vaccines to control *Haemophilus influenzae* type b, serogroups B and C meningococcus and some types of pneumococci have changed the landscape. The MenACWY vaccination programme for teenagers and young adults has also been introduced.

The major causes of bacterial meningitis in children and adolescents are *Neisseria meningitidis* and *Streptococcus pneumoniae.* Both are spread by person-to-person droplet transmission.

Viral meningitis is relatively common and tends to occur in the summer months. Presentation is with fever, neck stiffness, irritability and vomiting.

Tuberculous Meningitis

In tuberculous meningitis (TBM), the history will be quite different with an insidious onset of symptoms which may last weeks or months. There may be a history of exposure to a case of open tuberculosis (TB), background HIV disease or being from a refugee or unhoused background. Initial symptoms are weight loss, fever and apathy which evolve into neurological symptoms, raised intracranial pressure, cranial nerve

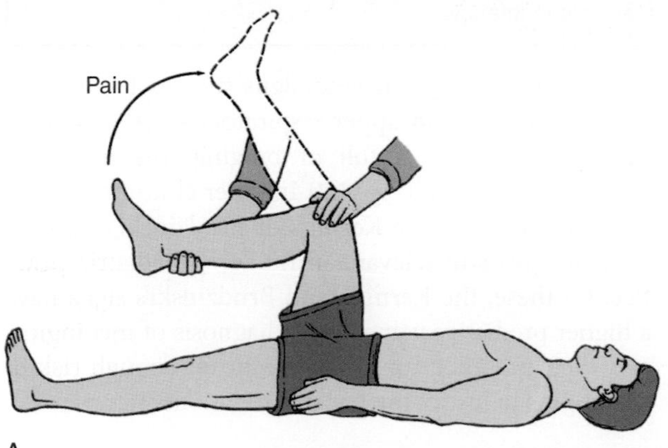

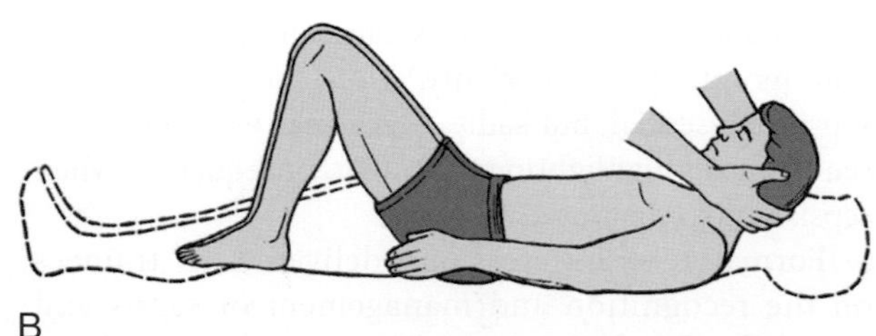

Fig. 3.3 Assessing a client with meningeal irritation. (A) Kernig's sign. (B) Brudzinski's sign. (Source: From Monahan FD, Sands JK, Neighbors M, et al. eds. Phipp's Medical-Surgical Nursing: Health and Illness Perspectives. 8th ed. St. Louis: Mosby; 2007)

BOX 3.1 CLINICAL HISTORY

A 2 Year Old Boy With Lethargy, a Poor Appetite and Neck Stiffness

A 2-year-old boy has presented to his family doctor on three occasions over the past 6 weeks with a history of intermittent fevers, recent weight loss, vomiting and marked lethargy. He lives with his parents and older sibling in a direct provision centre, as the family are seeking asylum following the conflict in Syria. His father smokes heavily and has a history of a recent productive cough.

His examination reveals a pale, lethargic and sick-looking toddler with a reluctance to move his neck freely. His vital signs are stable, and he is afebrile. His general neurological assessment reveals a right sixth nerve palsy, bilateral optic atrophy and hypertonia of the lower limbs with bilateral ankle clonus. He has several blood investigations performed and is noted to have significant hyponatraemia with a serum sodium of 128 mmol/L. He is admitted to hospital for investigation including neuroimaging and a subsequent lumbar puncture (LP). His MRI scan shows basal meningeal enhancement, and his CSF shows 150 white cells per high power field with a CSF protein of 1.5 g/dL and a CSF glucose of 0.5 mmol/L (blood glucose was 3.5 mmol/L). A diagnosis of tuberculous meningitis (TBM) is suspected, and he is empirically treated with quadruple therapy and oral prednisolone.

Clinical Pearls

TBM affects young children and carries a poor prognosis with 20% mortality and at least 50% of survivors have a persisting neurological deficit.[16] In South Africa, TBM is more common than either meningococcal or *Streptococcus pneumoniae* meningitis.

Presenting symptoms are often vague with nausea, vomiting, weight loss, lethargy and irritability, fever and seizures or focal neurological signs including cranial nerve palsies.

Early diagnosis is important, as TBM may present in three stages – stage one with nonspecific symptoms, stage two with the early development of neurological deficits (as above) or, finally, stage three with severe deficits including a depressed level of consciousness, papilloedema or marked hypertonia with ankle clonus.

A family history of tuberculosis is present in up to 50% of cases and up to 30% of children with TBM will have a positive tuberculin skin test.

Fundoscopy may show either optic atrophy or papilloedema, but many children have normal fundoscopy.

Hyponatraemia (as in this case) is relatively common in TBM.

If a child has suspected TBM, apart from MRI scanning and performing an LP, always request a chest X-ray and perform early morning gastric washings if there are changes on the CXR.

Typical CSF findings include lymphocytosis or leucocytosis, markedly elevated CSF protein and markedly low CSF glucose should be considered indicative of TBM until it is excluded. CSF culture is challenging, and nucleic acid amplification tests may hasten the diagnosis.

Treatment is with 2 months of isoniazid, rifampicin, pyrazinamide and ethambutol and daily prednisolone and a subsequent 10-month course of isoniazid and rifampicin according to local guidelines.[16]

Pitfalls to Avoid

The clinical features of TBM are often nonspecific in the early stages and empirical treatment may be required while awaiting test results.

BCG vaccination provides protection against TBM in high-risk populations.

Optic atrophy, focal neurological deficits and ankle clonus are key features in stage two.

Be aware of this diagnosis in high-risk groups.

palsies, neck stiffness and finally a depressed level of consciousness (Box 3.1).

In TBM, hyponatraemia is a frequent finding.[12] The Mantoux test may be positive, and an MRI scan may demonstrate meningeal inflammation at the base of the brain (Fig. 3.4). Cerebrospinal fluid (CSF) will classically show lymphocytosis, a high protein and a very low glucose. CSF cultures may take several weeks to come back, so PCR of CSF for *Mycobacterium tuberculosis* offers a timelier diagnosis in suspected cases.[13]

Herpes encephalitis (HSE) is the most common identifiable cause of viral encephalitis, and symptoms described by parents include a change in behaviour, excessive sleepiness or confusion.

Viral Encephalitis

Diagnosis of HSE is by finding herpes simplex DNA on polymerase chain reaction (PCR) testing of CSF. MRI is recommended (Fig. 3.5), and an EEG is also helpful.

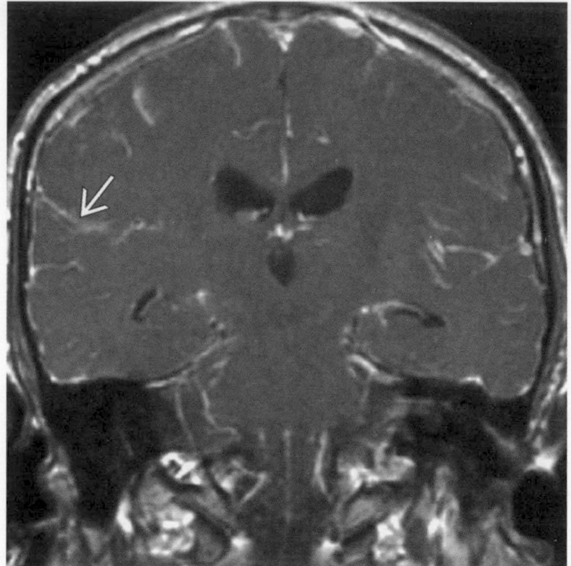

Fig. 3.4 Coronal T1 C+ MR shows diffuse leptomeningeal enhancement in a patient with TB meningitis. MR is particularly helpful in identifying the complications of meningitis including hydrocephalus, cerebritis, abscess, subdural empyema, ventriculitis and ischemia. (Source: *Diagnostic Imaging: Brain*, Fourth Edition, 2021.)

Prompt treatment with intravenous acyclovir is required (see case scenario below). Therefore, early diagnosis and prompt treatment are vital and offer the best chance to ameliorate an otherwise poor outcome (Box 3.2).

Encephalomyelitis

Acute disseminated encephalomyelitis (ADEM) is a post-infectious and immune-mediated inflammatory demyelinating disorder. Initially, symptoms include fever, lethargy, headache, vomiting and self-limiting neurological deficits.

> Symptoms of ADEM may be mild with a change in behaviour often picked up by the parents or severe with reduced consciousness.

Multifocal, hyperintense defects are evident on MRI of the brain with preferential involvement of the thalami and basal ganglia (Fig. 3.6). Spinal cord MRI may show lesions involving multiple segments with varying degrees of contrast enhancement.

Steroids are the recommended drug of choice in ADEM to reduce both the number of active lesions on MRI within days and help speed recovery.

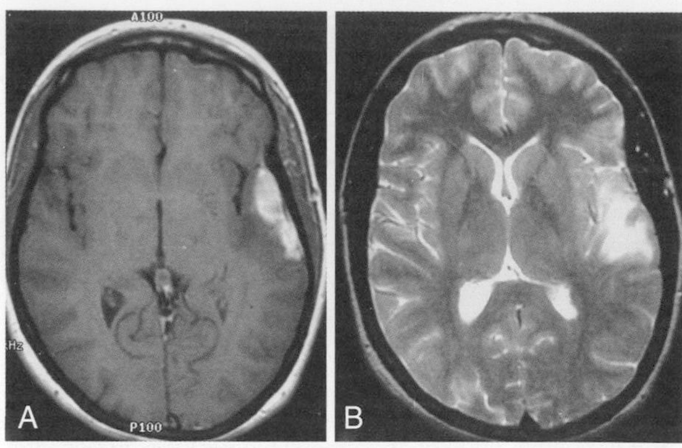

Fig. 3.5 Herpes encephalitis. (A) Spin echo, T1-weighted, non-contrast-enhanced axial image illustrating a lesion in the left anterior temporal lobe with a hypointense medial component and a hyperintense lateral component, which represents subacute parenchymal haemorrhage. (B) Fast spin echo, T2-weighted axial image showing the abnormal hyperintensity of this lesion, which represents a focus of encephalitis from herpes infection. (Source: *Youmans & Winn Neurological Surgery*, Eighth Edition, 2023.)

Performing a Lumbar Puncture (LP)

A good rule of thumb is that if you think of meningitis, an LP should be performed unless there are specific contraindications to doing so. Start antibiotics as per local or national guidelines as soon as the LP is done. The overall aims are first to identify children with meningitis, treat with minimal delay, use culture or PCR to help identify a pathogen and offer targeted treatment.

Across Europe and North America, there has been a 40% reduction in the number of LPs performed.[14] However, the LP remains a core procedural skill for paediatric trainees and is now performed in under 12-month-olds in most instances. Simulation has the potential to improve competency in the performance of an LP.

In recent studies from the United Kingdom, the median time from initial assessment in hospital to LP was 3 hours and many received antibiotics before the LP was performed.[15] Those who were admitted to intensive care most often had an LP deferred due to the severity of their illness.

Training programmes need to assess for procedural competence and identify opportunities using simulation to learn the procedure given the decline in clinical exposure over time.

Use a 22-gauge Quincke needle to perform an LP. Either poor positioning or poor anatomical knowledge

BOX 3.2 CLINICAL HISTORY

A 20 Month Old Presenting With Apparent Febrile Seizures

A developmentally appropriate 20-month-old female presented to hospital with a fever-related seizure lasting 20 minutes. There was a family history of febrile seizures, and the working diagnosis on admission was of a simple febrile seizure. Investigations including blood glucose and urinalysis were normal on admission. Blood cultures were negative.

Significant parental concerns were expressed to the nursing staff on several occasions during the first 48 hours following admission. She had a further febrile episode with a seven-minute-long seizure. Subsequently, drowsiness and lethargy were noted both by parents and nursing staff.

Three days following admission, a further focal seizure lasting 45 minutes occurred, and this led to further assessment and investigations.

A decision to perform an LP was taken with the following CSF results of 150 white cells, 210 red cells per high power field, CSF protein of 0.5 gm/dL and CSF glucose of 6.9 mmol/L. Cefotaxime and aciclovir were started intravenously.

A diagnosis of herpes encephalitis was confirmed, and she was subsequently transferred for further investigation and management to a tertiary neurology service. MRI imaging and EEG were performed with findings typical for herpes encephalitis

She had a subsequent relapse requiring further dose of aciclovir and developed frequent seizures requiring sodium valproate and lamotrigine.

On subsequent follow up, she had noted developmental regression and a striking hemiplegia and was referred to the local early intervention team for neuro-rehabilitation.

Key Clinical Pearls

Febrile seizures affect 1 in 20 infants and children. The definition of a febrile seizure is a seizure (usually generalised and tonic-clonic) associated with a temperature above 38.5°C in *the absence of CNS infection*. Therefore, both meningitis and encephalitis need to be considered especially if atypical, prolonged (more than 15 minutes) or focal seizures (as in this instance).

Fever and a focal seizure should merit consideration of herpes encephalitis and prompt commencement of aciclovir until it can be excluded.

Pitfalls to Avoid

Herpes encephalitis requires prompt treatment with aciclovir intravenously and should be suspected if focal features, an ongoing encephalopathy, or a prolonged seizure.

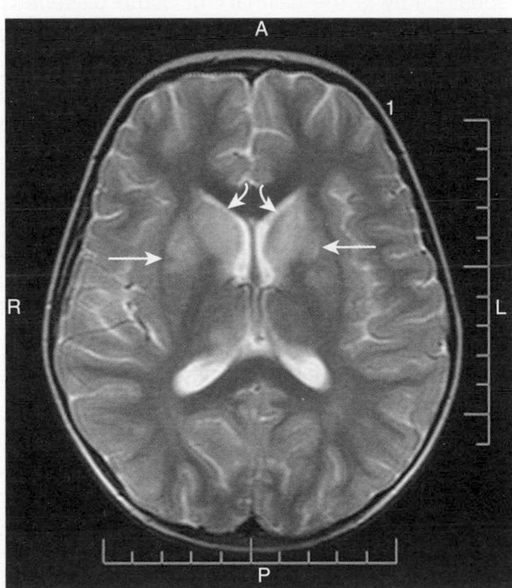

Fig. 3.6 Acute disseminated encephalomyelitis (ADEM). Axial T2-weighted magnetic resonance imaging shows symmetric increased signal in the head of the caudate nucleus (curved arrows) and anterior lentiform nuclei (straight arrows) associated with ADEM. (Source: *Fuhrman & Zimmerman's Pediatric Critical Care*, Sixth Edition, 2022.)

are the key reasons for failure to obtain CSF. The so-called Tuffier's line joins the superior aspect of both iliac crests and crosses the L4 spinous process in the midline. Insert the LP needle in a space inferior to this line in the midline (Fig. 3.7).

> CT brain is not reliable in identifying raised intracranial pressure so should not be solely used to decide whether a lumbar puncture is safe to perform.

Contraindications to performing an LP include cardiorespiratory compromise (e.g. due to sepsis with shock) and raised intracranial pressure (depressed conscious state, ongoing seizures with encephalopathy, sixth nerve palsy or papilloedema with hypertension and bradycardia). In children with haemophilia, disseminated intravascular coagulopathy or significant thrombocytopenia, the LP should be deferred until the bleeding disorder is corrected, and the patient should be empirically treated with antibiotics in the interim.[16]

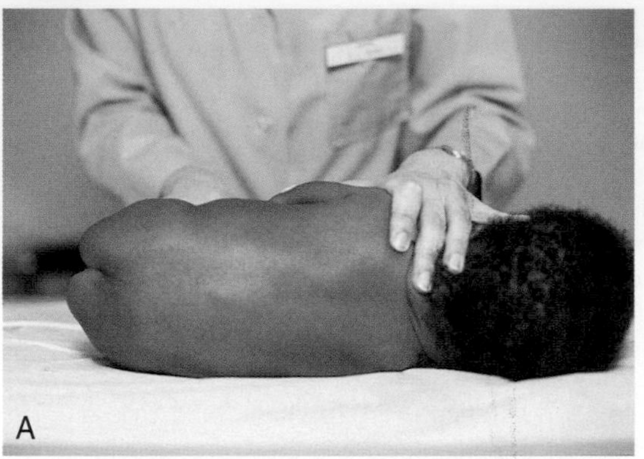

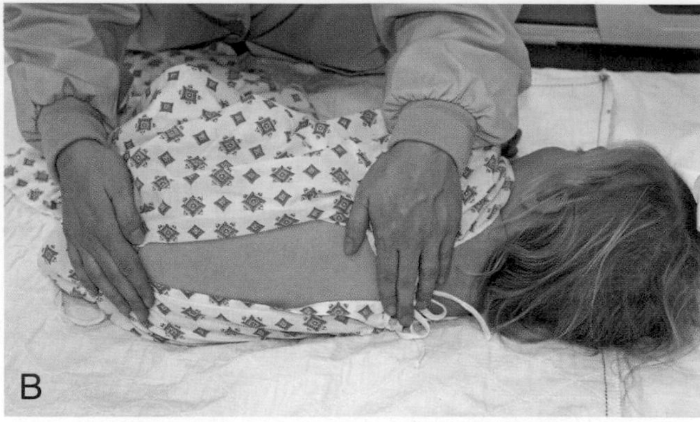

Fig. 3.7 (A) Modified side-lying position for lumbar puncture. (B) Older child in side-lying position. (A, From Wong DL, Perry SE, Hockenberry MJ, et al.: *Maternal-Child Nursing Care*, ed 3, St. Louis, 2006; Mosby.)

KEY LEARNING POINTS

Right at the core of acute paediatrics is a key conundrum – the chances of a serious illness in infants and children presenting to family practice are low, but the consequences of not recognising and treating specific illness can be devastating.

In any healthcare setting, prompt recognition of sepsis is essential to improve outcomes. With this in mind, parental level of concern is a key factor along with regular observation of vital signs and responding to concerns raised by nursing staff and excellent team communication.

The key skill to develop as an experienced clinician, whether in general practice or paediatric practice, is an awareness of the distinction between both instinctive and analytical cognition. Both are required to safely manage sick children, and the skill is knowing when to jump from instinctive to a more analytical approach.

Parents are incredibly important partners in the management of their acutely ill child both in terms of the history provided and in terms of their instincts about illness progression or resolution.

Meningitis continues to be the diagnosis that all family doctors fear missing the most and is the highest litigation payout condition in this group.

In suspected meningitis, drowsiness, somnolence, reduced tone and being nonreactive are all worrying symptoms. Also of concern is a change in crying pattern with moaning being a notable feature.

The three classical signs of meningism are neck stiffness (sometimes referred to as nuchal rigidity), Kernig's and Brudzinski's signs. These signs are not reliable in infants under 12 months of age.

Herpes encephalitis is rare and typically affects the temporal lobes of the brain. Children present with a significant alteration of consciousness, seizures or focal neurological signs.

Encephalopathy is the hallmark of acute disseminated encephalomyelitis (ADEM), and clinical presentation may vary from mild to severe.

In essence, PEWS scores convert clinical observations into a score and add in the concerns of nurses or family at the bedside and assist clinicians to recognise and treat a sick child before they deteriorate further. The trend of the PEWS score over time is key.

PEWS on its own is unlikely to be effective in improving outcomes and needs to be part of a system-wide approach to improve individual and team situational awareness.

Cold peripheries, marked tachycardia and prolonged capillary refill time are all key observations in assessing the sick infant or child for sepsis.

The 'Safe System' has six elements, and these are a safety culture, strong partnership with families, the ability to pick up the deteriorating child and respond to deterioration, a learning and nonpunitive culture and ongoing education and training.

REFERENCES

1. Fleming S, Gill PJ, Van den Bruel A, Thompson M. Capillary refill time in sick children: a clinical guide for general practice. *Br J Gen Pract*. 2016;66(652):587. doi:10.3399/bjgp16X687925.
2. Jones D, Dunn L, Watt I, Macleod U. Safety netting for primary care – evidence from a literature review. *British Journal of General Practice*. 2019. doi:10.3399/bjgp18X700193.

3. Roland D, Snelson E. 'So why didn't you think this baby was ill?' Decision-making in acute paediatrics. *Arch Dis Child Educ Pract Ed*. 2019;104(1):43–48. doi:10.1136/archdischild-2017-313199.
4. Clark A, Cannings-John R, Blyth M, Hay AD, Butler CC, Hughes K. Accuracy of the NICE traffic light system in children presenting to general practice: a retrospective cohort study. *Br J Gen Pract*. 2022;72(719):e398–e404. doi:10.3399/BJGP.2021.0633, Published 2022 May 26.
5. Blyth MH, Cannings-John R, Hay AD, Butler CC, Hughes K. Is the NICE traffic light system fit-for-purpose for children presenting with undifferentiated acute illness in primary care? *Arch Dis Child*. 2022;107(5):444–449. doi:10.1136/archdischild-2021-322768.
6. RCPCH. Safe system framework for children at risk of deterioration. Accessed online at: https://www.rcpch.ac.uk/resources/safe-system-framework-children-risk-deterioration#:~:text=This%20framework%20aims%20to%20improve,culture%20and%20support%20ongoing%20learning.
7. Chapman SM, Maconochie IK. Early warning scores in paediatrics: an overview. *Arch Dis Child*. 2019;104(4):395–399. doi:10.1136/archdischild-2018-314807.
8. Stewart CE, Radia T, Ghafoor K. Paediatric sepsis, the under-recognised killer: quality improvement initiative of outreach teaching in paediatric sepsis. *Arch Dis Child Educ Pract Ed*. 2017;102(5):278–280. doi:10.1136/archdischild-2016-312203.
9. Davis AL, Carcillo JA, Aneja RK, et al. American College of Critical Care Medicine Clinical Practice Parameters for Hemodynamic Support of Pediatric and Neonatal Septic Shock [published correction appears in Crit Care Med. 2017 Sep;45(9):e993. Kissoon, Niranjan Tex [corrected to Kissoon, Niranjan]; Weingarten-Abrams, Jacki [corrected to Weingarten-Arams, Jacki]]. *Crit Care Med*. 2017;45(6):1061–1093. doi:10.1097/CCM.0000000000002425.
10. McGregor C. Improving time to antibiotics and implementing the 'Sepsis 6'. *BMJ Qual Improv Rep*. 2014;2(2):u202548.w1443. doi:10.1136/bmjquality.u202548.w1443, Published 2014 Jan 14.
11. Tracy A, Waterfield T. How to use clinical signs of meningitis. *Arch Dis Child Educ Pract Ed*. 2020;105(1):46–49. doi:10.1136/archdischild-2018-31542.
12. Misra UK, Kalita J, Bhoi SK, Singh RK. A study of hyponatremia in tuberculous meningitis. *J Neurol Sci*. 2016;367:152–157. doi:10.1016/j.jns.2016.06.004.
13. Chiang SS, Khan FA, Milstein MB, et al. Treatment outcomes of childhood tuberculous meningitis: a systematic review and meta-analysis. *Lancet Infect Dis*. 2014;14(10):947–957. doi:10.1016/S1473-3099(14)70852-7.
14. Geanacopoulos AT, et al. Declines in the number of lumbar punctures performed at United States Children's Hospitals. *Journal of Pediatrics*. 2020:87–93. doi:10.1016/jpeds2020.10.034.
15. Lissauer S, Riordan A. Time to lumbar puncture: can we do any better? *Arch Dis Child*. 2018;103(12):1097–1098. doi:10.1136/archdischild-2017-314441.
16. Schulga P, Grattan R, Napier C, Babiker MO. How to use… lumbar puncture in children. *Arch Dis Child Educ Pract Ed*. 2015;100(5):264–271. doi:10.1136/archdischild-2014-307600.

ADDITIONAL READING

Bozzola E, et al. Management of paediatric post-infectious neurological syndromes. *Italian Journal of Paediatrics*. 2021;47:17. doi:10.1186/s13052-021-00968-y.

Corr M, Waterfield T, Shields M. Fifteen-minute consultation: Symptoms and signs of meningococcal disease. *Arch Dis Child Educ Pract Ed*. 2020;105(4):200–203. doi:10.1136/archdischild-2019-317722.

Defeating Meningitis by 2030. Accessed at https://www.who.int/initiatives/defeating-meningitis-by-2030

Edwards PJ, Silverston P, Sprackman J, Roland D. Safety-netting in the consultation. *BMJ*. 2022;378:e069094. doi:10.1136/bmj-2021-069094.

Fever in under 5s: assessment and initial management. NICE guideline [NG143] 2019. Accessed at https://www.nice.org.uk/guidance/ng143

Haj-Hassan TA, Thompson MJ, Mayon-White RT, et al. Which early 'red flag' symptoms identify children with meningococcal disease in primary care? *British Journal of General Practice*. 2011. doi:10.3399/bjgp11X561131.

Kawasaki T. Update on pediatric sepsis: a review. *J Intensive Care*. 2017;5:47. doi:10.1186/s40560-017-0240-1, Published 2017 Jul 20.

Sepsis: recognition, diagnosis and early management. NICE 2020. Accessed at https://www.guidelines.co.uk/infection/nice-sepsis-guideline/252817.article.

The Lancet. How best to assess children presenting to emergency care. *Lancet*. 2017;389(10076):1274. doi:10.1016/S0140-6736(17)30870-X.

The traffic light system. NICE Guideline 143, 2019. Accessed at https://www.nice.org.uk/guidance/ng143/resources/support-for-education-and-learning-educational-resource-traffic-light-table-pdf-6960664333.

Venkatesan P. Defeating meningitis by 2030: the WHO roadmap. *Lancet Infect Dis*. 2021;21(12):1635. doi:10.1016/S1473-3099(21)00712-X.

4

Managing the Febrile Infant or Child

Alf Nicholson, Karina Butler

CHAPTER OUTLINE

BACKGROUND

Fever is by far the commonest reason a young child is brought to their primary care doctor, and it requires a systematic approach. It is important in this post-COVID era that due consideration be given to all causes of fever.[1] High numbers of infants and children with fever are seen daily by family doctors who must decide on the spot about treatment or referral. They should always advise the parents to return for re-assessment if symptoms worsen.

If a febrile child visits an emergency department, a period of observation for up to 4 to 6 hours can be helpful, as signs can evolve in either direction in a relatively short period of time.

Latest evidence advises against use of paracetamol and ibuprofen together or being reassured that a temperature drop with antipyretics excludes sepsis.[2] One should check a urine sample for culture if febrile under 12 months of age, and there is no convincing focus of infection. After 1 to 2 hours, or sooner if indicated, reassess any infant or child with amber features on the NICE Traffic Light system (see Chapter 2).[3]

The triggering of cytokine receptors in response to the infection stimulates the production of prostaglandin E2 which causes the rise in temperature. Viruses and bacteria can cause a rise in body temperature. Viral infections can be associated with a high fever. Therefore, the height of fever does not tell you the type of infection. However, as fever in those aged under 3 months is associated with a higher risk of bacterial infection, a lower threshold to investigate and intervene with antibiotics is needed in this age group.

GETTING COMFORTABLE WITH RISK

There is an old saying that 'doctors do not take risks – patients do'. But there is little doubt that frontline family doctors, trainees and consultants in the emergency department (ED) are often concerned about the risks of discharging home an infant or young child with fever who might later, perhaps within 24 hours, re-present with serious bacterial infection, possibly meningitis. It certainly keeps us all awake at night (see Chapter 3 – recognising the sick child).

> Therefore, managing the febrile infant or child is all about accepting and managing risk.

The risk of invasive bacterial illness is highest in infants under 3 months of age, so added caution is advised. Over 3 months of age, the decision to refer or not, relates to the clinical presentation, characteristics of a rash if there is one, parental concerns and whether there have been prior visits to the surgery. Very few infants aged over 3 months require hospitalisation; however, when there is significant concern a period of observation is extremely important to detect early signs of clinical deterioration.

Traffic light systems (green, amber or red) may be helpful as are low-risk criteria for young infants, but both have limitations.[2,3] There has been a significant rise in febrile infants being referred to hospital despite a fall in rates of serious bacterial illness. A reduced tolerance of uncertainty on behalf of both parents and healthcare professionals is felt to be the reason for these increased referrals.

Key Points in the History

> In infants under 3 months of age, the risk of serious bacterial infection if presenting with fever is as high as 12%.

Infants Under 3 Months Require a Different Approach

In young infants, clinical examination alone is poorly predictive of serious bacterial infection. Symptoms may be non-specific and insidious in onset. They may present with a high or low temperature, poor feeding, irritability or lethargy and occasionally with circulatory collapse (Box 4.1).

BOX 4.1 CLINICAL HISTORY

A 6-Week-Old Infant With Fever

A 6-week-old male infant presents with a 24-hour history of excessive crying, low-grade fever and poor feeding. He was born by lower segment caesarean section, weighed 3.0 kg and was admitted to the special care unit for a short period due to transient tachypnoea. His chest X-ray at the time suggested transient tachypnoea of the newborn. He has been breastfed from birth, but his milk intake had dropped off over the previous 12 hours and his mother stated that he was not anxious to feed. He was admitted to hospital for observations and investigation. Subsequent blood cultures confirmed late-onset *Group B Streptococcus* (GBS) disease.

Pitfalls to Avoid

Infants under 3 months are different – Always be wary of a young infant under 3 months of age with a history of fever or documented fever on arrival. These infants are at risk for serious (invasive) bacterial infection, typically with GBS or Gram-negative organisms (*E. coli, Klebsiella* spp.) and much less commonly with *Listeria*.

Recognise sepsis – Suspect sepsis if an infant has a poor colour, prolonged capillary refill time, tachycardia (over 160 per minute), a drop in BP (under 30 mmHg if preterm), apnoea or tachypnoea (over 60 breaths per minute).

Act without delay – Prescribe them, get them, give them with the goal that the infant should receive intravenous antibiotics (ampicillin, gentamycin and cefotaxime) within *1 hour* of first contact or admission.

Several clinical guidelines, including the Rochester, Philadelphia, Boston and Pittsburgh criteria, are used by clinicians in an attempt to stratify febrile infants into high- or low-risk categories.[4–7]

> Any infant under 3 months of age with a documented fever should be referred to hospital for further assessment.

Infants aged 4 to 8 weeks with a fever have a 6% risk of serious bacterial illness. They may be observed in the ED setting for several hours if they fulfil the low-risk criteria (born at term, no underlying medical problem, a well appearance, no focus for bacterial infection on physical examination). In this well-appearing group, check the urine and blood cultures and perform a full blood count. The decision whether to perform a lumbar puncture

(LP) is a clinical decision based on the appearance of the infant informed by the results of the initial laboratory tests such as the white cell count or C-reactive protein (CRP). For the febrile young infant, the overall risk of bacterial meningitis is 1% to 2%, whereas the rate of a traumatic or blood-stained LP is 40%.[4]

Identifying young (aged under 3 months) febrile infants who are at low risk of serious bacterial illness and who may be safely managed without admission or antibiotic treatment is important. No single haematological or biochemical test reliably differentiates bacterial from viral infection. Blood tests such as the CRP and procalcitonin are superior in predicting serious bacterial illness than the white cell count.[5] Febrile infants under 3 months are at low risk of serious bacterial illness if they have a normal urinalysis and a procalcitonin level of under 1.71 ng/mL.[8] Experts caution in interpreting clinical prediction rules for young infants who have a very short history of fever (under 6 hours), as there may not have been enough time for the changes in parameters to take place.[4]

Overall, for febrile infants aged under 3 months (and in particular those aged under 8 weeks), investigations and observation in hospital are required with those aged under 4 weeks requiring a full septic screen and empirical antibiotics.

Looking for a Characteristic Rash Is Helpful

The overall incidence of invasive meningococcal disease (IMD) in England has dropped to one per 100,000.[9]

> As IMD is now so rarely seen, it may be difficult to recognise, especially early in the disease course.
>
> The characteristic purpuric or petechial rash is only evident in about half of the children with IMD prior to hospital admission, and classical meningism is often absent.[10]

There may be difficulties in distinguishing the early stages of IMD from a viral illness.

Four symptoms found to be highly specific for IMD are leg pains, photophobia, neck stiffness and confusion. These symptoms, if present in an acutely unwell febrile child, should be a cause for concern.[10]

Classical signs of meningitis (nuchal rigidity, Kernig's and Brudinski's) are *often absent in infancy*.

MAKING THE DIAGNOSIS IN PRIMARY CARE

Always be wary of a young infant under 3 months of age with a history of fever or documented fever on arrival. These should be referred to hospital. Febrile infants aged under 1 year with no obvious focus should have a urine sample taken (clean catch ideally), urinalysis performed and a sample sent for culture to confirm/exclude urinary tract infection (UTI).

In assessing a febrile infant or child, the key point in the history is the *response to stimulation*, as ill children tend to be under-responsive to caregivers.

> An infant or child with a fever who can generate a smile is less likely to be ill.

In older infants, suspect sepsis if an infant has a poor colour, prolonged capillary refill time, tachycardia (over 160 per minute), a drop in BP, apnoea or tachypnoea (over 60 breaths per minute). Early signs of septic shock include a capillary refill time of 3 seconds or more and tachycardia (age dependent but over 180 per minute significant). Later signs include cool or cold peripheries, a drop in blood pressure, an altered mental state with decreased conscious level and poor urinary output.[9]

> Lethargy, poor eye contact, altered mental status and a pale colour are all key and worrisome features that are unusual in children with minor illness.[11]

The tumbler test is helpful in defining the presence of a nonblanching rash and can be used by parents and healthcare professionals (Fig. 4.1). An ill infant or child with a fever and a spreading nonblanching rash (Fig. 4.2) must be assumed to have IMD until proven otherwise (Box 4.2). If meningococcal disease is suspected, then if readily available, pre-hospital parenteral penicillin or ceftriaxone should be administered without delay. This however should not be allowed to delay the urgent transfer to hospital, as that is the priority.

Invasive group A streptococcal infection, sometimes occurring in association with chickenpox, is characterised by a red macular rash with confluent areas and has re-emerged as an important cause of sepsis in children.[12]

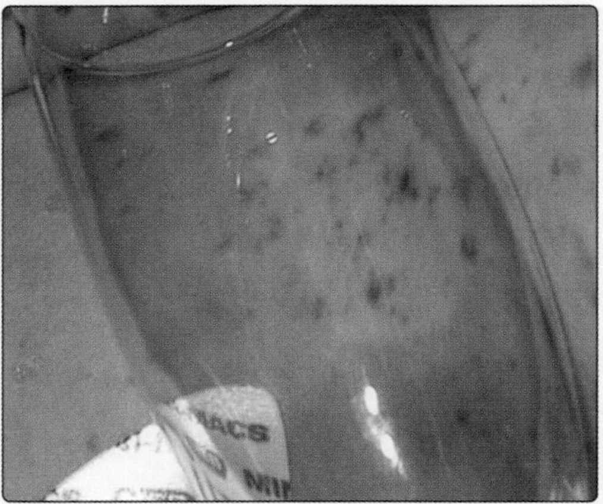

Fig. 4.1 Nonblanching rash in meningococcal disease. (Source: *Emergency Medicine: An Illustrated Colour Text*, 1st Edition, 2010.)

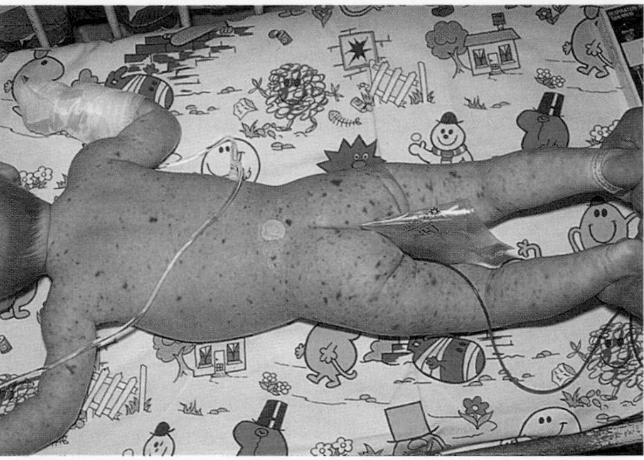

Fig. 4.2 Meningococcal septicaemia showing a purpuric rash. (Source: *Kumar & Clark's Medical Management and Therapeutics*, 2011.)

BOX 4.2 CLINICAL HISTORY

A 1 Year Old With Fever and an Evolving Rash

A 12-month-old female presents with a short history of fever and an evolving petechial rash to her family practice surgery. Her past and perinatal history are unremarkable. Her parents have been very reluctant to immunise her, and thus she had not received her primary vaccinations. Her examination revealed a high temperature, marked pallor, a capillary refill time of 4 seconds and a tachycardia of 180 per minute. She had several nonblanching spots over her chest and abdomen.

Mum and dad are present as the family doctor explains that the little girl will need an ambulance and emergency medication. The doctor confirms that she has no known allergies and promptly administers intramuscular benzylpenicillin. The ambulance arrives to transfer to hospital, and the family doctor calls ahead to inform the receiving team. The little girl required intensive care once she reached the hospital and stabilised, making a full recovery. *N. meningitidis* is confirmed by PCR testing and blood cultures.

Pitfalls to Avoid

Recognising Sepsis

In the early stages, meningococcal disease is hard to distinguish from a viral illness, and many do not have a classical petechial rash.

Children of African, Afro-Caribbean, Middle Eastern and South Asian origin pose additional challenges, as it can be harder to identify the typical rash associated with meningococcal disease on dark skin. If in doubt, ask the parent or guardian if they have noticed or can see any rash on the infant.

Signs of septic shock include a capillary refill time above 3 seconds, tachycardia (age dependent but over 180 per minute is significant) and later hypotension, cold hands and feet, a decreased conscious level and poor urinary output.

Signs of Meningitis

Classical signs of meningitis are *often absent* in infancy. Infants and children with meningitis may present with nonspecific symptoms and signs, including fever, irritability, vomiting and vague upper respiratory tract symptoms.

Timing of LP

Defer performing an LP if signs suggest raised intracranial pressure, shock, extensive or spreading purpura, respiratory insufficiency, coagulation results outside the normal range or a platelet count below 100.

CT brain is unreliable for identifying raised intracranial pressure.

If Recurrent Invasive Meningococcal Disease

Children and young people with recurrent episodes of meningococcal disease should be assessed for complement deficiency by a specialist in infectious disease or immunology.

If a child has a history of recent foreign travel, consider malaria or dengue depending on the geographic area visited, and request FBC and thick and thin malaria films. *Plasmodium falciparum* accounts for the majority of cases of malaria notified in the UK and is treated with artemether-lumefantrine (Riamet®). If signs of severe malaria, admit to hospital.

Searching for a Cause – Common Things Are Common

There are clear international guidelines that state that all infants under 1 year with a fever and no obvious source should have a urine sample collected and sent for culture and sensitivity. This may be challenging in a family practice surgery or emergency department setting. Clean catch urine is the preferred method of collection with a catheter specimen or suprapubic aspirate (with ultrasound guidance if available) preferred in a hospital setting in some countries.

> A urine bag specimen has a high rate of contamination and should be avoided.

Quite often an upper respiratory infection is likely where there is mild illness, rhinorrhoea and a mild cough with fever. Over the past 3 years, SARS-CoV-2 infection has been a common cause of mild nonspecific upper respiratory symptoms in young children, only rarely presenting as more severe disease warranting hospital admission.[1] Other members of the coronavirus family are common causes of mild upper respiratory infection in children.

Bronchiolitis is very common in winter in temperate climates and presents with tachypnoea, reduced feeding and a low-grade fever. Acute gastroenteritis is associated with mild fever, reduced oral intake, vomiting and the later development of diarrhoea. Hospitalisations due to rotavirus have declined markedly due to successful immunisation programmes. Over-diagnosis of acute otitis media (AOM) can lead to the unnecessary use of antibiotics. There are many risk factors for otitis media including male sex, indigenous ancestry, otitis media with effusion, a positive family history, passive smoking, low socio-economic status, daycare attendance and the use of pacifiers. Breastfeeding protects against otitis media.

> Acute otitis media (AOM) is very common (50% of children have had three episodes before their third birthday) and can be difficult to diagnose.

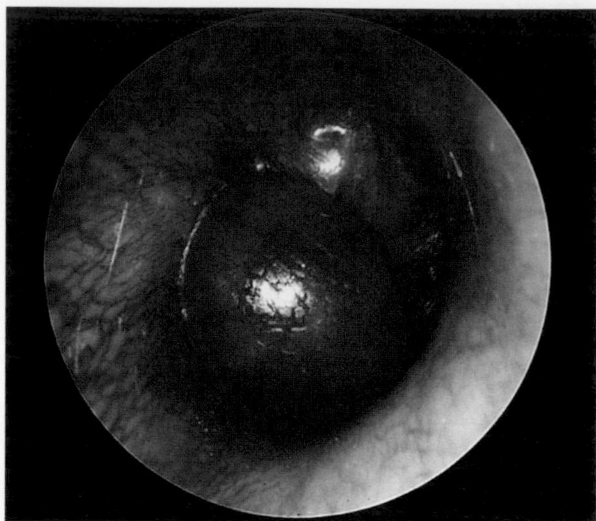

Fig. 4.3 Acute otitis media with bullous myringitis. This patient was febrile and extremely uncomfortable. On otoscopy, an erythematous bullous lesion is seen obscuring much of the tympanic membrane. This phenomenon, called bullous myringitis, is caused by the usual pathogens of otitis media in childhood. The bullous lesion often ruptures and drains spontaneously, providing immediate relief of pain. (Source: *Zitelli and Davis' Atlas of Pediatric Physical Diagnosis*, 8th Edition, 2023.)

Typically, the child has ear pain, fever and sleep disturbance. The presence of a middle ear effusion and a red bulging eardrum on otoscopy are helpful (Fig. 4.3).

> Acute otitis media in those aged 6 months and older is often self-limiting and should initially be managed with analgesics and an expectant approach.

Offer oral antibiotics to children aged under 24 months with bilateral otitis media or if there is an acute ear discharge due to perforation of the tympanic membrane.

Acute otitis media is managed by analgesia and watchful waiting and a delayed antibiotic prescription to be filled if symptoms are not improved within 3 days.[13] Prompt antibiotics are advised for infants under 6 months and those with immunodeficiency, craniofacial malformations or Down syndrome. Give amoxycillin for 5 to 10 days as the first line oral antibiotic with the backup of amoxycillin-clavulanate orally if the initial treatment is not working after 48 to 72 hours. Be wary of the child with a chronic or persistent ear discharge following a course of antibiotics where cholesteatoma (Fig. 4.4) may be the cause (Box 4.3).

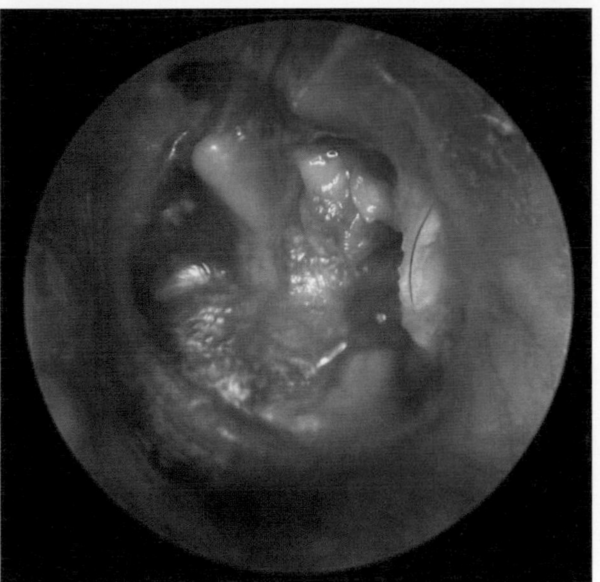

Fig. 4.4 A left tympanic membrane with cholesteatoma in the posterosuperior quadrant. (Source: *Hutchison's Clinical Methods: An Integrated Approach to Clinical Practice*, 25th Edition, 2023.)

Fever and a Rash

Your Greatest Worry – Invasive Meningococcal Disease

Experienced family doctors will have a keen awareness of the importance of a spreading petechial rash in an ill, febrile child.

> To check for IMD the infant or child has to be stripped down to observe the rash (eyeballing) is not sufficient.

As already outlined the early features of IMD, fever and erythematous maculopapular rash, are difficult to distinguish from a viral infection.

In a recent meta-analysis household overcrowding, passive smoking, a recent history of a respiratory tract infection and kissing all increased the risk of IMD.[14]

The Return of Invasive Group A Streptococcal (GAS) Illness

Whereas IMD has declined in recent years due to immunisation, we have seen a surge in invasive group A streptococcal (GAS) illness. The rash seen is quite distinct from that of meningococcal infection (Fig. 4.5).

BOX 4.3 CLINICAL HISTORY

A 10 Year Old With a Chronic Ear Discharge

A 10-year-old girl presents with a chronic ear discharge. She had no relevant past medical history but had been abroad on summer holidays and had presented with an ear discharge which was presumed to be otitis externa. Despite appropriate aural toilet, topical treatments and subsequent oral antibiotics, her ear discharge persisted. She had been seen by her family doctor on a few occasions, and she found visualisation of the tympanic membrane to be difficult. After 8 weeks, she was referred to a paediatric ENT clinic where it was noted that she had a significant conductive hearing loss in that ear. She went on to have an MRI scan that demonstrated a cholesteatoma which was surgically excised. Her parents were upset about the length of time it took to make the diagnosis.

Clinical Pearls

Cholesteatoma should be suspected where there is persistent or recurrent ear discharge. Cholesteatoma tends to occur in school-aged children and may have a slow onset with progressive hearing loss and an ear discharge. It may be misdiagnosed as recurrent otitis media or chronic otitis externa.

The classical appearance of cholesteatoma is of a yellow or white crust seen in the upper part of the tympanic membrane (Fig. 4.4). It may present with a facial palsy, and thus all new presentations of facial palsy should have an otoscopy with visualisation of the tympanic membrane.

Pitfalls to Avoid

Suspect cholesteatoma where a discharging ear fails to settle with treatment.

Visualisation may be quite challenging, as the external auditory canal may be filled with pus and be quite oedematous.

CT or MRI scanning is helpful and may demonstrate bony erosion due to the cholesteatoma.

If cholesteatoma is suspected, prompt ENT referral is recommended, and surgical excision is the definitive treatment and occasionally a mastoidectomy may also be required.

Rarely cholesteatoma may lead to complications such as a facial nerve palsy or a brain abscess.

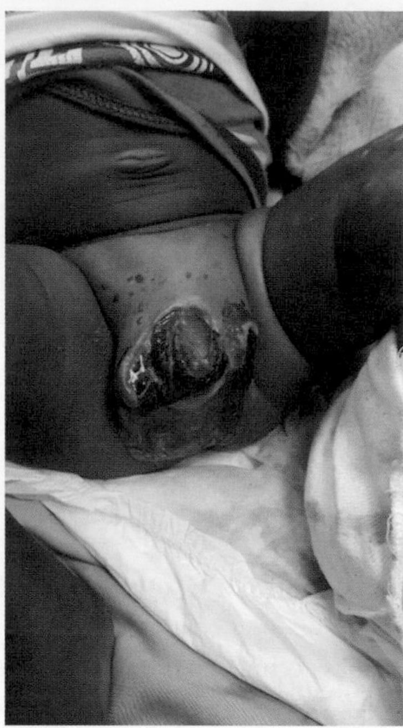

Fig. 4.5 Necrotising fasciitis in darker skin. (Source: Delport, J. E., Makamba, K. (2020). Necrotising fasciitis in a ten month old infant (Fig. 1). In: *Urology Case Reports*. Elsevier. © 2020 The Author(s).)

Diagnosis requires isolation of GAS from a normally sterile body site. There are three overlapping clinical presentations including focal disease (e.g. cellulitis, lymphadenitis, osteo-articular infection), bacteraemia and necrotising fasciitis.

> Some group A streptococcal strains, in addition to capacity for direct bacterial invasion, are associated with virulent toxin production and cause a toxic shock syndrome.

Toxic shock syndrome is associated with sudden rapid deterioration, hypotension, multiorgan failure and high mortality if not promptly treated.

Treatment of invasive GAS is with intravenous antibiotics such as penicillin or a cephalosporin. Clindamycin is generally added if there is serious infection or concern for toxin production. The combination of high-dose penicillin and clindamycin is the recommended treatment of necrotising fasciitis with the addition to intravenous gammaglobulin (IVIG). In toxic shock syndrome and in necrotising fasciitis, IVIG is postulated to reduce circulating toxin. Its use has been associated with a lower overall mortality.

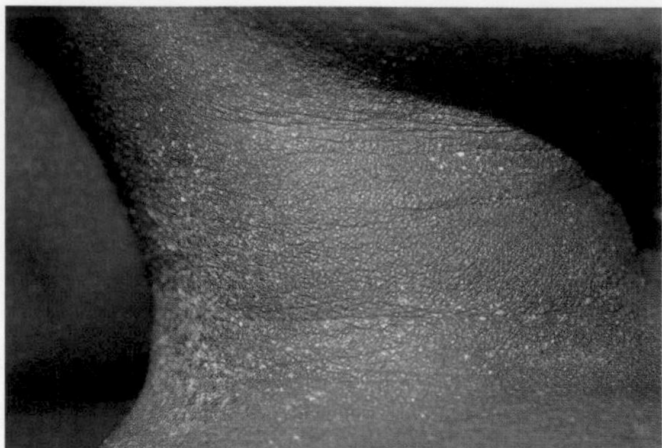

Fig. 4.6 Scarlet fever in a dark-skinned patient. The rash in this patient resembles 'goose flesh'. Note the early desquamation at some sites. (Source: *Paller and Mancini – Hurwitz Clinical Pediatric Dermatology: A Textbook of Skin Disorders of Childhood and Adolescence*, 6th Edition, 2022.)

Scarlet Fever – Making a Comeback

The rash of scarlet fever is due to a strain of group A streptococcus containing a bacteriophage that produces exotoxin A. The texture of the rash is like sandpaper (Fig. 4.6), and it blanches on pressure. The rash usually starts on the face and then spreads to become generalised after 24 hours.

> In scarlet fever the cheeks are red but there is a rim of circumoral pallor that is quite characteristic.

Erythema tends to be more marked at the anterior cubital fossae with linear, petechial appearance, so-called Pastia's lines. There is often a strawberry tongue (Fig. 4.7). Fading of the rash occurs within a few days. Fine desquamation begins after a week of onset starting on the face and progressing all over the body resembling mild sunburn.

The main differential diagnoses are staphylococcal toxic shock syndrome, Kawasaki disease and measles. Treatment is with oral penicillin for 10 days.

Erythema Multiforme – Dramatic but Benign

Erythema multiforme is a hypersensitivity eruption which may follow herpes simplex or other viral infection, *Mycoplasma pneumoniae* or medications. It is generally

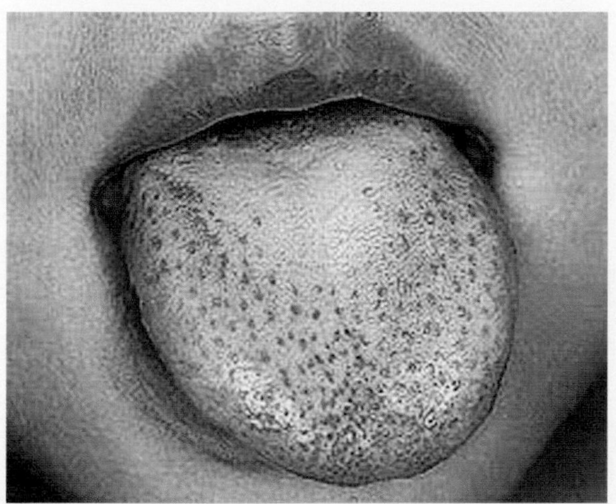

Fig. 4.7 Characteristic strawberry tongue of scarlet fever. (Ryan Pedigo, Amy Kaji. *Emergency Medicine Board Review*. Elsevier Inc. 2022.)

a relatively mild self-limiting condition associated with a low-grade fever. Skin lesions start as red macules or urticaria, and some later develop into characteristic target lesions (Fig. 4.8). Mucosal involvement is not uncommon.

The skin rash starts abruptly and symmetrically.

> With erythema multiforme parents are often concerned regarding a new striking rash on a background of apparent mild illness and fever.

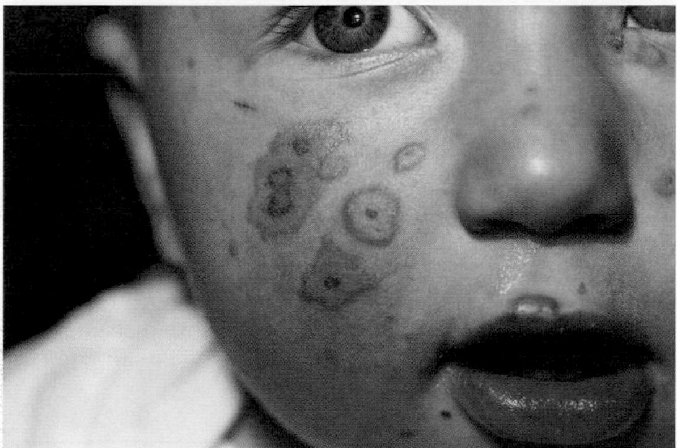

Fig. 4.8 Erythema multiforme. Classic target lesions and marginated wheals with central vesicles are characteristic. (Source: *Paller and Mancini – Hurwitz Clinical Pediatric Dermatology: A Textbook of Skin Disorders of Childhood and Adolescence*, 6th Edition, 2022.)

The skin lesions are usually round or oval, and all are present within the first few days. Management involves removal or treatment of the offending trigger, if identified, coupled with symptomatic support.

Varicella or Chickenpox – as Common as Ever with Rare Serious Complications in Unvaccinated Populations

Chickenpox is a common childhood exanthem caused by the varicella-zoster virus. The incubation period is approximately 14 days with a range of 9 to 21 days. Chickenpox has a characteristic spreading or cropping vesicular rash (Fig. 4.9).

> Chickenpox is highly contagious so secondary cases in the same family are very common.

Outbreaks are more common in late winter and spring. After initial presentation, the virus may remain latent in cranial nerves and dorsal root ganglia. Varicella may activate later in life in up to 30% of cases and present as shingles.

Severe disease is rare and is associated with pneumonia, neurological sequelae such as stroke or cerebellar ataxia (often delayed), hepatitis and the extremely important complication of secondary bacterial infection.

> Most cases of chickenpox are mild and self-limiting with a rash (initially described as 'dew drops on a pink rose petal') and a fever for 2 to 3 days.

Varicella immunisation is highly protective but not yet recommended in many European countries although used for many years in the United States. As a live vaccine, it is contraindicated in pregnant women and those who are immunosuppressed due to disease or its treatment.

Post-exposure prophylaxis with either varicella zoster immunoglobulin (VZIG) and by passive immunisation or with aciclovir is used for secondary prevention in high-risk children who have not had varicella or in whom varicella immunisation is contraindicated.

The rash of chickenpox first appears over the face, scalp and torso before spreading to the limbs.

Management of uncomplicated varicella is symptomatic with paracetamol, emollient lotions and

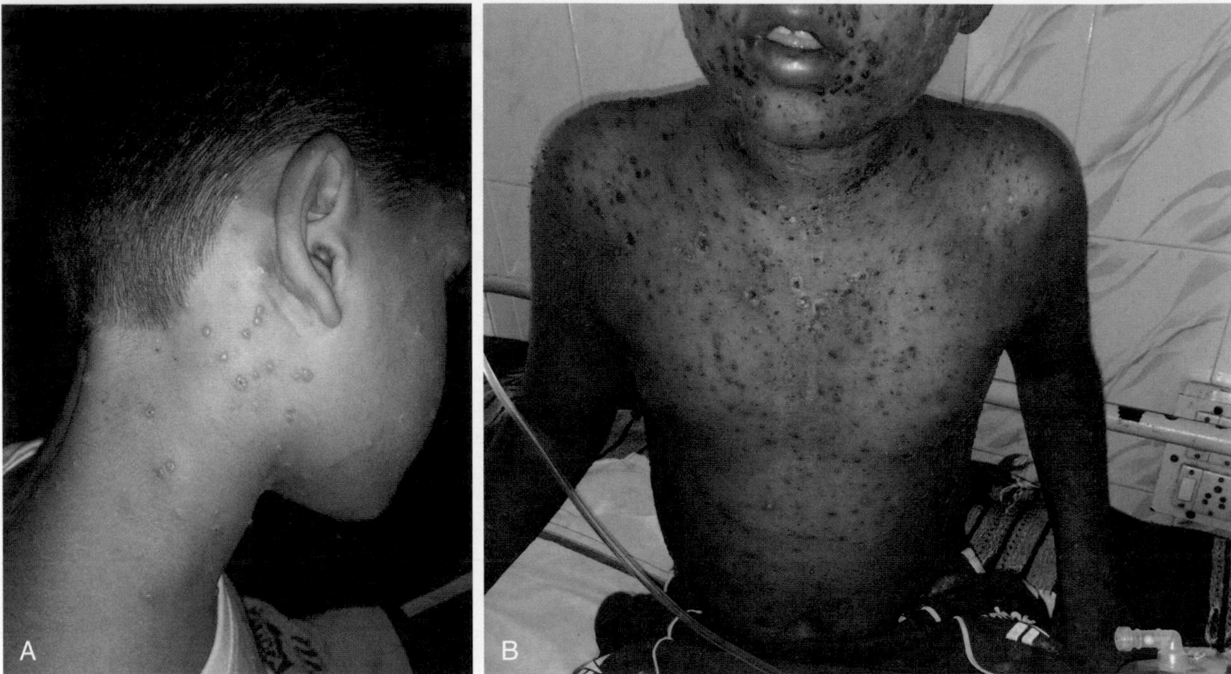

Fig. 4.9 (A, B) Pleomorphic lesions in varicella. (Aruchamy Lakshmanaswamy. *Textbook of Pediatrics, First Edition*, Elsevier Inc, 2022.)

antihistamines to relieve itching. Aspirin and nonsteroidal antiinflammatory drugs should be avoided.

> Chickenpox vesicles appear in crops and are usually completely crusted by 7 to 10 days.
> The diagnosis is usually a clinical one.

The key complication of chickenpox is secondary bacterial infection secondary to either *Staphylococcus aureus* or group A streptococcus (GAS).

> The key feature of secondary bacterial infection with chicken pox is a fever that persists beyond 3 days of the primary rash or that recurs.

The commonest complication of chickenpox is scarring which affects about one in five and most often affects the face. Varicella pneumonia is uncommon in children but does occur in adolescents and adults. Subclinical hepatitis with raised transaminases is quite common.

Varicella encephalitis presents with fever, headache and an altered sensorium and tends to present 2 to 6 days after the onset of the rash. Cerebellar ataxia is the most common neurological complication below 15 years of age (1 in 4000 children) and presents with a broad-based gait, tremor and rarely nystagmus.

Very rarely, children may develop intracranial vasculitis due to a post-varicella arteriopathy with the development of a paediatric stroke.

Dengue Fever – Common in Some Parts of the World

Dengue fever is an important airborne infection transmitted by four dengue virus serotypes transmitted by the *Aedes* genus of mosquito (Fig. 4.10).[15]

Dengue is endemic in over 120 countries, mainly in Southeast Asia, the Caribbean and Latin America. The incidence has increased strikingly over the past 50 years. Crowded urban tropical and subtropical climates provide the ideal backdrop for arboviral diseases and with global warming cases are now being reported in Europe.[16]

> Approximately one in four people who contract dengue are symptomatic

Symptoms may be mild or severe and last 2 to 7 days. Severe infection is more likely if there is a history of

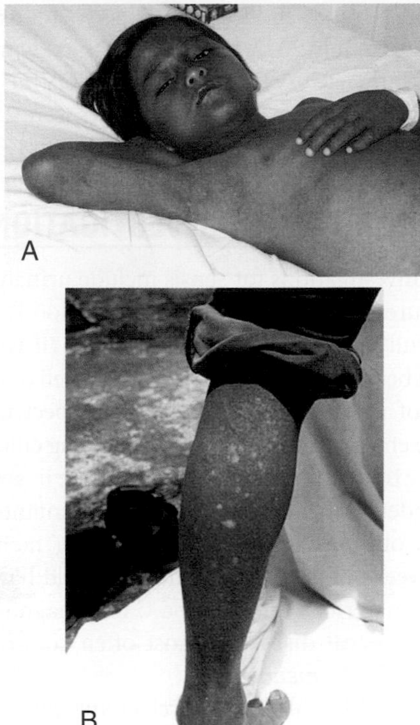

Fig. 4.10 Characteristic skin manifestations in convalescent dengue. (A) Early convalescent macular diffuse rash occurring in the first week after recovery. (B) Typical convalescent rash with 'islands of white in a sea of red'. (Source: From Vincent JL et al. *Textbook of Critical Care*, 6th Edition, Philadelphia: Saunders; 2011.)

prior infection with dengue virus, if under 1 year of age or if pregnant.

> Severe dengue disease is also associated with a marked thrombocytopenia, severe haemorrhage, organ impairment with shock and respiratory distress due to pulmonary oedema.

Diagnosis can be made using viral nucleic acid detection by polymerase chain reaction testing (PCR) or antigen testing; however, serology with detection of antidengue IgM is more commonly used. Elevation of IgM persists for 2 to 3 months. In secondary dengue infections, high titres of antidengue IgG occur soon after fever onset. Dengue haemorrhagic fever tends to occur in children during secondary dengue infection and in infants with a primary infection born to dengue-immune mothers. The main differentials are Zika and Chikungunya infections.

There is currently no specific approved antiviral agent for dengue, and treatment involves careful fluid management and the prompt identification of those with severe disease and associated shock. A new live attenuated Dengue vaccine, Dengvaxia, has been approved in several countries for use in children and adolescents who have had a previous infection. A number of other candidate vaccines are currently in trials.

SARS-COV-2 INFECTION

SARS-CoV-2 infection in healthy children is generally asymptomatic or a mild illness. Severe acute COVID-19 pneumonitis can occur. The risk of severe disease is higher for immunosuppressed children or those with underlying complex medical conditions. Symptomatic infection presents with fever, upper respiratory tract symptoms, cough and lethargy.[1] In young infants, the key symptoms seen are lethargy and poor feeding.

> Most children with COVID can be managed at home with supportive care.

The definitive test is real time reverse transcription PCR testing of a nasopharyngeal swab specimen. Antigen testing (lateral flow tests) of low nasal swabs, while somewhat less sensitive than PCR testing, has proved very useful in diagnosis and can be done in the home setting.

During the recent COVID-19 pandemic, a new condition termed paediatric multisystem inflammatory syndrome temporally associated with COVID-19 (PIMS-TS) (also known as MIS-C, multisystem inflammatory syndrome in children) has been described (Fig. 4.11).[17,18] PIMS-TS has been found to cluster more in certain ethnic groups than others, with reports noting that children of African American, Afro-Caribbean and Hispanic descent were more affected and had a more severe course than Caucasians.

Clinical manifestations include persistent fever, gastrointestinal symptoms (abdominal pain and diarrhoea), vomiting, nonpurulent conjunctivitis and an erythematous rash.[19]

> High rates of myocarditis and left ventricular dysfunction have been reported in PIMS-TS.

While there is much symptom overlap, the clinical features tend to cluster into one of three distinct groups:

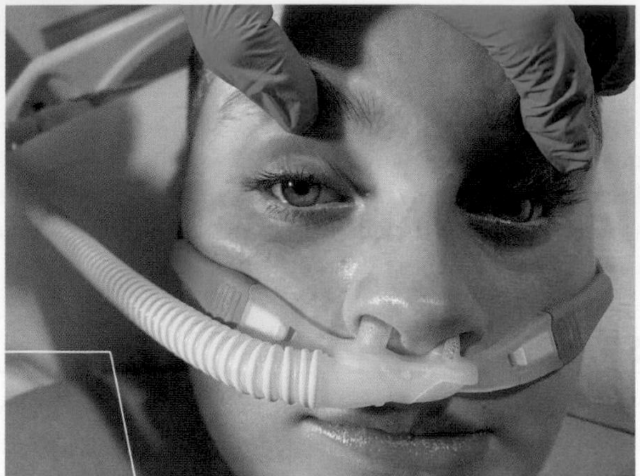

Fig. 4.11 Nonpurulent conjunctivitis with limbic sparing and red dry lips in an adolescent with multisystem inflammatory syndrome in children associated with severe acute respiratory syndrome coronavirus type-2. (Source: *Zitelli and Davis' Atlas of Pediatric Physical Diagnosis*, 8th Edition, 2023.)

A Kawasaki disease (KD)-like presentation, a sepsis or toxic shock syndrome (virtually clinically indistinguishable from other causes of sepsis) or a hyperinflammatory syndrome.

Manifestations of KD and PIMS may overlap in certain aspects, but differences can also be seen. In general PIM-TS patients are older and more likely to have prominent gastrointestinal symptoms (sometimes mimicking acute appendicitis) and to be hypotensive. Cardiac involvement is present in both diseases; however, higher rates of myocarditis and left ventricular dysfunction have been reported in PIMS-TS, and coronary artery dilatation and aneurysm formation are less common than in patients with classic KD. Lymphopenia is more common in PIMS-TS and may help differentiate these conditions.

Overall, SARS-CoV-2 infection is a mild viral illness in most children with key symptoms of fever and cough however severe disease and death can occur.

PIMS-TS is quite rare and long COVID (symptoms impacting on daily living that persist for at least 12 weeks after diagnosis) is less frequent in children than in adults.

COVID-19 vaccination has limited short-term impact in the prevention of SARS-CoV-2 infection but is very effective in reducing the risk of hospitalisation, severe disease and death in children as well as in adults. In the United States in July 2022, compared to those who are up to date with their COVID-19 vaccines, COVID-19 hospitalisations in children aged 5 to 11 years were 2.1 times higher and 2.4 times higher in those aged 12 to 17 years.[20]

INTERPRETATION OF INVESTIGATIONS

First-line investigations for sepsis include urinalysis and urine culture, stool culture (if diarrhoea), blood cultures, CRP and full blood count and procalcitonin (if available). LP should be performed if the infant is unwell or if under 3 months of age where intravenous broad-spectrum antibiotics are empirically started while awaiting cultures.

Urinary tract infection (UTI) affects one in six febrile infants under 4 weeks of age. Just 1 in 50 infants under 3 months old with UTI have co-existing meningitis. Under 4 weeks of age, febrile infants should have a full septic screen performed, even if a UTI is diagnosed.

Meningococcal disease is most often confirmed by PCR testing for *N. meningitidis*.

In KD an initial raised white cell count, elevated CRP and Erythrocyte Sedimentation Rate (ESR), thrombocytosis by day 14 of the illness are typically seen, and a sterile pyuria, mild transaminitis, low albumin and aseptic meningitis are other features commonly seen.[21] Echocardiography is essential to detect coronary artery aneurysms and coronary artery dilatation (Fig. 4.12).

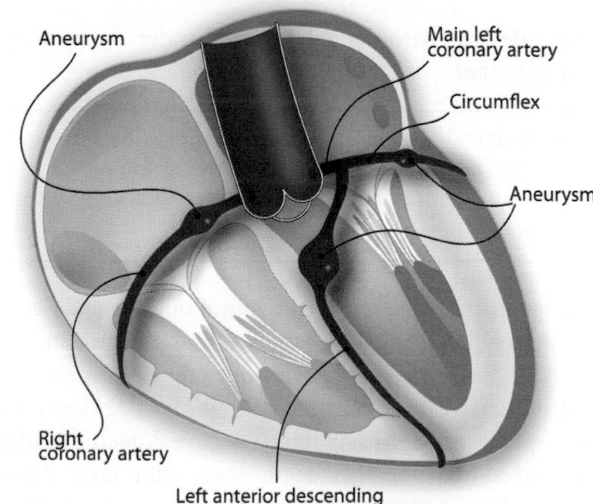

Fig. 4.12 Coronary aneurysms. (Courtesy Dr Bill Evans.)

REDUCING ANTIBIOTIC USE

Antibiotics are, of course, life-saving, but the more we prescribe them the less effective they become.

In the United States, up to a third of antibiotic prescriptions in an outpatient setting are felt to be unnecessary. Antibiotic prescribing is influenced by perceived parental expectations, clinician workload and habit. Antibiotic stewardship is defined as both the measurement and optimisation of antibiotic use both in hospital and the community.[22] Antibiotic resistance leads to poor prescribing and vice versa.

In paediatrics this poses unique challenges as a child with fever may have a serious bacterial infection that at first, is almost impossible to distinguish from a self-limiting viral illness. For those aged over 3 months presenting with fever, just 1% will have a serious bacterial infection.

In children with fever and no apparent source who are **clinically well**, antibiotics should not be prescribed.[21]

In those with acute otitis media, sore throat or cough, the best approach is delayed or no prescribing until after a thorough face-to-face clinical assessment of the child.

In the prescription of antibiotics, we should consider prescribing the shortest effective course and the most appropriate dose, complete the course, avoid antibiotics for self-limiting viral illnesses (not that easy) and avoid repeat prescriptions. In hospital practice, a review of all intravenous antimicrobial prescriptions after 48 to 72 hours should occur, evaluating the response to treatment and reviewing your choice of antibiotic in light of the microbiology results. Narrow-spectrum antibiotics should ideally be used. Always consider, if possible, once or twice daily dosing regimens, as this significantly improves compliance. Always consider and seek feedback regarding palatability, as it correlates well with adherence and completion of the course.

In addition, antibiotics can be associated with adverse effects ranging from a mild gastrointestinal upset to very serious *Clostridium difficile* infections.[23]

Antibiotic stewardship implies ensuring that antibiotics are only given when necessary, with the correct choice of antibiotic, in the right dose and for an appropriate length of time.

Most antibiotics are prescribed in the community, and while antibiotic stewardship efforts have focused in the past on antibiotic use in hospital, a far greater emphasis is now placed on outpatient and community use of antibiotics.

Why We Need to Reduce Antibiotic Use in the Community

Resistance

The overuse of antibiotics is associated with resistance both at a population and individual level.[22] Resistance patterns change in response to changes in antibiotic consumption in the community. Rarely, highly resistant strains of *Enterobacter* species have emerged, and these are increasingly challenging to treat.

Adverse Events Secondary to Antibiotic Use

Adverse events include relatively common gastrointestinal upset and rarely nephrotoxicity, secondary infections including *C. difficile* and sensory or motor disturbance or allergic reactions. Reducing the use of cephalosporins and fluoroquinolones helps to reduce *C. difficile* infections.

Effects on the Microbiome

Antibiotics can lead to a disturbance of the delicate balance of the gut microbiome that may persist for years. Disruption of the microbiome may contribute to the development of several conditions including coeliac disease, food allergies, juvenile idiopathic arthritis (JIA), inflammatory bowel disease and diabetes, and the risk increases if more antibiotic courses are given early in life.

Drivers of Inappropriate Antibiotic Prescribing

In the United States, acute respiratory infections are the main reason for the inappropriate use of antibiotics. Shortening the duration of antibiotic use is sensible and improves compliance. Happily, we have seen recent reductions in antibiotic use in children in the European

Union and the United States. This reduction may be due to changed prescribing habits among family doctors, public education of parents regarding the perils of antibiotic over-use and the introduction of the 13 valent pneumococcal conjugate vaccine.

In general, it is felt that prescription of antibiotics, especially in primary care, is as much a behaviour as a scientific decision. Family doctors require information on and oversight of their prescribing habits.

Workload and time constraints are also cited as reasons for antibiotic prescribing.[23] A Norwegian study found that antibiotic prescriptions were higher amongst family doctors with the highest number of visits to the surgery.[24]

Interventions to Reduce Antibiotic Prescribing

A multipronged approach appears to work best. Strategies include patient and doctor education, communication training, audits with feedback, delayed prescribing, clinical decision support for the GP and incentives to reduce antibiotic prescribing. Changing behaviour is the key strategy in antibiotic stewardship, and this applies to patient's families and to clinicians. Mass media campaigns such as the French 'antibiotics are not automatic' can work.

A key strategy for clinicians is to improve communication enabling a better understanding of parental concerns, the expected disease course and a backup plan if symptoms do not resolve. Most families can be satisfied without antibiotics if there is good communication.

Availability of inexpensive, rapid point-of-care tests with good sensitivity and specificity could help reduce antibiotic prescribing. Point-of-care testing (not least the rapid tests for streptococcal infection, nasopharyngeal aspirates for respiratory viruses and urinalysis) has been largely confined to an ED setting. The widespread use of home antigen testing for SARS-CoV-2 may represent a pivotal moment in empowering patient participation in self-diagnosis.

Active monitoring (or watchful waiting) is a very effective strategy and empowers parents to observe the progress of an illness and return or fill the antibiotic prescription if symptoms do not get better or progress.[22] Guidelines exist for this approach in otitis media in children. Delayed prescribing is a very effective strategy in reducing unnecessary antibiotic use.

The United States Centres for Disease Control and Prevention (CDC) offers excellent guidance about antibiotic stewardship.[25] Antibiotics are required when the clinical benefits outweigh the risks.

> The effective and appropriate use of antibiotics is an important element of best practice for family doctors.[24]

For Family Doctors and Those Working in Emergency or Paediatric Departments Dealing With Children

Try to avoid antibiotics for self-limiting illnesses.

Avoid prolonged intravenous use of antibiotics (over 72 hours) and switch earlier to oral antibiotics based on sensitivities.

Avoid empirical antibiotic treatment unless clearly indicated, as there is a balance to be reached.

Use antibiotics for the shortest possible course in accordance with local and national guidelines.

In hospital, seek advice from the infectious disease or microbiology teams in terms of reviewing the continued use of antibiotics in a particular child.

Regularly audit use of antibiotics to study prescribing trends in both hospital and the community.

Work closely and involve parents in a shared decision-making approach.

AN APPROACH TO PROLONGED FEVER

A prolonged unexplained fever is defined as a fever over 38°C daily for 14 days with still no diagnosis after an initial evaluation. The great majority have an infectious cause, some may have KD but a minority may have a rheumatological (systemic JIA, rheumatic fever or SLE) or malignant (leukaemia, lymphoma or neuroblastoma) cause.

The pattern of fever is important. A sustained fever with little variation throughout the day is characteristic of typhoid fever. In the case of typhoid, the fever is often associated with a relative bradycardia.

Intermittent fever, where the temperature drops to normal on at least one occasion each day, is characteristic of tuberculosis, abscesses, lymphoma, systemic JIA and some forms of malaria.

In relapsing fever, the child will have days without fever between febrile episodes and this pattern is seen in brucellosis, subacute bacterial endocarditis, lymphomas and malaria.[26]

Weight loss is important and is associated with chronic diseases such as inflammatory bowel disease, tuberculosis and lymphoma.

The six principal diagnostic criteria in KD are fever persisting at least 5 days, bilateral conjunctival injection,

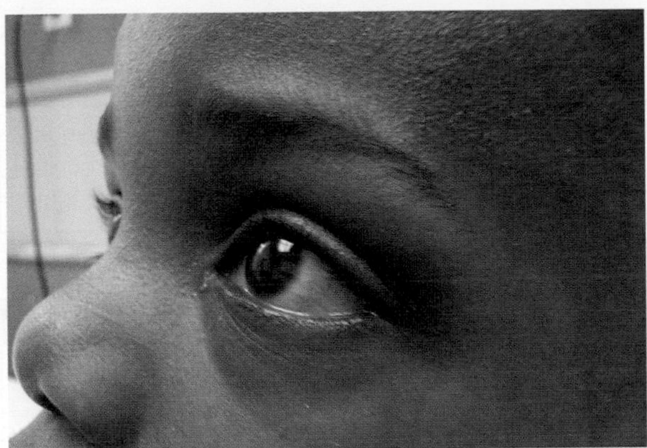

Fig. 4.13 Kawasaki disease. The conjunctivitis in this patient demonstrates the notable perilimbal sparing (halo of noninvolvement adjacent to the iris). (Source: *Paller and Mancini – Hurwitz Clinical Pediatric Dermatology: A Textbook of Skin Disorders of Childhood and Adolescence*, 6th Edition, 2022.)

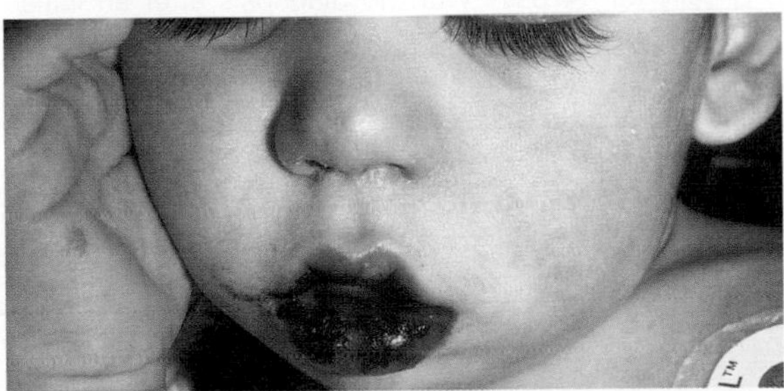

Fig. 4.14 Red, swollen, dry crusted lips in a child with Kawasaki disease. (Source: *Pediatric Dermatology DDX Deck*, 3rd Edition, 2021.)

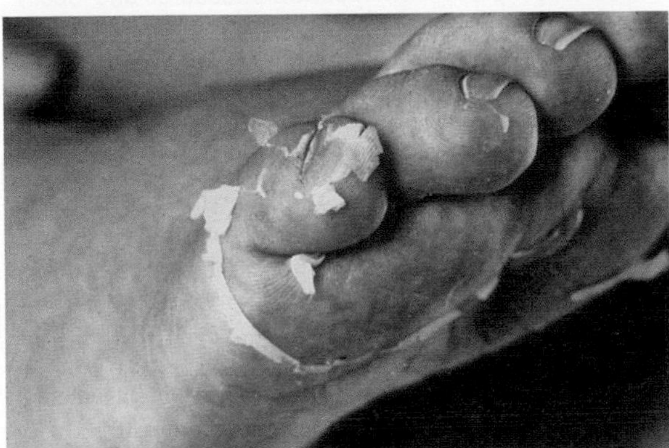

Fig. 4.15 'Candle-wax' peeling of skin typical of Kawasaki syndrome. (Source: Michalk, Schonau, *Differenzialdignose Padiatrie*, 5th Edition 2021 © Elsevier GmbH, Urban & Fischer, Munich.)

oral mucosal changes, polymorphous skin rash, peripheral extremity changes and cervical lymphadenopathy (Figs. 4.13–4.15). Five of these criteria must be met to diagnose KD. Atypical or incomplete is where less than five criteria are met.

Kawasaki Disease – Expect to See It and Be Ready to Treat It

KD is becoming more common worldwide (Box 4.4). It is now the most common cause of acquired heart disease (having taken over from rheumatic fever) worldwide.

BOX 4.4 CLINICAL HISTORY

An 18 Month Old With a Prolonged Fever

An 18-month-old male presents to their GP with fever and a diffuse macular rash. Initial assessment was within normal limits. The working diagnosis was a possible viral exanthem. His mother was given advice on what to expect and when to return. Over the next 5 days, he was very irritable, continued to have high intermittent fevers and a persistent macular rash prompting his mother to bring him back for review. He had no prior illness, a normal perinatal history and no history of recent foreign travel. On examination he is strikingly irritable. His temperature is 39°C and his heart rate is 170 beats per minute. He has a widespread macular rash and mild conjunctival injection. He is admitted for further assessment and investigation. His blood and CSF cultures are clear, and his urinalysis shows sterile pyuria. While in hospital over the next 48 hours his temperature fails to settle despite antipyretic measures.

Pitfalls to Avoid

Watch Out for Kawasaki Disease (KD)

In an irritable infant or young child with an unresolved fever (more than 5 days) and a rash, always consider the possibility of KD.

Nowadays KD is not as rare as might be thought. Early treatment with IVIG prevents the development of coronary artery aneurysms. The cause of KD is as yet unknown. It is now the leading cause of acquired heart disease in children.

Be aware of recent foreign travel

If a child has a history of recent foreign travel, consider malaria and request thick and thin malaria films. *Plasmodium falciparum* accounts for the majority of cases of malaria notified in the UK and is treated with Artemether-lumefantrine (Riamet®). If signs of severe malaria, admit to hospital.

Despite this, some healthcare professionals may be unaware of it and its potential to lead to long-term cardiac complications. Coronary aneurysm formation may occur in up to one-third of untreated cases. In treated KD, between 3% and 5% develop coronary aneurysms. A recent study from the British Paediatric Surveillance Unit (BPSU) found that infants and children treated 7 days following disease onset were at significantly increased risk of heart damage compared with those treated earlier.[27]

> Nowadays KD is more often seen than either meningitis or measles (in countries with high uptake of immunisation) so, is not as vanishingly rare as might be thought.

KEY LEARNING POINTS

Fever is the commonest reason a young child is brought to their family doctor and requires a systematic approach to its evaluation.

The risk of invasive bacterial illness is highest in infants under 3 months of age, so added caution is advised.

More febrile infants being referred to hospital despite a fall in rates of serious bacterial illness.

Infants under 4 weeks of age should be referred to hospital, have a full sepsis screen (including an LP) and commence intravenous antibiotics.

All infants under 1 year of age with a fever and no obvious source should have a urine sample collected and sent for culture and sensitivity.

Offer oral antibiotics to children aged under 24 months with bilateral otitis media or if an acute ear discharge due to perforation of the tympanic membrane. A red bulging eardrum is suggestive of otitis media.

As IMD is now so rarely seen, it may be difficult to recognise, especially in the early stages, when it closely resembles a viral illness.

Whereas IMD has declined in recent years due to immunisation, we have seen a surge in invasive group A streptococcal (GAS) illness and the rash seen is quite distinct.

In erythema multiforme, the rash starts abruptly and symmetrically. Parents are often concerned regarding a new striking rash on a background of apparent mild illness and fever. The skin lesions are usually round or oval and all are present within the first few days.

The scarlet fever rash is sandpaper-like in texture and blanches on pressure. The rash usually begins on the face and then spreads after 24 hours. The cheeks are red but there is a characteristic rim of circumoral pallor.

The rash of chickenpox first appears over the face, scalp and torso before spreading to the limbs. Vesicles appear in crops and are usually completely crusted by 7 to 10 days. The diagnosis is usually a clinical one.

Severe infection is more likely if there is a history of prior infection with dengue virus, if under 1 year of age or if pregnant.

Classical signs of meningitis are often absent in infancy. In older children, nuchal rigidity, a positive Kernig's or Brudzinski's sign are clinical signs still relevant in modern paediatric practice.

A prolonged unexplained fever is defined as a fever over 38°C daily for 14 days with no diagnosis after an initial evaluation.

Prescribe antibiotics for the shortest effective course, at the most appropriate dose and advise course completion. Avoid antibiotics for self-limiting viral illnesses (not that easy) and avoid repeat prescriptions.

Delayed prescribing for those assessed as being at low risk of serious invasive bacterial infection is a very effective strategy in reducing unnecessary antibiotic use.

In hospital use standardised antibiotic regimens and avoid third-generation cephalosporins if possible. Have clear 'stopping rules' whereby a review of antibiotic use is made after 48 to 72 hours.

Focus on general infection control measures and ideally conduct a weekly antibiotic stewardship round.

If a child has a history of recent foreign travel, consider malaria and request thick and thin malaria films. *Plasmodium falciparum* accounts for most cases of malaria notified in the UK and is treated with Artemether-lumefantrine (Riamet®) or other artemesin-based combinations.

KD is more often seen than either bacterial meningitis or measles in countries with high immunisation uptake.

REFERENCES

1. Ponmani C, Roland D. Fifteen-minute consultation: Does this child have COVID-19 (and does it matter)? *Arch Dis Child Educ Pract Ed.* 2021;106(5):278–283. doi:10.1136/archdischild-2020-320161.
2. Fever in under 5s: assessment and initial management NICE guideline [NG143] 2019. Accessed at https://www.nice.org.uk/guidance/ng143.
3. Traffic light system for identifying risk of serious illness in under 5s. NICE. Accessed at https://www.nice.org.uk/guidance/ng143/resources/

support-for-education-and-learning-educational-resource-traffic-light-table-pdf-6960664333.

4. Bonadio W. In search of an ideal protocol to distinguish risk for serious bacterial infection in febrile young infants. *J Pediatr*. 2021;231:32–34. doi:10.1016/j.jpeds.2020.10.069.
5. Velasco R, Gomez B, Benito J, Mintegi S. Accuracy of PECARN rule for predicting serious bacterial infection in infants with fever without a source. *Arch Dis Child*. 2021;106(2):143–148. doi:10.1136/archdischild-2020-318882. Children's Hospitals 2009–2019. *Journal of Paediatrics* 2021;231:87–93.
6. Jaskiewicz JA, McCarthy CA, Richardson AC, et al. Febrile infants at low risk for serious bacterial infection – an appraisal of the Rochester criteria and implications for management. Febrile Infant Collaborative Study Group. *Pediatrics*. 1994;94(3):390–396.
7. Huppler AR, Eickhoff JC, Wald ER. Performance of low-risk criteria in the evaluation of young infants with fever: review of the literature. *Pediatrics*. 2010;125(2):228–233. doi:10.1542/peds.2009-1070.
8. Pantell RH, Roberts KB, Adams WG, et al. Evaluation and Management of Well-Appearing Febrile Infants 8 to 60 Days Old [published correction appears in Pediatrics. 2021 Nov;148(5)]. *Pediatrics*. 2021;148(2):e2021052228. doi:10.1542/peds.2021-052228.
9. Meningitis (bacterial) and meningococcal septicaemia in under 16s: recognition, diagnosis and management. NICE Clinical guideline [CG102] 2010 (updated 2015). Accessed at https://www.nice.org.uk/guidance/cg102 and further update planned. Scope document Meningitis (bacterial) and meningococcal 2 septicaemia in children and young people: 3 recognition, diagnosis and management. Accessed at- https://www.nice.org.uk/guidance/GID-NG10149/documents/draft-scope
10. Haj-Hassan TA, Thompson MJ, Mayon-White RT, et al. Which early 'red flag' symptoms identify children with meningococcal disease in primary care? *Br J Gen Pract*. 2011;61(584):e97–e104. doi:10.3399/bjgp11X561131.
11. Brennan CA, Somerset M, Granier SK, Fahey TP, Heyderman RS. Management of diagnostic uncertainty in children with possible meningitis: a qualitative study. *Br J Gen Pract*. 2003;53(493):626–631.
12. Rodriguez-Santana Y, Sanchez-Almeida E, Garcia-Vera C. et al. Epidemiological and clinical characteristics, and the approach to infant chickenpox in primary care. *EJPE*. 2019;178:641–648.
13. Venekamp RP, Schilder AGM, van den Heuvel M, Hay AD. Acute otitis media in children [published correction appears in BMJ. 2020 Nov 23;371:m4550]. *BMJ*. 2020;371:m4238. doi:10.1136/bmj.m4238. Published 2020 Nov 18.
14. Spyromitrou-Xioufi P, Tsirigotaki M, Ladomenou F. Risk factors for meningococcal disease in children and adolescents: a systematic review and META-analysis. *Eur J Pediatr*. 2020;179(7):1017–1027. doi:10.1007/s00431-020-03658-9.
15. Guzman MG, Harris E. Dengue. *Lancet*. 2015;385(9966):453–465. doi:10.1016/S0140-6736(14)60572-9.
16. Wilder-Smith A, Lindsay SW, Scott TW, Ooi EE, Gubler DJ, Das P. The Lancet Commission on dengue and other Aedes-transmitted viral diseases. *Lancet*. 2020;395(10241):1890–1891. doi:10.1016/S0140-6736(20)31375-1.
17. Hoste L, Van Paemel R, Haerynck F. Multisystem inflammatory syndrome in children related to COVID-19: a systematic review. *Eur J Pediatr*. 2021;180(7):2019–2034. doi:10.1007/s00431-021-03993-5.
18. Stasiak A, Perdas E, Smolewska E. Risk factors of a severe course of pediatric multi-system inflammatory syndrome temporally associated with COVID-19 [published online ahead of print, 2022 Aug 10]. *Eur J Pediatr*. 2022:1–6. doi:10.1007/s00431-022-04584-8.
19. Schlapbach LJ, Andre MC, Grazioli S, et al. Best Practice Recommendations for the Diagnosis and Management of Children With Pediatric Inflammatory Multisystem Syndrome Temporally Associated With SARS-CoV-2 (PIMS-TS; Multisystem Inflammatory Syndrome in Children, MIS-C) in Switzerland. *Front Pediatr*. 2021;9:667507. doi:10.3389/fped.2021.667507. Published 2021 May 26.
20. CDC COVID Data Tracker. Accessed at https://covid.cdc.gov/covid-data-tracker/#covidnet-hospitalizations-vaccination
21. Gray H, Cornish J. Kawasaki disease: a need for earlier diagnosis and treatment. *Arch Dis Child*. 2019;104(7):615–616. doi:10.1136/archdischild-2018-316379.
22. Morley GL, Wacogne ID. UK recommendations for combating antimicrobial resistance: a review of 'antimicrobial stewardship: systems and processes for effective antimicrobial medicine use' (NICE guideline NG15, 2015) and related guidance [published online ahead of print, 2017 Aug 9]. *Arch Dis Child Educ Pract Ed*. 2017. doi:10.1136/archdischild-2016-311557. edpract-2016-311557.
23. King LM, Fleming-Dutra KE, Hicks LA. Advances in optimizing the prescription of antibiotics in outpatient settings. *BMJ*. 2018;363:k3047. doi:10.1136/bmj.k3047. Published 2018 Nov 12.
24. Gjelstad S, Dalen I, Lindbaek M. GPs' antibiotic prescription patterns for respiratory tract infections – still room for improvement. *Scand J Prim Health Care*. 2009;27(4):208–215. doi:10.3109/02813430903438718. PMID: 19929185; PMCID: PMC3413912.

25. CDC. Core Elements of Antibiotic Stewardship. Accessed at https://www.cdc.gov/antibiotic-use/core-elements/index.html
26. Lye PS, Densmore E. Fever. In: Kleigman RM, Lye PS, Bordini B, Toth H, Basel D, eds. *Nelson Pediatric Symptom-Based Diagnosis*. Elsevier; 2018:701–725.e2.
27. Kawasaki Disease. Results of the BPSU survey in UK and Ireland. April 2016 Archives of Disease in Childhood 101(Suppl 1). doi:10.1136/archdischild-2016-310863.7

ADDITIONAL READING

BMJ Best Practice. Acute varicella-zoster. April 2020. Accessed at https://bestpractice.bmj.com/topics/en-us/23/references

BMJ Best Practice. Evaluation of fever in children (updated 2019). Accessed at https://bestpractice.bmj.com/topics/en-us/692/references

Duke T, Wong NX. Antimicrobial resistance: think globally but act locally. *Arch Dis Child*. 2020;105(1):1–3. doi:10.1136/archdischild-2019-317953.

Fleming S, Gill PJ, Van den Bruel A, Thompson M. Capillary refill time in sick children: a clinical guide for general practice. *Br J Gen Pract*. 2016;66(652):587. doi:10.3399/bjgp16X687925.

Forbes H, Douglas I, Finn A, et al. Risk of herpes zoster after exposure to varicella to explore the exogenous boosting hypothesis: self controlled case series study using UK electronic healthcare data. *BMJ*. 2020;368:l6987. doi:10.1136/bmj.l6987. Published 2020 Jan 22.

Geanacopoulos AT, Porter JJ, Michelson KA, et al. Declines in the Number of Lumbar Punctures Performed at United States Children's Hospitals, 2009-2019. *J Pediatr*. 2021;231:87–93.e1. doi:10.1016/j.jpeds.2020.10.034.

Lissauer S, Riordan A. Time to lumbar puncture: can we do any better? *Arch Dis Child*. 2018;103(12):1097–1098. doi:10.1136/archdischild-2017-314441.

Lo J, et al. Multiple emergency department visits for a diagnosis of Kawasaki disease: an examination of risk factors and outcomes. *Journal of Paediatrics*. 2021;232:127–132.

NICE guideline [NG51] 2016 (updated 2017). Sepsis: recognition, diagnosis and early management Accessed at https://www.nice.org.uk/guidance/ng51

Tracy A, Waterfield T. How to use clinical signs of meningitis. *Arch Dis Child Educ Pract Ed*. 2020;105(1):46–49. doi:10.1136/archdischild-2018-315428.

WHO. Defeating Meningitis by 2030: A Global Road Map. Accessed at https://www.who.int/publications/i/item/9789240026407.

Yaeger JP, Jones J, Ertefaie A, Caserta MT, van Wijngaarden E, Fiscella K. Using Clinical History Factors to Identify Bacterial Infections in Young Febrile Infants. *J Pediatr*. 2021;232:192–199.e2. doi:10.1016/j.jpeds.2020.12.079.

5

The Newborn and Six-week Examinations

John Murphy

CHAPTER OUTLINE

The newborn and 6-week examinations are equally important. These examinations are often performed by paediatric trainees in the newborn period and largely by primary care doctors or nurses at the 6-week check. They are key opportunities to identify problems at an early stage in an infant's life. There is a different emphasis between the two examinations. The newborn examination is to a greater extent concerned with the detection of serious underlying problems including congenital anomalies. On the other hand, the 6-week check has more of an emphasis on the infant's growth and early development.

When undertaking the newborn examination, always note whether the infant is alert and stable. Ask about feeding, and the passage of urine and meconium.

In conducting a full head-to-toe examination prior to the infant going home, we recommend giving additional focus to the following areas:

- assessment for jaundice
- the assessment for a red reflex (absence of a red reflex may indicate a congenital cataract or retinoblastoma)
- checking for a cleft palate
- cardiac examination (looking for cyanosis, normal femoral pulses and the presence of murmurs)
- examination of the hips looking for hip instability
- looking for anal patency
- assessment of tone (now even more important in the light of new treatments for spinal muscular atrophy).[1]

These should also be looked out for at the 6-week check where again a complete examination is necessary with a clear focus on diagnoses that can be missed.

The 6-week examination is an opportunity to check on the infant's progress, whether they are meeting the expected targets in terms of weight gain, head circumference, length and reaching early developmental milestones. By this stage, most of the major abnormalities will have been detected or have declared themselves. Cardiac murmurs may now be evident as pulmonary vascular resistance falls.

This chapter will focus on these elements that can easily be missed on examination and may present at different ages using clinical case scenarios as a learning tool (Boxes 5.1–5.15).

THE FIRST FEW DAYS OF LIFE

BOX 5.1 CLINICAL HISTORY

A Newborn With Apparent Cyanosis

A paediatric trainee doctor was called to the postnatal ward as the mother became concerned about the colour of her 1-day-old infant. She informed the nurse who thought that the infant was cyanosed. Pulse oximetry was performed with an oxygen saturation reading of 70%. She called the on-call registrar, who confirmed the cyanosis, and she also noted a soft murmur. The infant was promptly transferred to the neonatal intensive care unit. Over the next hour, the infant's condition deteriorated with worsening cyanosis. The cardiology specialist service was contacted for advice, and the infant was intubated and ventilated and commenced on intravenous prostaglandin E1 infusion pending a definitive diagnosis. Both chest X-ray and ECG were performed. The infant was transferred to a tertiary paediatric cardiology centre where a diagnosis of transposition of the great vessels was made, and the infant was taken for an emergency balloon atrial septostomy in view of inadequate atrial mixing (Fig. 5.1).

Clinical Pearls

When an infant presents with suspected cyanotic congenital heart disease, urgent assessment and treatment is required. An immediate blood gas should be performed. A metabolic acidosis is indicative that the infant is already decompensating.

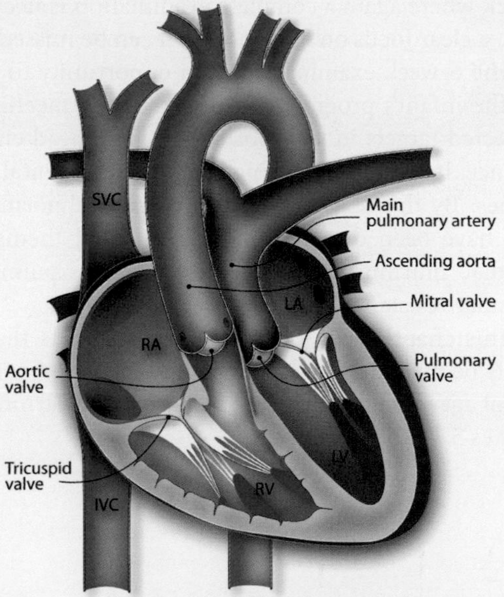

D-Transposition of the great arteries

Fig. 5.1 Transposition of the great arteries. (Courtesy of Dr W. Evans.)

The hyperoxia test helps differentiate cardiac from respiratory causes of cyanosis in the newborn period. The infant should be placed in 100% oxygen for 15 minutes and the pre- and post-ductal saturation documented. Failure of the oxygen saturation to rise above 92% and an arterial blood gas showing an arterial PaO_2 of less than 20 kPa indicates a high likelihood of cyanotic heart disease.[2]

Cyanotic congenital heart disease needs to be distinguished from persistent pulmonary hypertension of the newborn (PPHN) which is usually related to perinatal asphyxia, meconium aspiration syndrome, sepsis or idiopathic respiratory distress syndrome. In PPHN, the preductal oxygen saturation (measured in the upper limbs) can be somewhat higher than the postductal saturation (measured in the lower limbs). This observation of saturations being lower in the lower limbs with pulmonary hypertension is due to reversal of arterial flow in the PDA contributing desaturated blood to the descending aorta.

The presence of cyanosis or the observation of weak or absent femoral pulses are the most useful clinical indications to start a prostaglandin E1 (PG E1) infusion. There are nearly no cyanotic congenital heart lesions for which PG E1 is contraindicated besides obstructed total anomalous pulmonary venous drainage and, in balance, the risk-to-benefit ratio favours commencement of PGE1 pending a definitive cardiac diagnosis being made. However, it is unlikely to be effective in improving oxygen saturation in cases of transposition with an intact atrial septum. Transposition of the great arteries with an intact atrial and ventricular septum manifests as profound cyanosis immediately after birth that is refractory to all respiratory interventions.

Echocardiography provides the definitive diagnosis with increasingly diagnoses being made antenatally following routine 20-week fetal anomaly scans.

Pitfalls to Avoid

Cyanosis may be more challenging to pick up clinically on the newborn examination, especially in darker-skinned infants, and thus both antenatal scans and newborn pulse oximetry have helped to detect cases prior to further clinical deterioration.

If cyanotic congenital heart disease is suspected, start a prostaglandin E1 infusion to keep the ductus open, maintain oxygen saturations in the mid-'80s and seek prompt transfer to a paediatric cardiology tertiary centre. Be prepared for the risk of apnoea with PGE1 that might require respiratory intervention.

Always check the blood gases looking for acidosis.

BOX 5.2 CLINICAL HISTORY

Delayed Passage of Meconium

A newborn infant is diagnosed with Down syndrome at birth. On day 2, the junior paediatric trainee was asked to review because the infant had not passed meconium since birth. The infant was tolerating feeds, and the abdomen was clinically normal. The mother was very anxious to go home. This was agreed, but she was advised to return if the infant had not passed a stool over the next 24 to 36 hours. The parents returned to the hospital on day 7 of age because of concerns about the infant being listless and not feeding.

On review, the infant was clinically unwell. He had a low-grade fever, pallor and a prolonged capillary refill time; the abdomen was markedly distended (Fig. 5.2), and there was watery diarrhoea. The plain abdominal X-rays showed intestinal obstruction, the pattern in keeping with a possible diagnosis of Hirschsprung's disease (HD).[3] The infant's immediate critical condition was consistent with Hirschsprung's-associated-enterocolitis (HAEC). His initial treatment included assisted ventilation, fluid replacement, pressors, nil orally and intravenous antibiotics. Subsequent investigations, contrast enema and suction rectal biopsy confirmed HD. He was treated with daily bowel washouts (using normal saline via a rectal tube) and anal (Hegar) dilators to facilitate bowel emptying and he was booked to have a pull-through operation at 6 months of age.

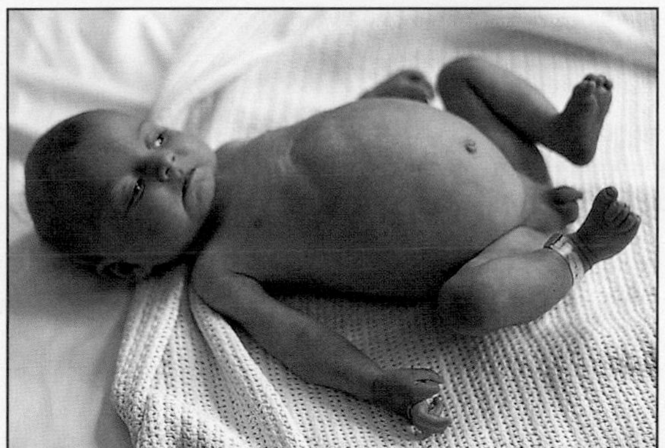

Fig. 5.2 Abdominal distension from Hirschsprung disease. (Tom Lissauer, Will Carroll. *Illustrated Textbook of Paediatrics*, Sixth Edition, 2020, Elsevier Ltd.)

Clinical Pearls

There was a missed opportunity to make an earlier diagnosis in this case. The infant's failure to pass meconium by 24 hours was an important pointer to possible underlying bowel pathology. The second piece of information was that the infant had Down syndrome, which has a clear association with HD. The third point was that the instructions given to the mother when going home were vague. At a minimum, the medical staff should have phoned her the following day and advised her to return as there had been no passage of meconium.

HD is characterised by the absence of the Auerbach and Meissner ganglion plexuses along a variable length of the distal bowel. The ganglion cells facilitate bowel relaxation therefore, in their absence, there is increased tonicity of the distal colon resulting in a functional obstruction. On a contrast enema there may be a transition zone, with a visible change in calibre, with dilated normal colon above and a narrow segment of aganglionic colon below.

Pitfalls to Avoid

Most infants have passed meconium by 24 hours of age. Delay in the passage of stools beyond that time point is a marker for bowel pathology. Senior staff should be notified, and investigations to determine the cause should be commenced.

Hirschsprung's associated enterocolitis (HAEC) is a recognised complication when the diagnosis of HD is delayed, but it may also occur after diagnosis either prior to or after a technically successful pull-through procedure. The likelihood of HAEC rises rapidly after day 7 of age. HAEC is caused by the increasing intra-luminal colonic pressure over the first week with bacterial proliferation, translocation and evolving sepsis.

HAEC typically presents with fever, diarrhoea and abdominal distension. HAEC is a life-threatening complication that requires aggressive rectal washouts to decompress the bowel and systemic antibiotics to treat sepsis.

BOX 5.3 CLINICAL HISTORY

Grass Green Vomiting in a Newborn

The postnatal ward staff midwife asks for a review of a 2-day-old infant who has had a single episode of bile-stained vomiting. The infant is breastfeeding well and has passed meconium on three occasions. The clinical examination of the abdomen is normal, and the anus is patent. The senior trainee advises to observe the infant and to report any further episodes of bile-stained vomiting. There are no further episodes, and the infant is discharged home the following morning.

Two weeks later the infant presents with pallor, abdominal distension and blood per rectum. An urgent abdominal X-ray showed intestinal obstruction with fluid levels. An emergency abdominal ultrasound and Doppler demonstrated a positive whirlpool sign, which indicates volvulus in the likely setting of a malrotation (see images, Chapter 18). Following intubation, ventilation and resuscitation, an emergency laparotomy was performed. The small bowel was untwisted, the Ladd's bands were divided and a section of ischaemic bowel was resected. An ileostomy was performed. The ileostomy was closed some months later with a good result.

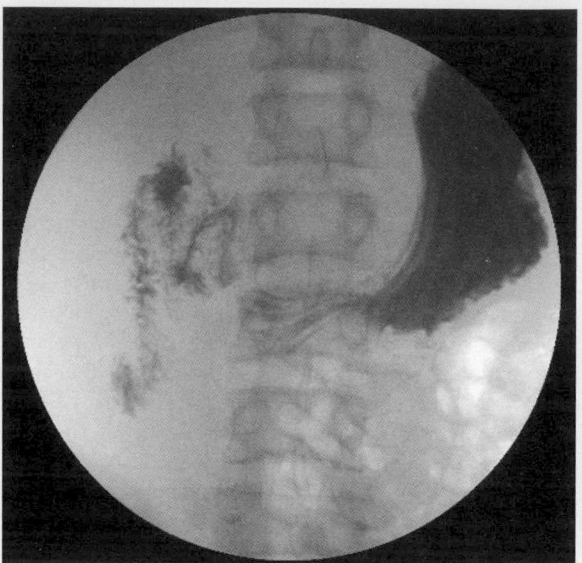

Fig. 5.3 Contrast fluoroscopy (upper gastrointestinal series) demonstrating malrotation. Note the small bowel fills with contrast all to the right of midline and does not cross over the left upper quadrant where the ligament of Treitz would be normally located. (Bordini BJ, et al. *Nelson Pediatric Symptom-Based Diagnosis: Common Diseases and Their Mimics*, Second Edition, 2023, Elsevier Inc.)

Clinical Pearls

The newborn infant who presents with an isolated episode of bile-stained vomiting remains a challenge.[4] One should always be aware of a young infant under 12 weeks of age with bilious or grass-green vomits. Bile-stained vomiting in the newborn period is *always* significant and merits immediate investigation for a surgical cause. Any infant or child with malrotation is at risk of midgut volvulus, which is a surgical emergency possibly leading to loss of the entire small bowel due to ischaemia, infarction and necrosis. The surgical treatment for malrotation is known as a Ladd's procedure.

The gold standard to make the diagnosis of malrotation is to undertake an upper gastrointestinal (GI) contrast study in every case. In malrotation the duodeno-jejunal (DJ) flexure fails to cross the mid-line to the left side of the patient and to rise to the level of the pylorus (Fig. 5.3). Doppler ultrasound shows the superior mesenteric vein wrapped in a clockwise direction around the superior mesenteric artery indicating midgut volvulus.

An upper GI contrast study should be arranged at the earliest opportunity. On the other hand, if there is a clinical concern about an acute abdomen in a newborn infant with bilious vomiting, a midgut volvulus must be suspected, and an urgent surgical referral should be made, with the possibility of an immediate laparotomy being required with or without a contrast study or even an abdominal X-ray prior to proceeding to surgery. Time is of the essence to avoid catastrophic loss of small bowel.

Pitfalls to Avoid

Never ignore bile-stained vomiting, even if it is a single episode. Bilious vomiting should always prompt an urgent upper GI contrast study even in an otherwise well infant. In young infants, malrotation is frequently associated with volvulus.

An upper GI contrast study must be undertaken in every case unless an immediate laparotomy is indicated due to the clinical status of the infant. It is the only way to exclude a malrotation of the small bowel. Plain X-rays are unhelpful, and a relatively normal study may be falsely reassuring. The plain films can be normal unless there is a volvulus causing obstruction and showing fluid levels. Abdominal ultrasound may be more useful.[5]

BOX 5.4 CLINICAL HISTORY

A Newborn Infant With Reduced Femoral Pulses

A newborn infant has a routine neonatal examination on day one as the parents had requested an early discharge within 24 hours of the birth. At the discharge examination the junior trainee was uncertain about the palpation of the femoral pulses but, on checking the pulses by a senior colleague, the junior trainee and mother were both reassured and the infant was discharged home.

On day four of life, the parents noticed that the infant was feeding poorly and had a poor colour. They contacted their Health Visitor who correctly advised that the infant be brought back to the hospital urgently.

When seen at the hospital, the infant was clinically quite unwell. She was pale with a prolonged capillary time of 4 seconds. Her heart rate was 180/min, and her respiratory rate was 70/min, her oxygen saturation was 92%. On cardiac examination, the femoral pulses were not palpable and there was an obvious left parasternal heave. A faint interscapular murmur was auscultated posteriorly, and an enlarged liver of 4 cm was palpated. A differential gradient of 20 mmHg was noted in the systolic BP measurements from the right upper and lower limb assessment. A clinical diagnosis of coarctation of the aorta was made.

The immediate management consisted of intubation and ventilation, a fluid bolus for volume resuscitation and the commencement of intravenous prostaglandin infusion. The infant was then transferred to the tertiary cardiac centre.

At the cardiac centre, the diagnosis of coarctation of the aorta was confirmed. Surgical repair of the coarctation was performed through a left lateral thoracoscopic approach. The infant had features of acute renal failure and required dialysis for a period of 4 days. The infant made a good postoperative recovery and was discharged home.

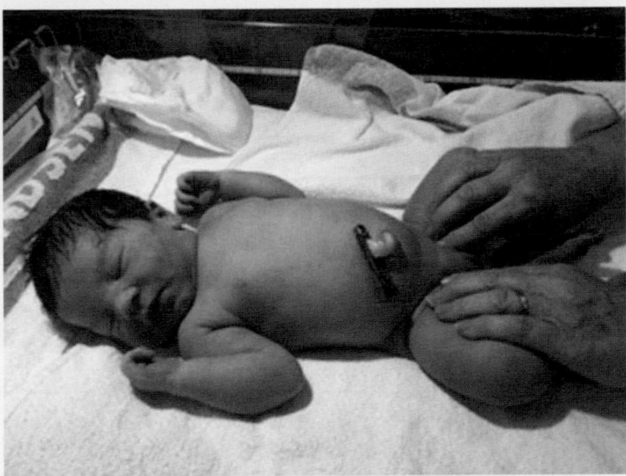

Fig. 5.4 Femoral pulses. (Sharon McDonald, Lorna Davies. *Examination of the Newborn and Neonatal Health; A Multidimensional Approach*, Second Edition, 2021, Elsevier Inc.)

Clinical Pearls

Coarctation of the aorta is one of the most commonly 'missed' congenital heart disease defects.

The key finding on physical examination is the absence or reduction of femoral pulses. We all know that feeling for femoral pulse is challenging for inexperienced doctors and thus coarctation is easily missed on the newborn examination. Palpation for femoral pulses is best performed with the thighs semiflexed. The pulse is mid-way between the symphysis pubis and the anterior iliac crest (Fig. 5.4).

Infants with coarctation are often asymptomatic until the ductus arteriosus closes (usually 48–72 hours). All newborn examinations tend to take place within the first 48 hours of age, and this poses very significant challenges in terms of picking up coarctation as classical signs of coarctation (hypertension of the upper limbs and absent femoral pulses) may not be evident until 5 days of age.

Most infants with severe coarctation develop heart failure symptoms by the end of the first week of life, and these symptoms may be poor feeding, tachypnoea, cool legs and feet and an overall poor colour.[6] Coarctation causes failure to thrive both due to breathlessness leading to poor feeding and increased energy requirements due to the added work of breathing.

In coarctation of the aorta there may be a left parasternal impulse, due to the dominance of the right ventricle. We have found this a very helpful pointer when there is a concern about the femoral pulses. The presence of a left parasternal heave substantially increases the likelihood of cardiac pathology.

The four limb blood pressures can be measured when there is concern about the femoral pulses. Upper limb hypertension has been found in 97% of infants with coarctation, and a systolic blood pressure that is over 20 mm Hg higher in the arms than the legs is evidence of a coarctation (specificity 92%). However, a negative finding does not exclude the diagnosis.[6]

Another useful tip would be to bring the infant back in 24 to 48 hours for a review. This is particularly helpful for infants who are discharged within the first 24 hours. In cases of coarctation the pulses may have become definitely impalpable.

Continued

BOX 5.4 CLINICAL HISTORY—CONT'D

Pitfalls to Avoid

Pulse oximetry struggles to consistently detect left heart obstructive disease, such as coarctation of the aorta, interrupted aortic arch and hypoplastic left heart syndrome, as initially these may not be associated with abnormal saturations.[7,8]

Always palpate the praecordium looking for a left parasternal heave. The presence of a parasternal heave increases the likelihood of congenital heart disease.

Be extra vigilant when the examination is carried out less than 24 hours after the birth.

If coarctation is suspected, urgent cardiology referral is indicated.

BOX 5.5 CLINICAL HISTORY

Overstretched Again

A young trainee had ten newborn examinations to be performed and, in addition, had multiple calls from the newborn nursery. During one of the newborn examinations, the trainee noted that there was meconium present on the infant's nappy and presumed that the anus was patent. The infant was discharged home and 3 days later the parents brought the infant to the hospital because he was listless and vomiting. He was now markedly ill with a prolonged capillary refill time, a distended tense abdomen and the anus was clearly not patent (Fig. 5.5).

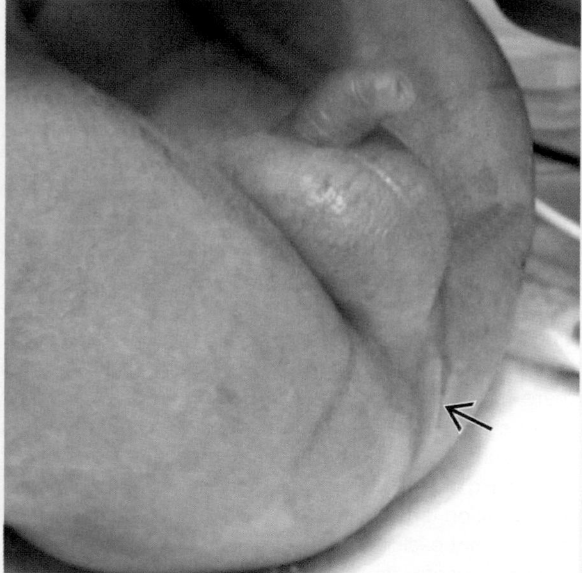

Fig. 5.5 Clinical photograph shows a newborn male patient with anal atresia. In this case, the genitalia are normal, but vertebral body anomalies were suspected on ultrasound. (Kennedy A, et al. *Diagnostic Imaging: Obstetrics*, Fourth Edition, 2021, Elsevier; Inc.)

Abdominal X-rays showed distended bowel loops and free air under the diaphragm. The clinical diagnosis was imperforate anus (ARM) with bowel perforation.

The infant was intubated, ventilated and given fluid boluses and intravenous antibiotics. When his condition was stabilised, a laparotomy was performed. The colonic perforation was repaired, peritoneal lavage undertaken and a double-barrel colostomy performed. The infant made a satisfactory recovery. He underwent a distal loopogram, where contrast is instilled into the distal limb of his colostomy (mucous fistula) to define the exact anatomy of his potential recto-urethral or recto-perineal fistula on an elective basis. After appropriate counselling of his parents regarding the risks and long-term management of their child's condition, he was booked for surgery. The definitive repair of his imperforate anus (Posterior Sagittal AnoRectoPlasty – PSARP) was performed at 6 months of age. He underwent a period of anal dilatations postoperatively to prevent anal stenosis or stricture formation, and 3 months later his colostomy was closed.

Clinical Pearls

Confirmation that the anus is patent is an important part of the abdominal examination of the newborn infant. The anus must be examined carefully and positively identified. Gently separate the buttocks and wipe away any meconium. Satisfy yourself that the anus is in the correct position and that it looks normal.

This examination of the anus is not as easy as it would initially appear. Previous studies have reported that as many as 25% of cases are missed on newborn examination.

In this instance, an imperforate anus was not identified because the doctor presumed that the presence of meconium meant that the anus must be patent.[9] This was incorrect. In cases of ARM there is usually a recto-urethral (prostatic or bulbar), recto-vesical or recto-perineal fistula in males or a recto-vestibular (vaginal) fistula in females, which may permit the passage of some meconium. In infants with Down syndrome, who have an ARM, they are significantly less likely to have a fistula and therefore are unlikely to pass any meconium in the newborn period.

In approximately half of cases of ARM there are associated anomalies which may form part of the VACTERL association – V (vertebral), A (anal), C (cardiac), T (tracheaoesophageal), R (renal), L (limb defects). To make the diagnosis of VACTERL, at least three defects must be present.

Pitfalls to Avoid

The anus must always be positively identified.

Doctors need to be very vigilant as an ARM can be easily missed if one is in a hurry.

BOX 5.6 CLINICAL HISTORY

Creamy Discharge From the Eyes

A 5-day-old infant returns to the maternity hospital due to bilateral sticky eyes. The infant's mother is 20 years of age and had an uneventful pregnancy and delivery. The infant had quite puffy eyelids in the newborn period and was discharged on day 2.

The day 5 examination of the infant revealed a profuse bilateral creamy discharge and thus the attending doctor wisely admitted the infant (Fig. 5.6). Eye swabs subsequently demonstrated *Chlamydia trachomatis*.

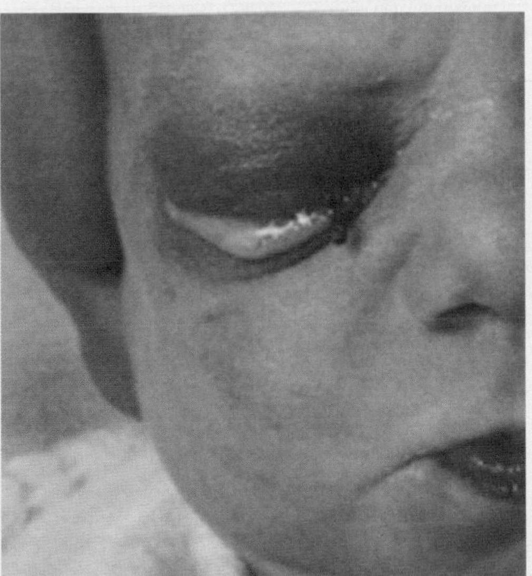

Fig. 5.6 Gonococcal ophthalmia neonatorum. (Source: From McMillan A, Scott GR. *Sexually Transmitted Infections: A Colour Guide*. Churchill Livingstone, Elsevier Ltd; 2000.)

Clinical Pearls

Bilateral persistent creamy discharge from both eyes should be easily distinguishable from a so-called sticky eye.

Perinatal transmission of *C. trachomatis* and *Neisseria gonorrhoeae* can result in neonatal conjunctivitis known as ophthalmia neonatorum.[10] The infant requires a 14-day course of oral erythromycin and a single dose of azithromycin for both parents.

The ongoing incidence of ophthalmia neonatorum caused by *C. trachomatis* or *N. gonorrhoeae* can be addressed by routine maternal prenatal screening for and treatment of sexually transmitted infections and by postpartum neonatal ocular prophylaxis against *N. gonorrhoeae*.[10]

Pitfalls to Avoid

A creamy or bloody eye discharge, particularly if bilateral, may indicate ophthalmia neonatorum and relevant swabs (testing for DNA by polymerase chain reaction) should be taken and treatment started.

THE FIRST FEW WEEKS OF LIFE

BOX 5.7 CLINICAL HISTORY

Vomiting in Early Infancy

A mother brings her 2-week-old male infant to the family doctor because he has been vomiting some of his feeds. The amount that he is vomiting is small. He remains keen to feed and he is passing bowel motions. He is back to his birth weight. Physical examination is normal. The doctor concludes that the vomits are due to reflux and reassures the mother.

The mother rings the family practice a week later. The infant is vomiting larger amounts of feeds. There is a different doctor on duty. He checks the infant's record and notes that his colleague has previously made a diagnosis of gastro-oesophageal reflux. He prescribes a course of omeprazole over the phone and sends the electronic script to the family's pharmacy for collection.

Some 5 days later, the mother contacts the practice stating that the infant is vomiting after most feeds and that he is constipated. The first doctor takes the call. He advises the mother to double the dose of omeprazole and to contact the surgery again if the infant has not improved in 3 days. The mother becomes more concerned and takes the infant to hospital.

The infant is now thin, with loose skin folds, with cold peripheries and a depressed anterior fontanelle. He is 200 g below his birth weight. There are visible peristaltic waves across the upper abdomen (Fig. 5.7). A diagnosis of pyloric stenosis with dehydration is made. The diagnosis is confirmed on ultrasound. Following rehydration and correction of his electrolyte abnormalities, a pyloromyotomy is performed. He is discharged home 2 days later once his normal feeding pattern has resumed with no vomiting.

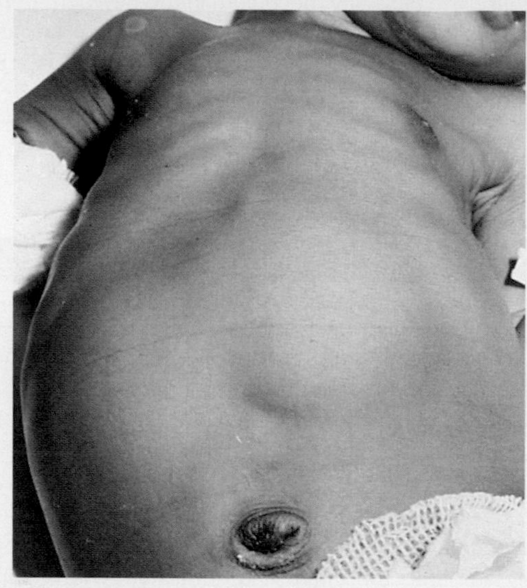

Fig. 5.7 Pyloric stenosis may cause epigastric distention by the obstructed stomach. This patient also demonstrates a visible wave of peristalsis, which moves from left to right. (Source: *Zitelli and Davis' Atlas of Pediatric Physical Diagnosis*, 8th Edition. 2023.)

Clinical Pearls

The important point to remember about pyloric stenosis is that it is an acquired condition. It is not present at birth.[11]

The first symptom of vomiting can appear after 10 days of age when the pyloric sphincter starts to hypertrophy. Pyloric stenosis can occur between 10 days and 10 weeks but is usually diagnosed at around 4 to 6 weeks of age. In the first few days the vomiting is mild and intermittent with an otherwise well infant who is still hungry to feed.

The other important point is that it is a progressive condition. The vomits become larger and more frequent over a matter of days. The infant may become constipated because of poor intake despite being alert and hungry. This observation can be falsely reassuring for a doctor who is not familiar with the condition. The degree of fluid and electrolyte disturbance is proportionate to the duration of symptoms prior to presentation.

In this case, the initial diagnosis of gastro-oesophageal (GE) reflux was acceptable. However, when the mother rang back the following week and reported that the vomiting was worse, the infant should have been seen and examined. This case highlights the risk of evaluating newborns over the phone and the utmost importance of clinical examination in infants.

Weight loss is very uncommon in cases of reflux unless it is very severe. In simple terms, a combination of vomiting and weight loss always spells trouble. The diagnosis of pyloric stenosis can be readily confirmed or excluded by an ultrasound. The clinical confirmation by a test feed and palpating the pyloric tumour is now infrequently performed by paediatricians. The classic biochemical abnormality found in pyloric stenosis is hypochloraemic, hypokalaemic metabolic alkalosis. This is never a surgical emergency, and in fact, surgery will not be contemplated until the biochemical derangement has been corrected with a combination of keeping the infant nil orally with a nasogastric tube on drainage and aggressive fluid resuscitation ensuring adequate amounts of sodium chloride and potassium are administered to take account of the deficit, the ongoing losses (from the nasogastric tube) and maintenance fluid requirements. Failure to correct the metabolic alkalosis prior to undertaking a general anaesthetic and pyloromyotomy risks the development of profound postoperative apnoeas.

Pitfalls to Avoid

Remember that pyloric stenosis is a progressive condition, and the vomiting gets worse over time. In this case the vomiting was mild at the initial encounter, but it got progressively worse over a period of days.

Always weigh small infants who are vomiting. If they are losing weight, there is something wrong.

The description of an infant being active and hungry is a 'false friend' in the case of pyloric stenosis. It can mistakenly reassure the doctor that the infant is well.

BOX 5.8 CLINICAL HISTORY

Feeding Issues in a 4 Week Old

An infant had an apparently normal newborn examination and was discharged home. At 4 weeks of age, the parents returned with concerns that there was milk coming down the infant's nostrils on feeding and that she had several choking episodes. The parents had found the choking episodes to be quite alarming, as the infant had gone blue and needed to be picked up immediately.

When the infant was examined, she was found to have a cleft of her soft palate and was referred to the specialist cleft palate team. The mother was provided with the correct feeding advice including a Haberman teat. Further investigations were instituted. The infant was subsequently found to have a 22q.11 deletion. The cleft palate was repaired at 9 months.

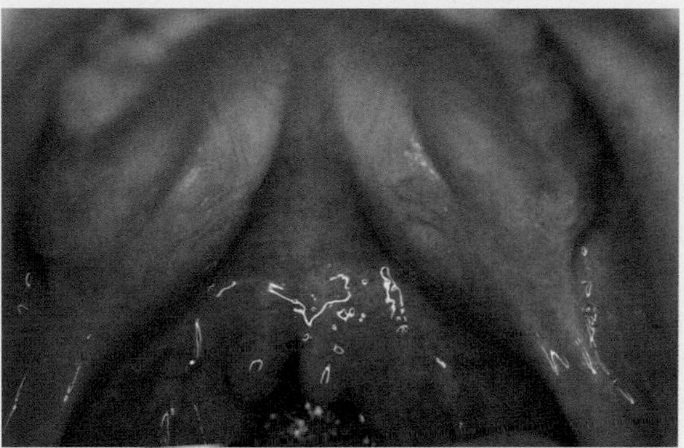

Fig. 5.8 Submucous palatal cleft. A cleft of the midline palatal bone exists, but the overlying mucosa is intact. A bifid uvula is also present. (Source: *Oral and Maxillofacial Pathology*, 3rd Edition. 2009.)

Clinical Pearls

In 2015, the Royal College of Paediatrics and Child Health (RCPCH) felt compelled to issue a short document titled 'identification of cleft palate in the newborn' following reports that up to 1 in 6 newborns with cleft palate were *not* picked up on the initial examination.[12]

The recommendation is that a wooden spatula and torch be used when visualising the palate. If this is not done, cases will be missed. The eye can see a cleft lip, the finger can feel a cleft of the hard palate, but a tongue depressor and light source are needed to identify a cleft of the soft palate. The examiner must also be satisfied that the uvula has been visualised. A bifid uvula can be a marker for a submucous cleft (Fig. 5.8).[13]

The consequences of delayed diagnosis are significant, and the infant may have feeding issues and may have difficulties with latching on if being breastfed. These feeding issues are very distressing, and the infant may be quite unsettled and gain weight poorly. There may also be a history of milk coming down the infant's nostrils.

The other issue is that a cleft palate may be a marker for another condition as occurred in the above case. The infant in this case had a 22q.11 deletion, which is associated with frequent infections, hypocalcaemia, cardiac anomalies, cognitive problems and a 30% risk of schizophrenia in later life.

Some cases of cleft palate are associated with Stickler's syndrome, a connective tissue disorder. Features of this disorder include myopia, hearing problems and musculoskeletal difficulties due to hypotonia.

Pitfalls to Avoid

Always use a tongue depressor and a torch when examining the palate. The palate must be fully visualised, and the presence of the uvula confirmed. The red flag is the milk coming down the nostril on feeding. In missed cases this is more likely to happen after the infant goes home as the volumes being taken by the infant increase. If an infant presents to primary care in the early days after birth with history of struggling with feeds or any choking with feeds, it is good practice to check the infant's palate.

When dealing with an infant with a cleft palate, it is important to consider an underlying causation such as 22q.11 deletion or Stickler's syndrome.

BOX 5.9 CLINICAL HISTORY

A Very Floppy Infant

An infant girl is born at term and following a normal day two examination, she is discharged home from the nursery. At 4 weeks of age the parents bring her to the family doctor because she is slow at taking her bottle feeds. The doctor remarks that she is a happy, alert infant. He offers feeding advice including the use of a more free-flowing teat. When she was brought by the parents for her 6-week check they again reported poor feeding. She was seen by another family doctor in the practice who recommended a referral to the community dietician.

At 4 months of age the infant develops a respiratory illness with rapid breathing, diminished feeding and is admitted to hospital. On admission she was found to be profoundly hypotonic, with extreme head lag (Fig. 5.9). The tendon reflexes were absent, there was tongue fasciculation and a bell-shaped chest. A clinical diagnosis of spinal muscular atrophy (SMA) was made and subsequently confirmed on genetic testing. Following the establishment of the diagnosis, she was commenced on Nusinersen.

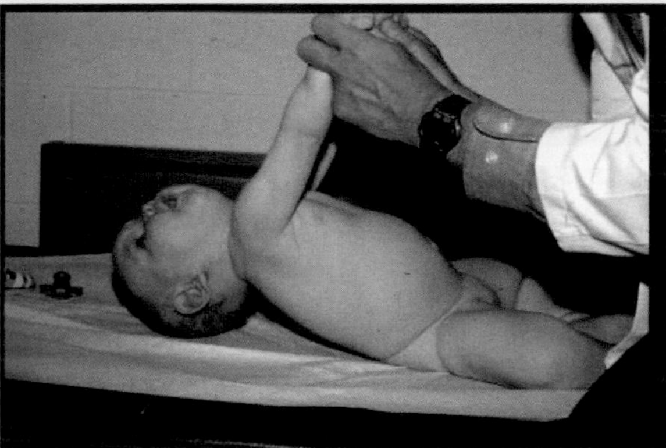

Fig. 5.9 SMA type 1 infant with typically marked head lag and noticeable proximal weakness when pulled to a sit. Slight sternal retraction is also seen. *SMA*, Spinal muscular atrophy. (Juan M. Pascual, Roger N. Rosenberg. *Rosenberg's Molecular and Genetic Basis of Neurological and Psychiatric Disease*, Sixth Edition. Elsevier Inc. 2020.)

Clinical Pearls

SMA is a rare condition associated with profound hypotonia, reduced or absent deep tendon reflexes and often tongue fasciculations. The advent of new treatments such as Nusinersen and gene therapy has changed the landscape and puts a premium on earlier diagnosis. Thus, examination of tone is important to diagnose SMA earlier.[1]

It is well beyond the scope of a family doctor to make the diagnosis of SMA, which is a rare neurological disorder. It is important to consider the potential significance of the combination of poor feeding and poor weight gain. This combination is always worrying and is indicative of an underlying problem. When examining an infant with such a presentation, examination with attention to the tone is essential.

Infants with SMA may have a frog-like posture and marked head lag. All doctors who regularly examine young infants should acquaint themselves on the features of hypotonia.

In SMA, the survival motor neurone (SMN) protein is deficient. This protein is necessary for lower motor neurone function. In its absence the lower motor neurone atrophies. Nusinersen increases the production of the SMN protein.

Pitfalls to Avoid

Be aware when an infant presents with a combination of poor feeding and poor weight gain, marked hypotonia and areflexia may indicate spinal muscular atrophy. The poor feeding is due to hypotonia of the oral musculature.

If an infant is found to be markedly hypotonic and has absent deep tendon reflexes (usually easy to elicit in early infancy) then referral to a specialist paediatric neurology service is warranted.

BOX 5.10 CLINICAL HISTORY

An Inguinal Swelling

A primary care trainee is performing the 6-week examination. The mother points out a lump in the baby boy's groin. She is unsure how long it has been there. On inspection, there is a soft and non-tender lump in the right groin. The infant is not distressed. The trainee is relatively inexperienced and is unsure whether it is a hernia or a hydrocoele. She plans for her trainer to see the infant the following week when he is back from leave. The practice becomes very busy, and the appointment is put back for another 2 weeks.

In the interim, the infant became unsettled with constant crying and vomiting. His parents brought him to the regional paediatric emergency department. On examination, he has a right-sided irreducible groin swelling in keeping with an incarcerated inguinal hernia. The hernia was reduced under sedation and was surgically repaired 48 hours later.

Clinical Pearls

It is important for all doctors who deal with children to be able to distinguish between a hernia and a hydrocoele.

This distinction is important as an inguinal hernia needs a surgical referral and repair, while a hydrocoele may spontaneously resolve within the first 2-years of life. A persistent hydrocoele does not carry any risk to the infant nor does it adversely affect the testicle on that side or even cause symptoms. It is generally the unsightly cosmetic appearance of a large hydrocoele that would prompt consideration of hydrocoele repair electively after 2 years of age.

The ability to make the correct diagnosis requires clinical acumen and experience. It is a commonly encountered problem with up to 3% of term male infants developing a hernia, and up to 20% of preterm infants.[14] On the other hand, approximately 10% of infants will develop a hydrocoele.

The history is a very helpful aid. The hydrocoele will usually have been present since birth, while the hernia will have developed sometime after birth, except in very premature infants, where it may be noted in the nursery. The hydrocoele is more likely to be present constantly but can vary in size throughout the day depending on whether it is a communicating or a noncommunicating hydrocoele (Fig. 5.10). The hernia will generally come and go. It is most likely to appear when the infant is crying or straining at stool and may reduce spontaneously when he or she is quiet (Fig. 5.11).

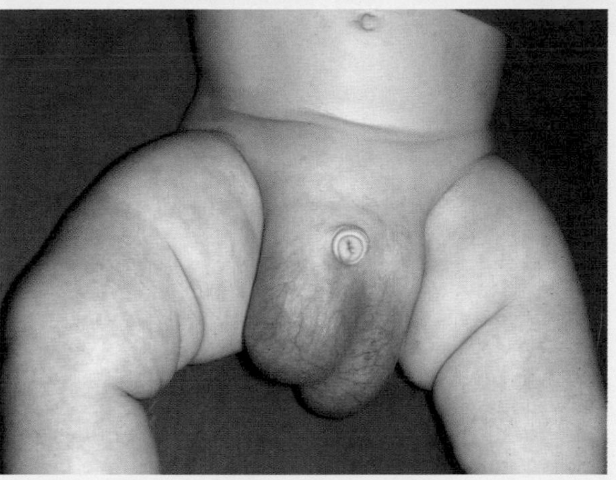

Fig. 5.10 Hydrocoeles. This 11-month-old boy had an enlarged scrotum confirmed by transillumination to be the result of hydrocoeles. (Arulampalam THA, et al. *Essential Surgery: Problems, Diagnosis and Management*, Sixth Edition. 2020, Elsevier Ltd.)

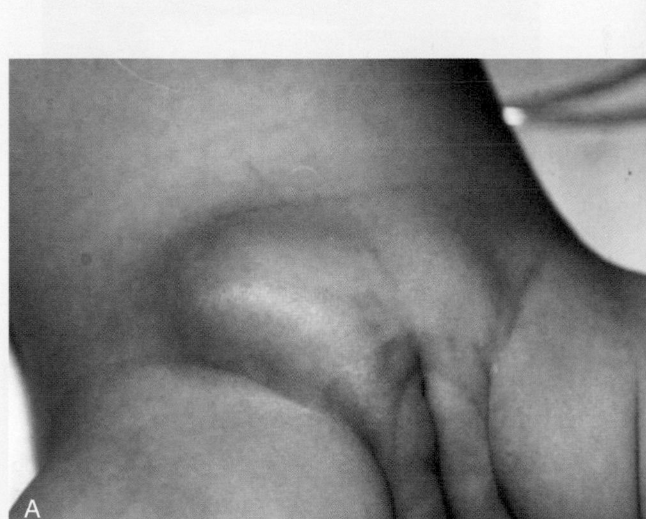

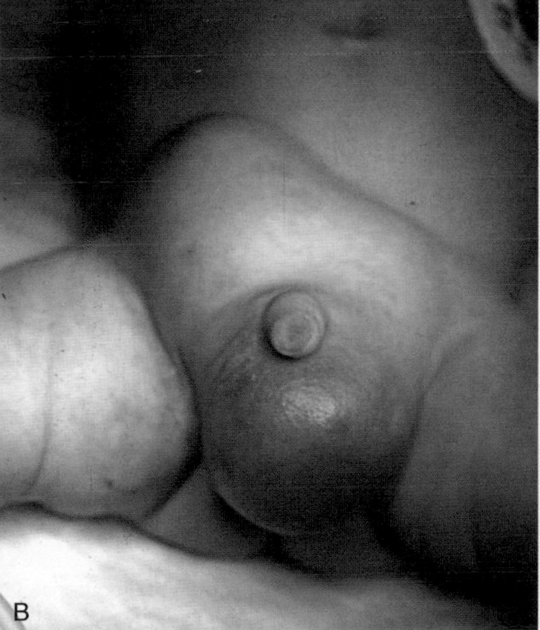

Fig. 5.11 Inguinal hernia in an infant. Right inguinal hernias in a female (A) and male (B) infant. Note the asymmetry in the groin area with the prominent bulge indicating the hernia. (Source: Reproduced with permission from Gleason CA, Juul SE. *Avery's Diseases of the Newborn*, 10th Edition. Elsevier; 2020.)

Continued

BOX 5.10 CLINICAL HISTORY—CONT'D

In the case of a hydrocoele, one can 'get above' the swelling. This means that the examiner can feel a narrow spermatic cord above the testicle and hydrocoele, and therefore it is not a swelling that is arising from inside the abdomen (as would be expected in a hernia). The exception to this 'rule' is the encysted hydrocoele of the cord, where there may be a swelling that one cannot easily get above and which cannot be reduced. Ultrasound may be of benefit in this case to determine that the content of the encysted hydrocoele is simple fluid rather than bowel. The groin and/or scrotal swelling found in an inguinal hernia, on the other hand, should be continuous with the groin. In experienced hands, the contents of a hernia can be reduced back into the abdomen by gentle squeezing of the lump from distal to proximal, and it is often accompanied by a gurgling sensation if the contents are bowel. If omentum or fat is reduced, this sensation may not be noted. In females with inguinal hernias, it is not uncommon for the hernia to contain an ovary. This is often described as feeling like a small firm olive or grape in the groin, and it is frequently irreducible which does not necessarily prompt an emergency operation but does warrant surgical review.

If the doctor is uncertain whether it is a hernia or a hydrocoele, an ultrasound of the groin and/or scrotum can be helpful to resolve the issue.

Hernias are more common on the right side (60% right, 25% left and 15% bilateral).

Pitfalls to Avoid

Refer cases of inguinal hernia promptly to a surgeon, as delays increase the rate of incarceration. The frequency of incarceration can be as high as 30% in infants less than 12 months of age.

One of the complications of hernia incarceration in male infants is damage to the adjacent spermatic cord. Venous compression can compromise the circulation to the testis leading ultimately to testicular atrophy. The risk of testicular atrophy following an incarcerated inguinal hernia is approximately 3%.

BOX 5.11 CLINICAL HISTORY

An 8 Week Old With Prolonged Jaundice

An 8-week-old infant, who is breastfed, presents to primary care with prolonged jaundice, and is thought to have breast milk jaundice. His stools are pale (Fig. 5.12), and his urine is dark yellow in colour. His sclerae are mildly icteric. He is immediately referred for paediatric assessment. Further testing shows a raised conjugated bilirubin.

Clinical Pearls

Always ask about stool and urine colour in an infant with prolonged jaundice and seek a measurement of the conjugated bilirubin.

Biliary atresia may present simply as a prolongation of physiological jaundice. Infants with biliary atresia are often superficially well with normal early growth although an enlarged liver may be felt.

Pale stools are evident by 2 weeks and are the rule by 4 weeks of age.[15]

The pickup is time-critical, and the traditional target was to perform a Kasai portoenterostomy before 60 days of age, but it is increasingly evident that it should be done as soon as possible to maximise the chances of success.

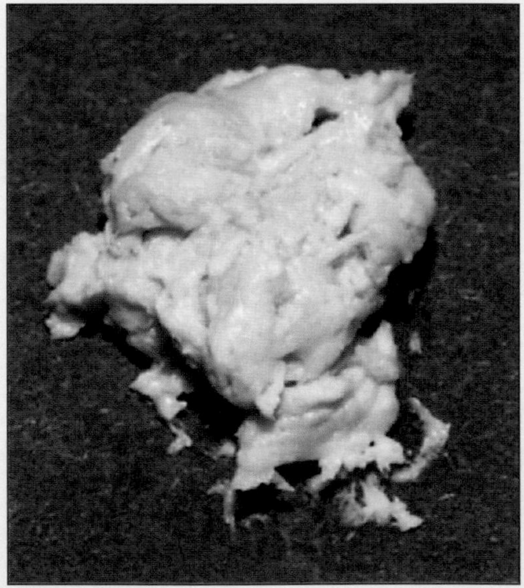

Fig. 5.12 Pale stool secondary to biliary atresia. (Lissauer T, Carroll W. *Illustrated Textbook of Paediatrics*, 6th edn. Elsevier; 2022.)

In general terms, the major cause for delay is the failure to appreciate the significance of prolonged jaundice. The use of the Stool Colour Chart (SCC) has been successful in countries including Japan and has led to an earlier diagnosis of biliary atresia. As clinical detection has not worked, some experts now recommend universal screening for biliary atresia.[16]

In any term infant with jaundice that persists beyond 2 weeks of age, ask about the colour of the stools and urine, and consider referral if concerns for urgent measurement of the conjugated bilirubin level (which should be under 20 μmol/L).

Late diagnosis of biliary atresia may be associated with irreversible liver cirrhosis, a risk of ascending cholangitis post-Kasai procedure and subsequent requirement for liver transplantation (Fig. 5.13).

Infants with prolonged physiological jaundice or breast milk jaundice will have a rise in unconjugated bilirubin whereas those with liver disease, including biliary atresia, will have a raised conjugated bilirubin.

Pitfalls to Avoid

While most infants with jaundice over 2 weeks of age will have breastmilk jaundice, always ask about a history of dark urine and pale stools and, if evident, refer for measurement of conjugated bilirubin at your local hospital.

Speed is of the essence in diagnosing biliary atresia as delays may lead to irreversible cirrhosis.

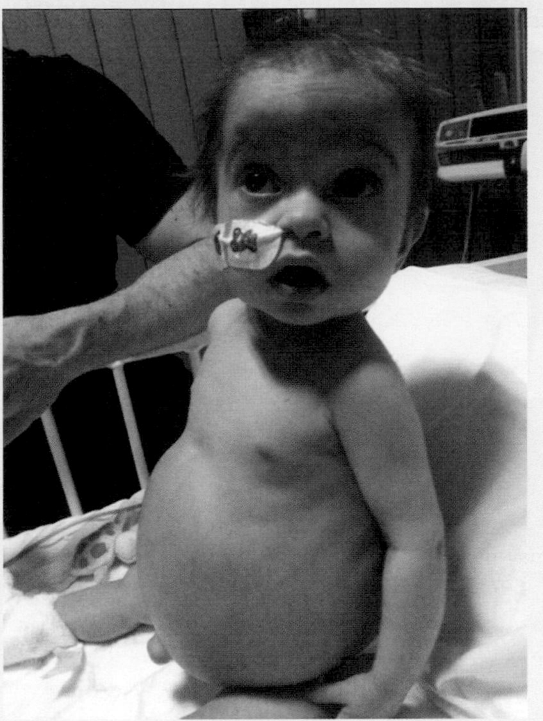

Fig. 5.13 A child with biliary atresia with a failed Kasai procedure. Shown is jaundice, a distended abdomen attributed to ascites, with protrusion of the umbilicus, and prominent abdominal veins. The abdomen is distended by ascites; the child's arms and legs show cachexia because of her severe liver disease, despite receiving supplemental nasogastric tube feeding. (Baumann U, et al. *Pediatric Liver Transplantation: A Clinical Guide*. 2021, Elsevier Inc.)

BOX 5.12 CLINICAL HISTORY

An Absent Red Reflex

An infant undergoes an eye examination at the day two newborn check. The paediatric trainee doctor finds it difficult to get the infant to open his eyes. The examination is passed as normal, and the infant is discharged home.

The infant subsequently attends the primary care clinic for the '6-week check' at 12 weeks old. The delay in coming to the practice was due to the family being away on holidays. The mother mentions to the doctor that the infant appears not to look at her. On examination it is found that the infant is following objects but the 'red reflex' is absent (Fig. 5.14). Bilateral cataracts were diagnosed, and an urgent referral was made to a paediatric ophthalmologist who confirmed the diagnosis. The cataracts were removed as a matter of urgency. The infant, however, was left with a significant visual impairment.

Clinical Pearls

The examination of the eyes is somewhat challenging in newborns, and one can be distracted by subconjunctival haemorrhage or a sticky eye. Eyelid swelling at birth is not infrequent and can make eye opening difficult, especially if the infant is distressed.[17]

Continued

BOX 5.12 CLINICAL HISTORY—CONT'D

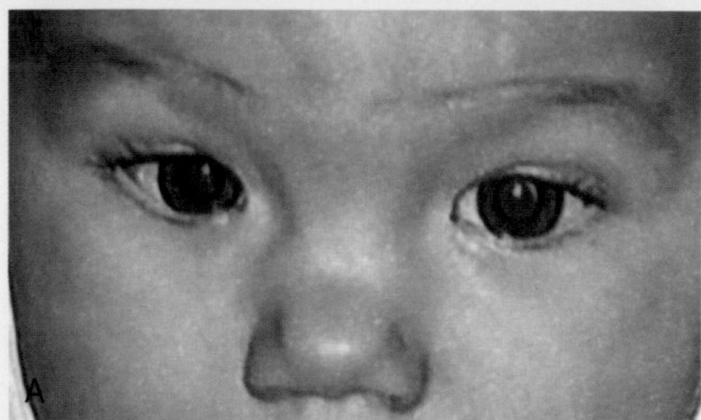

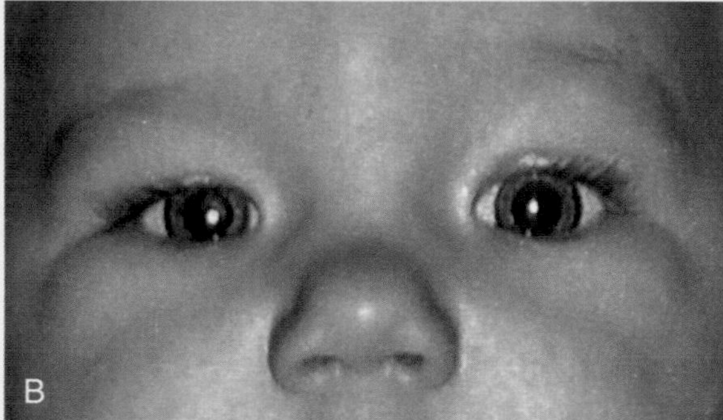

Fig. 5.14 (A) Photograph of an infant taken when 4 months of age showing normal red reflexes in both eyes. (B) Photograph of the same infant 2 months later showing loss of the red reflex in the right eye. At the time of cataract surgery, the right eye was found to have a dense central cataract and persistent foetal vasculature. (Source: From Lambert SR, Lyons CJ, eds. *Taylor & Hoyt's Pediatric Ophthalmology and Strabismus*, 5th Edition. Elsevier; 2017:353, Fig. 37.22.)

Position the infant comfortably on the mother's lap. Offering a feed or gently singing may promote eye opening in the infant and allow the red reflex to be assessed using an ophthalmoscope.

The key item in the newborn eye examination involves visualisation of the retina. The presence of the 'red reflex' confirms that the lens is clear. When a cataract is present, the lens is opaque (Fig. 5.15), and the 'red reflex' is absent. A congenital cataract is the leading cause of visual deprivation in infants. The sooner the cataract is removed, the better the outcome. The upper time limit is thought to be 8 weeks of age, after that the infant's vision will be compromised.

The screening is more challenging in Asian and African infants because they have a pigmented rather than a red retina.

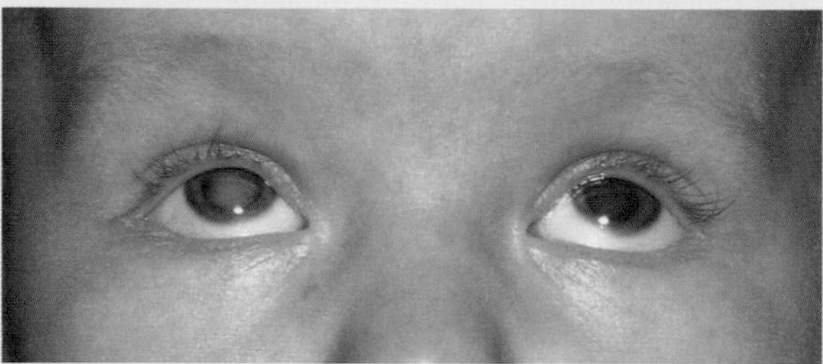

Fig. 5.15 Nuclear cataracts. This 4-month-old child presented with nystagmus and bilateral nuclear cataracts. His parents had noted that he would stare at room lights. After bilateral lensectomies and contact lens correction, his nystagmus improved. After long-term follow-up, his best-corrected visual acuity is 20/25 when both eyes are tested together, but 20/50 when each of his eyes is tested separately due to latent nystagmus. (Christopher J. Lyons, Scott R. Lambert. *Taylor and Hoyt's Pediatric Opthalmology and Strabismus*, Sixth Edition, 2023, Elsevier Ltd.)

It is one of the conditions that should be specifically examined for at the 6-week check. At that stage the clues are not fixing and following, with possibly a squint or nystagmus. Also, it is easier to visualise the retina at that age.

Urgent ophthalmology referral is required if there is an absent red reflex, a white pupillary reflex or leukocoria.

Congenital cataracts are managed by prompt cataract surgery with later contact lenses, intraocular lens implantation and spectacles.[17]

Pitfalls to Avoid

Every infant must be screened for a congenital cataract at the newborn examination. If there is uncertainty, do not take a chance and pass as normal. A further review with a re-examination is recommended, and if still unsure, get an ophthalmology opinion. Keep the possibility of a cataract in mind when doing the 6-week check.

A red reflex assessment needs both patience and experience to perform and is quite challenging in newborns.

Many causes of blindness (cataracts, retinopathy of prematurity and glaucoma in particular) are treatable if diagnosed early. Early detection of retinoblastoma improves the outcome.[18] One should suspect a significant impairment of visual acuity in an infant who does not fix, follow or smile by 6 to 8 weeks of age or an obvious strabismus at a young age or nystagmus or 'roving' eye movements.

LATER PRESENTATIONS IN INFANCY AND PRE-SCHOOL YEARS

BOX 5.13 CLINICAL HISTORY

An Infant With Delayed Motor Milestones

A male infant is born at term but is noted to be small for dates with a birth weight of 2.1 kg. There was meconium staining of liquor prior to delivery, but he cried at birth and was observed with more frequent feeds and regular checks of his blood glucose all of which were normal. He was discharged home after 7 days.

He was reviewed by his family doctor for his six-week check and was noted to be exhibiting good catch-up growth and was feeding well. He was smiling and was very bright and alert. His examination was felt to be normal apart from moderate head lag. He had further immunisation visits to his family doctor where his ongoing poor head control was noted, and thus, he was referred for paediatric physiotherapy assessment. At 6 months of age, he was unable to sit with support and appeared to have a mild hand preference, favouring his right hand.

By 9 months of age his parents were quite concerned, as he was still not sitting up and now had a definite right-hand preference. He was referred to a developmental paediatrician who noted poor overall truncal tone with a tight left Achilles tendon and increased tone of the left upper and lower limb with exaggerated deep tendon reflexes on that side. A diagnosis of hemiplegic cerebral palsy was made, and he was referred for investigations including an MRI brain scan and a full multidisciplinary team assessment (Fig. 5.16).

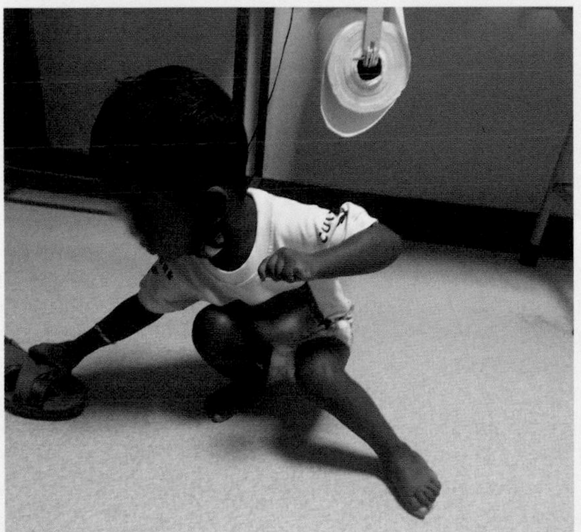

Fig. 5.16 Left hemiplegia – typical hand posture – can't bear weight on left foot – left leg spastic – cant flex. (Illingworth RS, et al. *Illingworth's The Development of the Infant and Young Child: Normal and Abnormal*, Eleventh Edition, 2021, Elsevier Inc.)

Clinical Pearls

Cerebral palsy (CP) is a clinical diagnosis with the parents reporting that the infant fails to meet motor milestones in the presence of either abnormal movements or tone. Feeding difficulties are also frequently reported.

If suspected as a primary care doctor, it is important to clearly outline your concerns and also to emphasise both the varied presentations and functional outcomes. Once CP is suspected, onward referral is advised, and an MRI brain scan is important in the workup.

The Gross Motor Functional Classification System (GMFCS) is a very helpful indicator of motor function.[19]

The aim of current multidisciplinary management of cerebral palsy (CP) is in essence to minimise the impact of secondary musculoskeletal complications.

The goals of physiotherapy, occupational therapy and speech therapy are to allow the child to reach their developmental potential by providing equipment and support, to facilitate participation in home and school and to both prevent and detect secondary complications. Therapists rely on parent-delivered interventions, so support must be given to the training of parents and other caregivers.

In a case of hemiplegic CP (such as this) the child may require orthotics, botulinum toxin injections and potentially later release of the Achilles tendon to relieve tightening.

Pitfalls to Avoid

Normal variants such as bottom shufflers and rollers are not a source of concern in general terms and parents can be rightly reassured.

As always, be guided by parental concerns, and if they are very concerned, you should be too.

Consider the following Red flags requiring referral to paediatric services include:[20]

Loss of developmental skills at any age

Persistently low tone or increased muscle tone

Hand preference under 18 months (may indicate hemiplegia)

Persistent toe walking (consider spastic diplegia) or dragging of one foot (consider hemiplegia)

Head circumference above 97% or below 0.4%

If an infant cannot sit unsupported by 12 months or walk by 18 months in boys or inability to run by 2 years 6 months

Inability to reach out for objects by 6 months or inability to hold an object placed in the infant's hand by 5 months

Finally, in the majority of cases of CP, no history of perinatal asphyxia is evident.

BOX 5.14 CLINICAL HISTORY

A 10 Month Old With a Late Pick Up of DDH

A female infant was born at term as a vertex delivery with no complications. At the newborn examination the hips were examined and found to be normal. Subsequently the hips were also passed as normal at 6 weeks. At 10 months of age, the nurse at the local community clinic noticed that the infant was dragging her left lower limb when crawling. She was referred to the orthopaedic services. Subsequent examination and investigations found the infant had a dislocated left hip. She required an open hip reduction.

On discussion with the parents, it emerged that the mother had a dislocated hip which was treated when she was an infant. This relevant information had not been elicited by the doctor who performed the infant's day two examination.

Clinical Pearls

The Barlow Test is a recommended screening test for DDH in the first few weeks of life. With the infant on their back, flex the knees and grasp the legs with the thumbs along the inner side of the thighs and the middle finger over the greater trochanter. Adduct the hip and apply light downward pressure on the knee. If the hip is unstable, it will pop out of the acetabulum.

The Ortolani test is another screening test. Hold the legs as previously for the Barlow test. Abduct the leg while the middle finger presses upwards on the greater trochanter. If the hip is dislocated a 'clunk' will be felt (Fig. 5.17).[21]

A positive Ortolani or Barlow test, or an unstable hip joint, requires early investigation and treatment.

The examination of the newborn hips is very much a skill that must be demonstrated and learned. It is our experience that the most important part of the examination is to place the middle finger over the greater trochanter. This plays a key part in detecting the dislocated hip (Ortolani's sign) and the dislocatable hip (Barlow's sign). These signs are time-limited and cannot be elicited at 6 weeks of age because of muscle tightness around the hip joint. At this later time point, the main finding is limited hip abduction on the affected side.

It is accepted that not all dislocated hips can be detected at the clinical examination after birth or 6 to 8 weeks.[22,23]

It is well established that infants with breech presentation and those with a positive family history of hip dysplasia are at an increased risk of DDH. A positive family history is defined as the situation where a first-degree relative (parent or sibling) had DDH. The breech and positive family group account for 20% of births. Infants in the at-risk group for DDH should have a hip ultrasound performed at 6 weeks of age. The purpose and timing of this scan is to identify cases of DDH that were not detectable at birth.

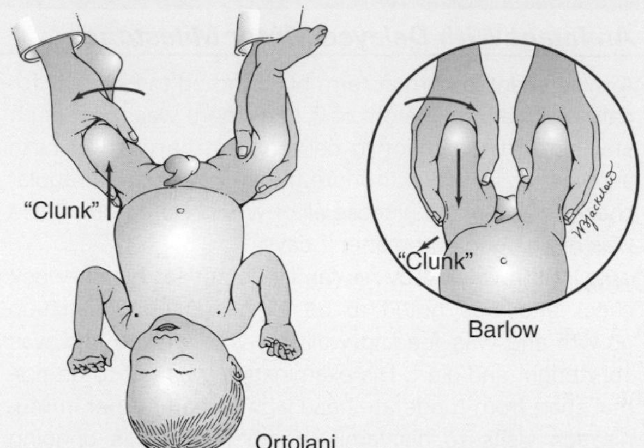

Fig. 5.17 Evaluation for congenital dislocation of the hip. (A) Barlow manoeuvre (left side). With one hand pressing the symphysis in front and the sacral spine in back, lateral pressure is applied to the thigh with the thumb of the other hand while pressure is applied with the palm to the knee on the side being examined. The hip that has been flexed to 90 degrees is then adducted. A positive sign is a sensation of abnormal movement, indicating dislocation of the femoral head from the acetabulum. The hands are reversed for examining the other hip. This sign and the Ortolani sign may be found only in the first weeks of life. (B) Ortolani manoeuvre (right side). Sign of jerking into correct position. After Barlow manoeuvre (A), the hip should be abducted to about 80 degrees while the femur is lifted anteriorly with the fingers along the thigh. A positive sign is a sensation of a jerk or snap with reduction into the joint socket. (Source: From Dains J, Baumann L, Scheibel P. *Advanced Health Assessment and Clinical Diagnosis in Primary Care*, 6th Edition. Elsevier; 2019.)

The other important step in the care pathway is to ensure that the hip ultrasound scan result is seen promptly by the referring doctor, and that the infant is referred to orthopaedics when there is an abnormal finding.

Unfortunately, the 6-week check is unreliable in detecting DDH. Asymmetrical skin folds,[24] limb shortening and limited abduction of the hips are not reliable indicators of DDH.

Ultrasound is helpful for high-risk cases or to confirm an abnormal hip examination.[25]

Most cases of DDH are treated with an abduction harness called a Pavlik harness, and surgery is only required for those with severe DDH and those who have failed treatment with a harness or in older children with a late diagnosis of DDH.

Pitfalls to Avoid

The Ortolani and Barlow tests often fail to identify DDH at birth.

The timing of the 6-week check is unfortunate in that there may be a resolution of hip instability, and unilateral limitation of hip abduction has yet to appear (not until 3 months of age).

BOX 5.15 CLINICAL HISTORY

Difficult to Palpate Testes

A 4-year-old boy is referred to the surgical outpatients with a right-sided undescended testis. On examination the right side of the scrotum is smaller than the left. There is no testis palpable on the right side of the scrotal sac. The left testis is normally placed. An orchidopexy is performed, and the testis is secured in the scrotum. The testis is small in size when compared with the left testis.

Clinical Pearls

An undescended testis is determined when the testis cannot be manipulated, tension-free into the base of the scrotum (Fig. 5.18). A retractile testis can be manually manipulated to the base of the scrotum, and it stays there, or it may re-ascend after manipulation with the initiation of the cremasteric reflex.[26]

About 6% of boys have an undescended testis (UDT) at birth. Risk factors include prematurity and a birth weight less than 2.5 kg.[26]

Newborn males should be carefully checked to ensure that both testes are fully descended. The neonatal period is a very good time to undertake this examination, as the scrotal sac is relatively large, and there is no cremasteric reflex.

If one or both testes are not fully descended at 6 months of age, then surgical intervention by a general paediatric surgeon or a paediatric urologist should take place ideally prior to 1 year of age.

Prompt referral from primary care is required if the testes are undescended and there is also hypospadias (consider disorders of sexual development), bilateral impalpable testes or if testicular pain develops with or without erythema, where torsion needs to be considered.

If a single UDT is detected at the newborn or 6-week check with none of the above concerns, it is important to arrange a review at 3 months of age as this allows for natural descent of the testis to potentially occur. The incidence falls from 6% at birth to 2% at 3 months. Consider referral of infants with UDT at 3 months of age (corrected if preterm) or older children with UDT for a surgical assessment.[12]

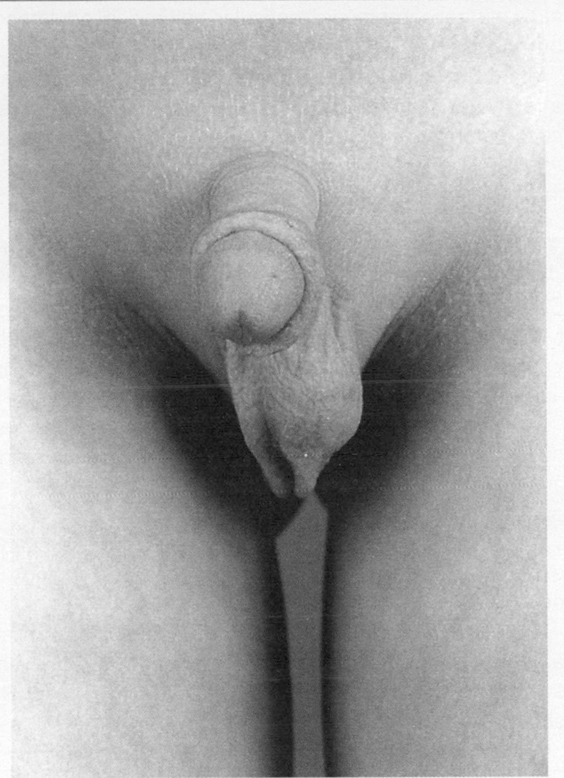

Fig. 5.18 Right undescended testis. (David Isaacs, Mike South. *Practical Paediatrics*, Seventh Edition. 2012, Elsevier Ltd.)

In 80% of cases the testis is palpable along the inguinal canal, and in 20% of cases it is not palpable because it is intra-abdominal or absent (atrophic).

Diagnostic laparotomy is now the investigation of choice if the testis is impalpable.

If the testis is palpable along the inguinal canal, there is a 50% chance that it will migrate into the scrotum. If the testis has not descended by 6 months old, it is unlikely to descend.

Continued

BOX 5.15 CLINICAL HISTORY—CONT'D

Treatment is by orchidopexy as a day case procedure with international guidelines recommending surgery between 6 and 18 months of age. Orchidopexy should be performed before 18 months to reduce the risk of infertility and to facilitate the detection of a testicular malignancy in later life.

The incidence of testicular cancer is about 6.9 per 100,000 and even with timely orchidopexy, the cancer risk is three times the baseline prevalence for adult men. Regular testicular self-examination is recommended once the child reaches adolescence. There is good evidence that early surgery improves testicular volume in adulthood, but the potential fertility benefits are still uncertain.[26]

Infants with bilateral undescended testis should raise a red flag particularly if there is a hypospadias. In these circumstances, a virilised female needs to be considered. A quick and useful test is an ultrasound to exclude the presence of a uterus. A karyotype should be undertaken, and congenital adrenal hyperplasia excluded.

Pitfalls to Avoid

It is important to diagnose an undescended testis at the newborn examination. At this point the exam is easiest because the scrotum is thin-walled, and there is no cremasteric reflex.

Try to determine whether the UDT is palpable along the inguinal canal, as this is an important determinant of the subsequent outcome.

All UDTs should ideally be operated on by at least 18 months of age.

Bilateral UDTs with hypospadias are a real concern. It raises the possibility of a virilised female. An immediate ultrasound looking for the presence of a uterus is a very helpful pointer.

KEY LEARNING POINTS

Coarctation of the aorta is the MOST COMMONLY MISSED congenital heart disease and may present later with signs of heart failure (rapid respirations, tachycardia and an enlarged liver) and poor weight gain.

Cyanosis may be difficult to pick up clinically on the newborn examination, and thus both antenatal scans and newborn pulse oximetry have helped to pick up cases prior to further clinical deterioration.

A red reflex assessment needs both patience and experience to perform and is quite challenging in newborns.

A creamy or bloody eye discharge, particularly if bilateral, may indicate ophthalmia neonatorum and relevant swabs (testing for DNA by polymerase chain reaction) should be taken and treatment started.

Delayed passage of meconium beyond 24 hours is always significant and requires assessment.

Bilious vomiting should always prompt urgent surgical consultation even in an otherwise well infant.

Always conduct a visual examination to ensure that the hard palate is normal using a torch and a tongue depressor to ensure that all the palate is seen.

A bimanual approach with warm hands will pick up UDT which should be treated surgically before 18 months of age, and primary care doctors play a significant role in screening in infancy, in particular at the 6-week check.

While most infants with jaundice over 2 weeks of age will have breastmilk jaundice, always ask about a history of dark urine and pale stools. Speed is of the essence in diagnosing biliary atresia, as delays may lead to irreversible cirrhosis.

REFERENCES

1. Institute for Quality and Efficiency in Health Care (IQWiG). *Newborn screening for 5q-linked spinal muscular atrophy: IQWiG Reports – Commission No. S18-02.* Cologne (Germany): Institute for Quality and Efficiency in Health Care (IQWiG); April 22, 2020.
2. Ismail AQT, Cawsey M, Ewer AK. Newborn pulse oximetry screening in practice. *Arch Dis Child Educ Pract Ed.* 2017;102(3):155–161. doi:10.1136/archdischild-2016-311047.
3. Arshad A, Powell C, Tighe MP. Hirschsprung's disease. *BMJ.* 2012;345:e5521. doi:10.1136/bmj.e5521.
4. Lin ZL, Zhu JH. A neonate with bilious emesis. *BMJ.* 2019;365:l1351. doi:10.1136/bmj.l1351.
5. Nguyen HN, Kulkarni M, Jose J, et al. Ultrasound for the diagnosis of malrotation and volvulus in children and adolescents: a systematic review and meta-analysis. *Arch Dis Child.* 2021;106(12):1171–1178. doi:10.1136/archdischild-2020-321082.
6. Punukollu M, Harnden A, Tulloh R. Coarctation of the aorta in the newborn. *BMJ.* 2011;343:d6838. doi:10.1136/bmj.d6838.

7. Searle J, Thakkar DD, Banerjee J. Does pulsatility index add value to newborn pulse oximetry screening for critical congenital heart disease? *Arch Dis Child*. 2019;104(5):504–506. doi:10.1136/archdischild-2018-315891.
8. Thangaratinam S, Brown K, Zamora J, Khan KS, Ewer AK. Pulse oximetry screening for critical congenital heart defects in asymptomatic newborn babies: a systematic review and meta-analysis. *Lancet*. 2012;379(9835):2459–2464. doi:10.1016/S0140-6736(12)60107-X.
9. HSE Ireland. The newborn clinical examination handbook. Accessed online at http://www.mychild.ie.
10. Tan AK. Ophthalmia Neonatorum. *N Engl J Med*. 2019;380(2):e2. doi:10.1056/NEJMicm1808613.
11. Pandya S, Heiss K. Pyloric stenosis in pediatric surgery: an evidence-based review. *Surg Clin North Am*. 2012;92(3):527–viii. doi:10.1016/j.suc.2012.03.006.
12. RCPCH. Palate examination: Identification of cleft palate in the newborn. Accessed online at https://www.rcpch.ac.uk/sites/default/files/2018-04/2015_palate_examination_-_best_practice_guide.pdf.
13. Bargas O. Submucosal Cleft Palate. *N Engl J Med*. 2020;382(22):e77. doi:10.1056/NEJMicm1913924.
14. Abdulhai S, Glenn IC, Ponsky TA. Inguinal Hernia. *Clin Perinatol*. 2017;44(4):865–877. doi:10.1016/j.clp.2017.08.005.
15. Hartley J, Harnden A, Kelly D. Biliary atresia. *BMJ*. 2010;340:c2383. doi:10.1136/bmj.c2383.
16. McKiernan PJ. Prompt diagnosis of biliary atresia: education has not succeeded, time to move to universal screening. *Arch Dis Child*. 2020;105(8):709–710. doi:10.1136/archdischild-2020-319351.
17. Russell HC, McDougall V, Dutton GN. Congenital cataract. *BMJ*. 2011;342:d3075. doi:10.1136/bmj.d3075.
18. Dimaras H, Kimani K, Dimba EA, et al. Retinoblastoma. *Lancet*. 2012;379(9824):1436–1446. doi:10.1016/S0140-6736(11)61137-9.
19. Palisano RJ, Rosenbaum P, Bartlett D, Livingston MH. Content validity of the expanded and revised Gross Motor Function Classification System. *Dev Med Child Neurol*. 2008;50(10):744–750. doi:10.1111/j.1469-8749.2008.03089.x.
20. Bellman M, Byrne O, Sege R. Developmental assessment of children. *BMJ*. 2013;346:e8687. doi:10.1136/bmj.e8687.
21. Mubarak SJ. In search of Ortolani: the man and the method. *J Pediatr Orthop*. 2015;35(2):210–216. doi:10.1097/BPO.0000000000000250.
22. Reidy M, Collins C, MacLean JGB, Campbell D. Examining the effectiveness of examination at 6-8 weeks for developmental dysplasia: testing the safety net. *Arch Dis Child*. 2019;104(10):953–955. doi:10.1136/archdischild-2018-316520.
23. Davies R, Talbot C, Paton R. Evaluation of primary care 6- to 8-week hip check for diagnosis of developmental dysplasia of the hip: a 15-year observational cohort study. *Br J Gen Pract*. 2020;70(693):e230–e235. doi:10.3399/bjgp20x708269.
24. Anderton MJ, Hastie GR, Paton RW. The positive predictive value of asymmetrical skin creases in the diagnosis of pathological developmental dysplasia of the hip. *Bone Joint J*. 2018;100-B(5):675–679. doi:10.1302/0301-620X.100B5.BJJ-2017-0994.R2.
25. Yu RX, Gunaseelan L, Malik AS, et al. Utility of Clinical and Ultrasonographic Hip Screening in Neonates for Developmental Dysplasia of the Hip. *Cureus*. 2021;13(10):e18516. doi:10.7759/cureus.18516.
26. Cho A, Thomas J, Perera R, Cherian A. Undescended testis. *BMJ*. 2019;364:l926. doi:10.1136/bmj.l926.

ADDITIONAL READING

HSE Ireland. Growth monitoring. Accessed online at http://www.hse.ie/eng/health/child/growthmonitoring/

Murphy D, Bishop H, Edgar A. Leukocoria and retinoblastoma–pitfalls of the digital age? *Lancet*. 2012;379(9835):2465. doi:10.1016/S0140-6736(11)61644-9.

6

Important Rashes to Recognise in Infants and Children

Fiona Browne, Kevin Dunne

CHAPTER OUTLINE

Primary care doctors, nurse practitioners, paediatric trainees and consultants are often presented with a wide spectrum of rashes. Many relate to intercurrent viral illnesses, but we remain aware of the potential sinister causes of a non-blanching rash, not least invasive meningococcal disease[1] (see Chapter 3, the sick child).

This chapter will highlight rashes of concern in which recognition and referral is advised. Common viral exanthems are relatively easy to recognise and will not be discussed further in this chapter (see Chapter 4, approaching the febrile infant or child). We also describe a number of newborn rashes where prompt recognition is important.

The approach to the diagnosis of a rash is to firstly describe the site and distribution of the rash and then to place the rash into a number of defined categories including macular (where the rash is flat and not palpable), papular where the rash is raised in small palpable bumps less than 5 mm papulosquamous (as in psoriasis), vesicular in which small fluid-filled blisters are seen (examples include varicella and herpes simplex) and bullous in which larger fluid-filled blisters are seen (such as bullous impetigo).

> Paediatric dermatological emergencies are relatively uncommon but important to recognise.

In assessing a rash, always estimate the body surface area involved and whether there is associated systemic involvement. The Nikolsky sign (Fig. 6.1) is where the skin is gently rubbed and if this promotes separation of the uppermost layer of the skin, the sign is deemed positive. This sign is associated with skin fragility as seen in staphylococcal scalded skin syndrome and toxic epidermal necrolysis (TEN).

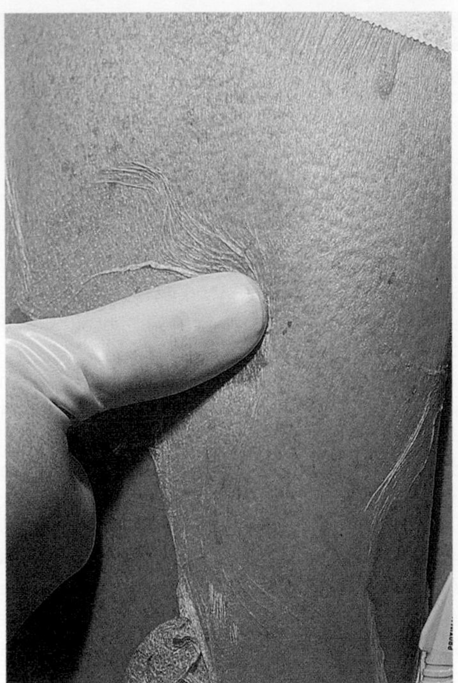

Fig. 6.1 Nickolsky's sign. (Source: Thomas P. Habif. *Maladies cutanées: Diagnostic et traitement*, 2e édition, 2012, Elsevier Masson SAS.)

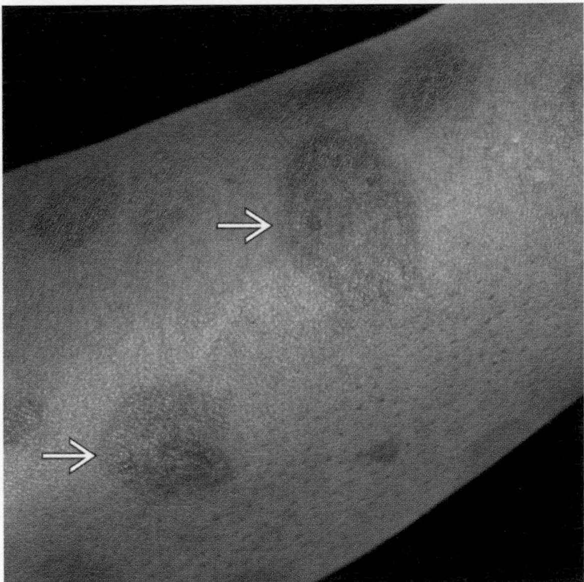

Fig. 6.2 Erythema multiforme. (Source: Lester D.R. Thompson, Brenda L. Nelson, Susan Müller. *Diagnostic Pathology: Head and Neck*. Third ed. Elsevier; 2022.)

IMPORTANT RASHES TO RECOGNISE AS A PRIMARY CARE DOCTOR

Erythema Multiforme

A common presentation to primary care doctors is erythema multiforme (Fig. 6.2) with a typical erythematous papule with a dusky centre, surrounding pale ring of oedema and outer halo of erythema (described as a target lesion) and a rapid evolution which is frightening to parents. The rash is most evident on the arms, the palms and the soles of the feet. Treatment should be aimed at management of underlying trigger (HSV, Mycoplasma, withdrawal of culprit drug trigger).

Erythema Migrans

This rash of Lyme disease (Fig. 6.3) is red or bluish-red and expands over a period of days or weeks (Box 6.1). Less than 50% can recall a prior tick bite. Untreated erythema migrans may persist for several weeks.

Ten percent develop neurological complications with early manifestations being a lymphocytic meningitis or cranial nerve palsies. The most common complication in children is a facial nerve palsy.[2]

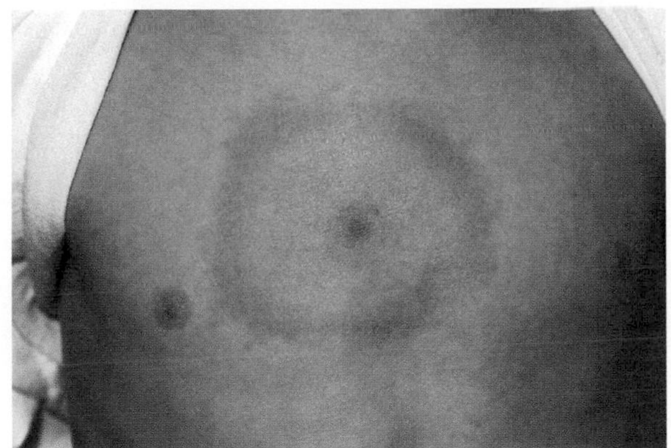

Fig. 6.3 Erythema migrans of Lyme disease. Expanding, erythematous, annular patch of early localised Lyme disease. A small red papule is seen centrally at the site of the tick bite. (Source: *Paller and Mancini – Hurwitz Clinical Pediatric Dermatology: A Textbook of Skin Disorders of Childhood and Adolescence*. 6th ed. 2022.)

Fungal Infections

Tinea capitis is very common and presents with both scaling and a well-defined area of alopecia with broken hair follicles (Fig. 6.4). Most children with tinea capitis will also have posterior cervical lymphadenopathy. Treat tinea capitis with systemic antifungals.

BOX 6.1 CLINICAL HISTORY

An 8 Year Old With a Rash and Subsequently a Facial Palsy

An 8-year-old girl presented to her primary care doctor with red macular rash on her left arm which slowly expanded over a two-week period. Her mother was unable to point to a history of tick bite, but the family had been on a camping trip 6 weeks before presentation. She then was noted to have facial asymmetry and a facial nerve palsy was confirmed on examination. Three months later she developed marked swelling of the left knee without evidence of a fever. Based on the original rash (felt to be erythema migrans), the facial nerve palsy and monoarthritis, a diagnosis of Lyme disease was made and confirmed on serology.

Clinical Pearls

Lyme disease is tick-borne due to *Borrelia burgdorferi* in North America and *Borrelia afzelii* or *garini* in Europe.

Establishing the diagnosis can be challenging and recognition of the classical erythema migrans rash is important.

During early Lyme infection, acute atrioventricular conductive events may occur and Lyme carditis is usually self-limiting.

Treat erythema migrans with amoxycillin, cephalosporins or doxycycline. Treatment with either amoxycillin for 14 days or doxycycline for 10 days is recommended.

Pitfalls to Avoid

Neurological manifestations of Lyme disease require 14 days treatment with ceftriaxone, and Lyme arthritis may be very slow to improve even with prolonged courses of antibiotics.

Debate still rages as to whether Lyme disease can lead to disabling fatigue and neurocognitive disturbances or so-called 'chronic Lyme'.

Acrodermatitis chronica atrophicans is quite rare and is described as a chronic red skin lesion that may become atrophic.

At least five randomised controlled trials have provided little support for prolonged antibiotics in children or adults with persistent symptoms attributable to Lyme disease.[2]

Lyme arthritis is delayed (3–6 months) and largely involves the knee joint.

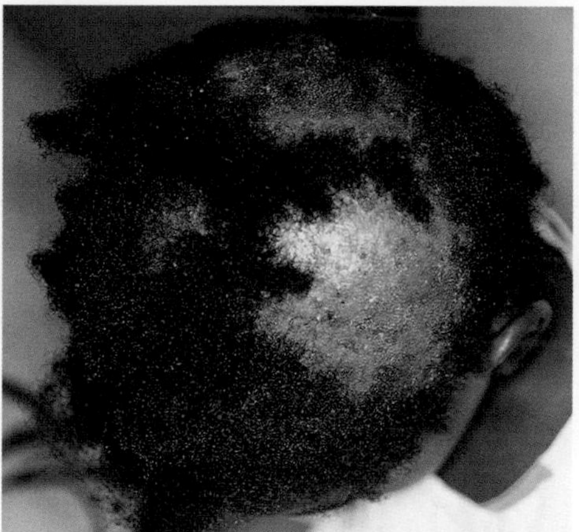

Fig. 6.4 Tinea capitis. (Source: From Bolognia J, Jorizzo J, Rapini R. *Dermatology*. St. Louis, MO: Mosby; 2003.)

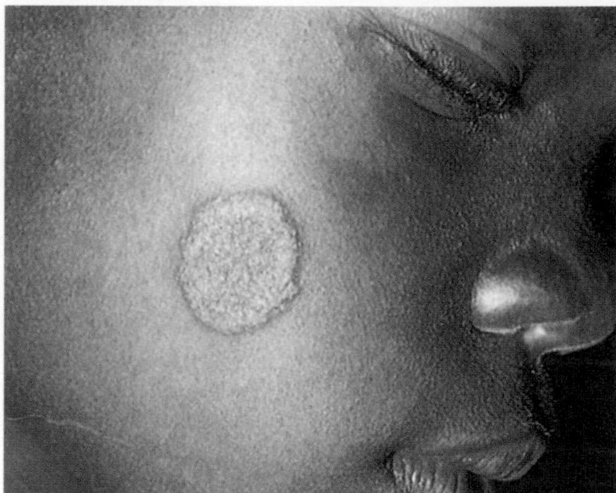

Fig. 6.5 Tinea corporis, or ringworm of the body, presents anywhere on the body of an adult or child but is more commonly seen on the chest, abdomen, back of the arms, face and dorsum of the feet. The circular lesions with clear centres can form singly or in clusters and represent a fungal infection that is both contagious and treatable. Tinea pedis (not shown), also known as ringworm of the feet or 'athlete's foot', occurs most often between the toes, but also along the sides of the feet and the soles (easily spread and treatable). (Source: From Hurwitz S. *Clinical Pediatric Dermatology: A Textbook of Skin Disorders of Childhood and Adolescence*. 2nd ed. Philadelphia: WB Saunders; 1993.)

In tinea corporis, the characteristic lesion is a red annular patch with a raised border and central clearing and some scaling along the border (Fig. 6.5). Treat tinea corporis (commonly referred to as ringworm) with topical antifungals.

Redness Around the Eye

Preseptal or periorbital cellulitis (Fig. 6.6) is important to diagnose with typically redness around the eye with associated fever, and the red skin is warm to touch. The child needs to be referred to hospital if preseptal cellulitis is suspected.[3]

Delay in diagnosis may lead to progression to orbital cellulitis (Fig. 6.7) where movements of the eye are painful or limited, there is proptosis and the eyelid is markedly swollen.[4] Orbital cellulitis requires prompt intravenous antibiotics and ophthalmology review. Orbital abscesses may need to be drained.

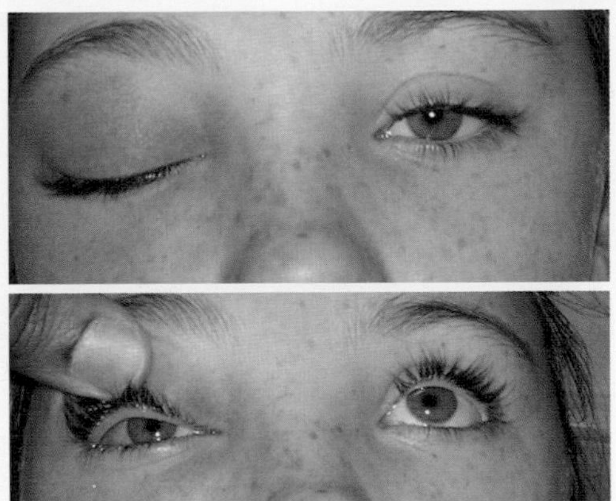

Fig. 6.7 A 12-year-old boy with orbital cellulitis. Note the poor elevation of the affected eye. (Source: From Hoyt C. *Pediatric Ophthalmology and Strabismus*. 4th ed. Philadelphia: Saunders; 2012 [fig. 13.10].)

Redness Around the Anal Margin

Perianal infection due to *Streptococcus pyogenes* is typified by a bright red rash in the perianal area with frequent fissuring, itching and associated reluctance to pass bowel motions. Typically, the rash is striking with a 'raw beef' appearance and a well-demarcated edge (Fig. 6.8). Group A Streptococcus can be cultured from a swab of the perianal area. Treatment is with oral co-amoxiclav for seven to 10 days.

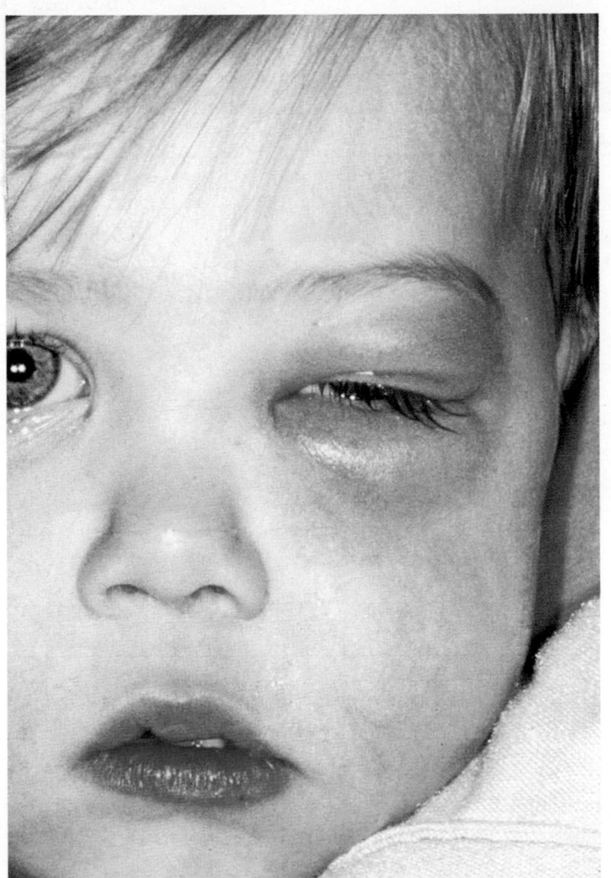

Fig. 6.6 Preseptal cellulitis. This is an infection of the periorbital tissue anterior to the orbital septum. Visual acuity, pupil reactivity and ocular motility are normal. (Source: *Cornea Atlas: Expert Consult* – Online and Print. 3rd ed. 2014.)

Henoch-Schonlein Purpura

Purpuric rashes may be relatively benign as in Henoch-Schonlein purpura (HSP) (Box 6.2) with a typical distribution of the rash (Fig. 6.9) or rapidly evolving as in invasive meningococcal disease. A rapid evolution of a petechial or nonblanching rash in a febrile child (see Chapter 4) is always of concern.

Acute Flare of Atopic Dermatitis

Be wary of an infant with an acute flare of atopic dermatitis.[5] This often results from infection with *Staphylococcus aureus* (Fig. 6.10) or herpes simplex (Fig. 6.11).

> Bacterial infection is suggested by weeping and crusted skin lesions or, in herpes simplex, a rapid deterioration of the rash with numerous vesicles and pustules.

In atopic dermatitis, the features suggestive of bacterial infection include weeping, crusting, a rapid worsening of the rash and a failure to respond to treatment (Box 6.3). Scabies remains a differential if severe pruritus (Box 6.4; Fig. 6.12).

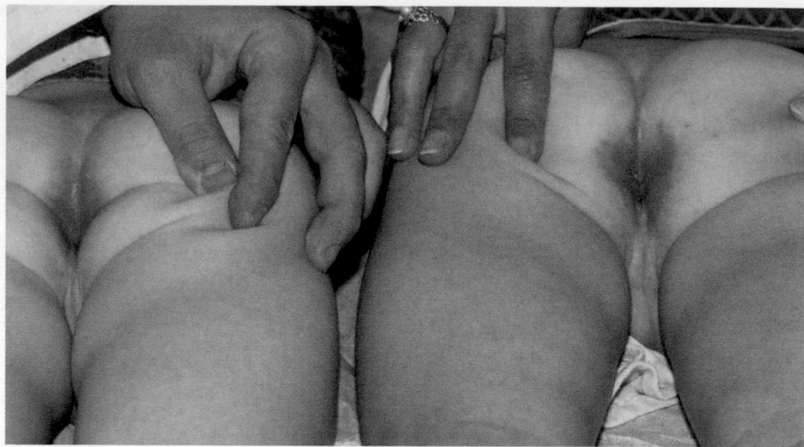

Fig. 6.8 Brilliant erythematous perianal dermatitis due to *Streptococcus pyogenes* brothers, reflecting the contagious nature of this infection. (Source: Kimberlin D, et al. *Principles and Practice of Pediatric Infectious Diseases*. 6th edition, 2022, Elsevier Inc.)

BOX 6.2 **CLINICAL HISTORY**

A 6-Year-Old Girl With a Purpuric Rash Over Her Legs

A 6-year-old girl presents to her family doctor with a 3-day history of a nonblanching rash over both her legs. She had significant crampy abdominal pain and bilateral pain and swelling of her ankles. Her examination revealed palpable purpura over both legs and buttocks. Her full blood count was normal, and her urinalysis showed microscopic haematuria and proteinuria. Her faecal occult blood test was positive, and she went on to have an abdominal ultrasound which excluded intussusception.

A diagnosis of Henoch-Schonlein purpura (HSP) was made.

Clinical Pearls

HSP (also known as Immunoglobulin A vasculitis) is common, self-limiting and resolves usually within 4 weeks.

The palpable purpura in HSP is distributed symmetrically and occurs mainly over the legs and buttocks.

Always check urinalysis looking for both haematuria and proteinuria.

The rash usually subsides after 14 days but may evolve into a bullous rash with later necrosis.

Pitfalls to Avoid

The initial rash may be macular and urticarial, and later it evolves into palpable purpura.

As a priority, outrule meningococcal sepsis, coagulopathies and thrombocytopenia.

Renal complications with a purpuric rash can also occur in Wegener's granulomatosis, polyarteritis nodosa and Churg-Strauss syndrome.

Renal biopsy is rarely indicated.

Oral corticosteroids are occasionally required but need to be tapered down very slowly to avoid recurrences of abdominal pain.

The severe abdominal cramps may predate the rash and thus may present not unlike an acute appendicitis.

BULLOUS RASHES OF CONCERN

Bullous impetigo is relatively common and initially presents with transparent flaccid bullae and honey-coloured crusting. Bullous impetigo is mainly seen in infancy and starts as small vesicles that coalesce into larger bullae (Fig. 6.13). It tends to affect the axillae, neck and groin creases and can resemble staphylococcal scalded skin

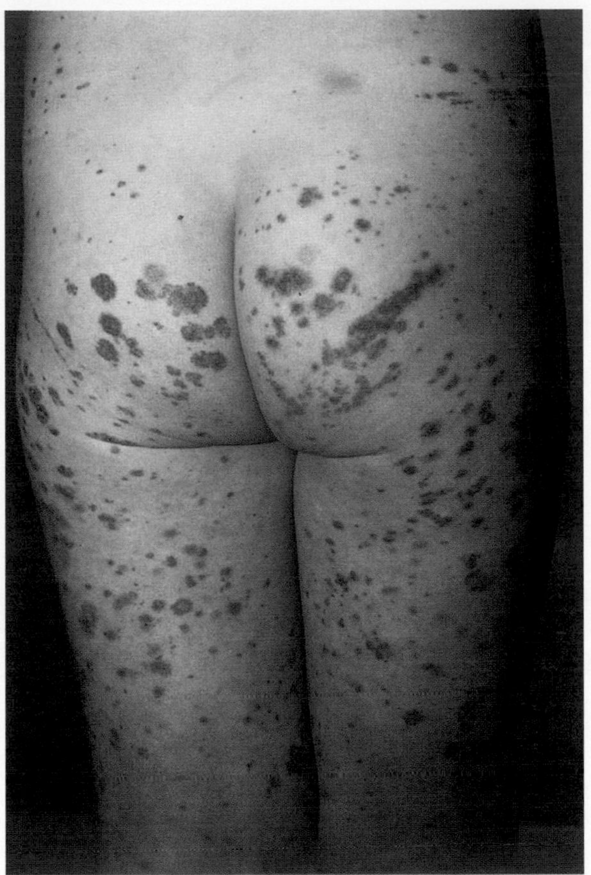

Fig. 6.9 A 6-year-old girl with Henoch-Schonlein purpura showing purpura over buttocks and lower limbs. (Source: Hewitt M, Adappa R. *Applied Knowledge in Paediatrics: MRCPCH Mastercourse*. 1st ed. Elsevier; 2022.)

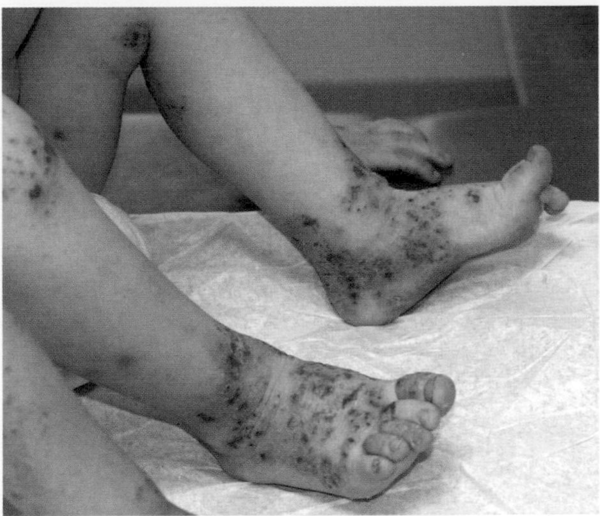

Fig. 6.10 Atopic dermatitis with *Staphylococcus* superinfection. (Soure: Marcdante KJ, et al. *Nelson Essentials of Pediatrics*. Ninth Edition, 2023, Elsevier Inc.)

syndrome (SSS) clinically. Bullous impetigo results from local *Staphylococcus aureus* infection which may be cultured from bullae.

Staphylococcal scalded skin syndrome (Fig. 6.14) is most often seen in preschool children and infants and is due to toxigenic strains of *Staphylococcus aureus*. There may be a generalised red rash with fever and irritability. Flaccid bullae may be seen. Prompt referral to hospital is indicated.[6]

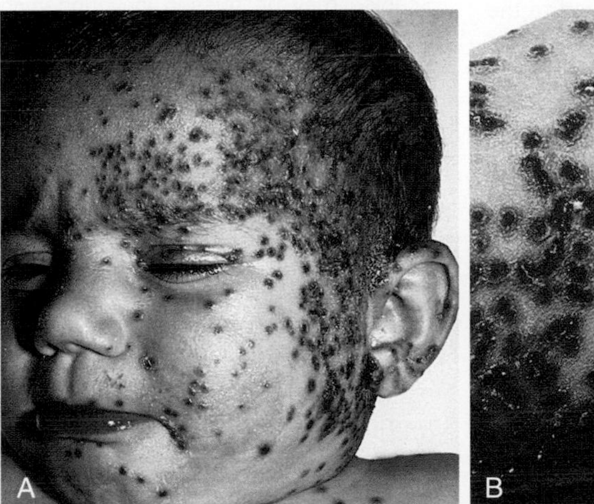

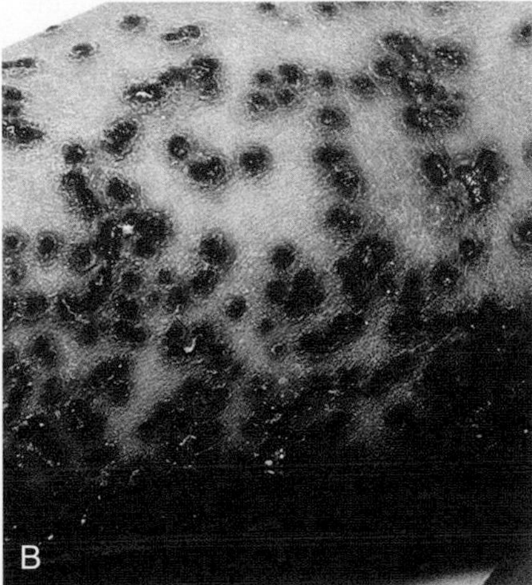

Fig. 6.11 Eczema herpeticum infection in a patient with atopic dermatitis. Numerous punched-out vesicles and erosions involving the face (A) and extremities (B). (Source: From Papulosquamous eruptions. In: Cohen BA, ed. *Pediatric Dermatology*. Philadelphia: Saunders; 2013:68–103.)

BOX 6.3 **CLINICAL HISTORY**

An 18 Month Old With a Sudden Flare Up of Atopic Dermatitis

An 18-month-old male toddler presents to his family doctor with a widespread rash on a background of atopic dermatitis. The rash has evolved rapidly over the past 2 days and now covers the face, neck and trunk. On examination there were multiple tiny vesicles over the back and chest. A diagnosis of eczema herpeticum was made, and he was commenced on aciclovir therapy. His rash improved over the next 3 days.

Clinical Pearls

Early diagnosis and treatment of eczema herpeticum is essential. Infection with herpes simplex virus leads to the rapid evolution of numerous vesicles, and the flare up is often quite dramatic.

Eczema herpeticum tends to occur in children under 3 years of age with a background history of atopic dermatitis, a superimposed vesicular rash and a history of exposure to herpes virus. Facial and neck involvement is typical.

The child is often systemically unwell with a high fever and lymphadenopathy.

Prompt treatment with aciclovir is required. Continue treatment for 7 to 10 days.

Pitfalls to Avoid

A rapid deterioration of atopic dermatitis is often due to infection.

If HSV suspected, hospital referral is indicated with early ophthalmology review for possible eye involvement.

BOX 6.4 **CLINICAL HISTORY**

A Toddler With a Widespread Itchy Rash and Background Atopic Dermatitis

An 18-month-old toddler presented with a 1-month history of an itchy rash mainly involving the limbs and the trunk. He had a past medical history of atopic dermatitis treated by emollients and topical steroids. His mother felt that this rash was perhaps related to some dietary changes and wondered about food allergies. His family doctor had seen him on several occasions and prescribed topical steroids and oral antibiotics for the rash. His examination revealed a very widespread rash with crusting over the web spaces between the fingers and toes and multiple eruptions over the soles of both feet. The toddler was otherwise well. He was referred to the dermatology clinic where a diagnosis of scabies infestation was made.

Clinical Pearls

Scabies and atopic dermatitis are the most common rashes causing itch in infancy and early childhood. In infants, scabies often involves the head and neck region and the soles of the feet. The rash may not involve the interdigital areas and may present with a variety of skin lesions, including papules, vesicles and plaques.

Transmission of scabies is by human-to-human contact with the clinical features occurring between 4 and 28 days of exposure.

Treatment is by the application of a parasiticide cream (5% permethrin) to the whole body, including the head, neck and palms and soles, with a repeat application 7 days later.

Pitfalls to Avoid

Scabies may be missed in younger children where the diagnosis of atopic dermatitis is assumed.

All close contacts of the index case should also be treated at the same time. Machine wash bedclothes at 60°C to eradicate fomites from bed linen.

Many children with scabies itch for some time following treatment, and this is managed by topical emollients and antihistamines.

Recurrence is mainly due to re-infection, and this may occur within weeks or months.

In staphylococcal scalded skin syndrome, an erythematous rash progresses to a generalised epidermal exfoliation with a fever, skin tenderness and an unwell child.

The rash often commences on the head and skin folds and spreads rapidly over a 48-hour period. Flaccid bullae develop and the Nikolsky sign is positive.

The mucous membranes are spared in SSS, and blood cultures may be positive for *Staphylococcus aureus*.

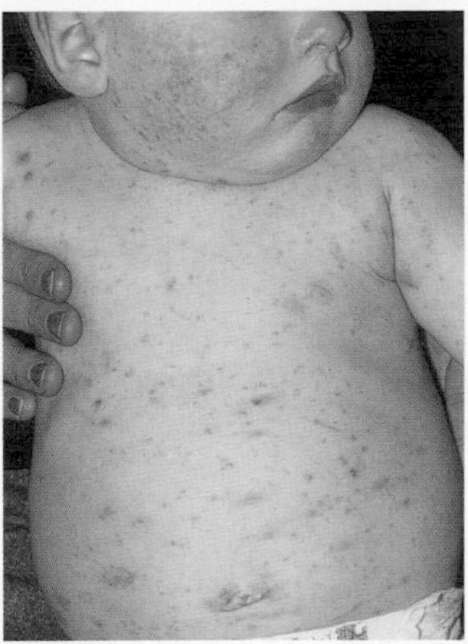

Fig. 6.12 Scabies in an infant. Diffuse pruritic, eczematous lesions on an infant are often confused with eczema. (Source: From White GM, Cox NH, eds. *Diseases of the Skin: A Color Atlas and Text.* 2nd ed. St Louis: Mosby; 2006.)

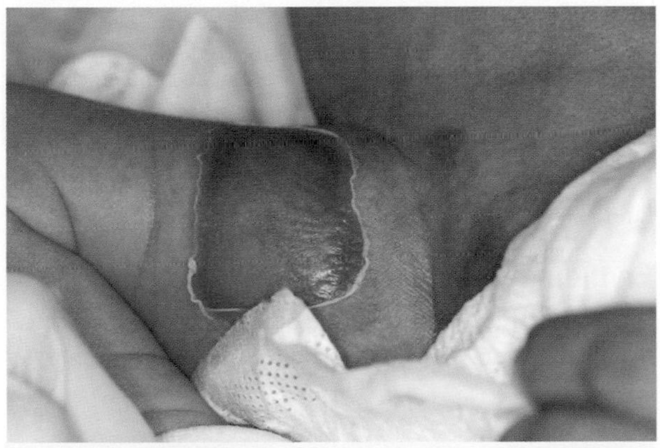

Fig. 6.13 Bullous impetigo. This 11-day-old boy developed flaccid vesicles and bullae that ruptured easily, leaving behind tender red patches with peripheral collarettes as seen here. *Staphylococcus aureus* grew in culture from the skin swab. (Source: *Paller and Mancini – Hurwitz Clinical Pediatric Dermatology: A Textbook of Skin Disorders of Childhood and Adolescence.* 6th ed. 2022.)

Epidermolysis bullosa (EB) is rare and may either be localised (usually hands and feet blisters with minimal trauma) or generalised. Bullae are present from birth and, in some subtypes, multisystem involvement is present. Diagnosis is confirmed through genetic testing and skin biopsies.

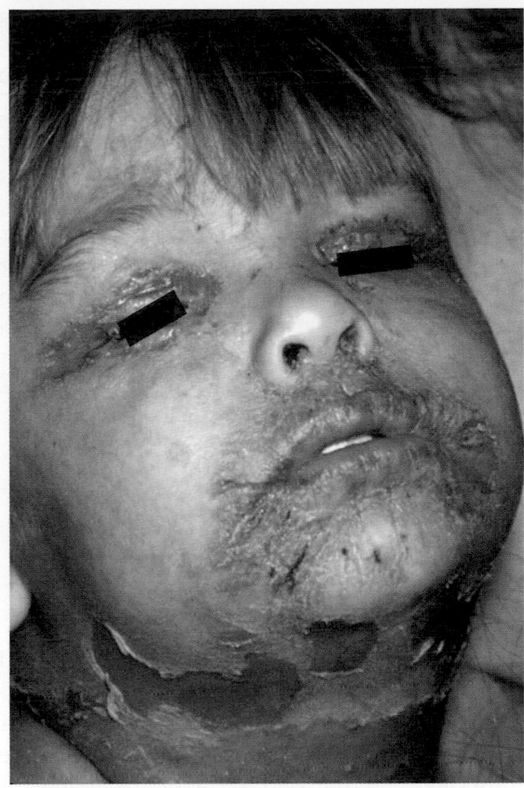

Fig. 6.14 Staphylococcal scalded skin syndrome – a toxin-mediated eruption characterised by erythema, skin separation (split is at granular layer and not full-thickness epidermis) and focus of infection – nares. (Source: *Lookingbill and Marks' Principles of Dermatology.* 6th ed. 2019.)

Stevens-Johnson Syndrome and Toxic Epidermal Necrolysis

Rarely one may see Stevens-Johnson syndrome (Box 6.5) or toxic epidermal necrolysis (TEN), and both may relate to medications in adults, but in children the trigger is more often a viral respiratory infection.

> In both SJS and TEN. the child is very unwell with significant mucosal involvement of the eyes, mouth, nose and genitalia. Prompt referral to hospital is required.

RASHES AND SYSTEMIC DISEASE

Rash of Systemic Juvenile Idiopathic Arthritis

Children with systemic juvenile idiopathic arthritis (JIA) typically have one to two temperature spikes per day with a rapid return to normal temperature. In tandem with

BOX 6.5 **CLINICAL HISTORY**

A 10 Year Old With Rapid Evolution of a Widespread Blistering Rash

A 10-year-old girl has a diagnosis of epilepsy and was commenced on lamotrigine therapy 4 weeks prior to presentation to her family doctor with a florid rash. She had a 2-day history of fever and general malaise. Her examination showed a widespread rash covering over 15% of the total body surface area. There was widespread blistering and the Nikolsky sign was positive. She had significant oral ulceration and was now having great difficulty taking fluids. She looked quite unwell and was referred directly to hospital by her family doctor. A diagnosis of Stevens-Johnson syndrome (SJS) was made.

Clinical Pearls

SJS and TEN are both type four hypersensitivity reactions which may be due to drugs (in particular antiepileptic drugs) or following *Mycoplasma* infection.

They are both serious illnesses often requiring paediatric intensive care admission.

TEN has a higher degree of body surface involvement (>30%) than SJS and a higher mortality.

Mucous membrane involvement is often painful and may be haemorrhagic.[1]

The rash progresses rapidly with formation of bullae and the skin may detach in large sheets.

Pitfalls to Avoid

Take a thorough history always asking about possible drug exposure and discontinue the drug if suspected.

Seek an early ophthalmology review if ocular involvement and always refer for dermatology input.

Plan for paediatric intensive care transfer if significant body surface area involvement.

the fever spike, a pink macular rash appears (Fig. 6.15), and this rash disappears again once the temperature settles. Generalised lymphadenopathy and an enlarged liver and spleen are also seen. During the course of the temperature spike, children with systemic JIA do look quite unwell, but they rapidly perk up once the temperature settles. Children with systemic JIA are at increased risk of macrophage activation syndrome leading to disseminated intravascular coagulation.[7]

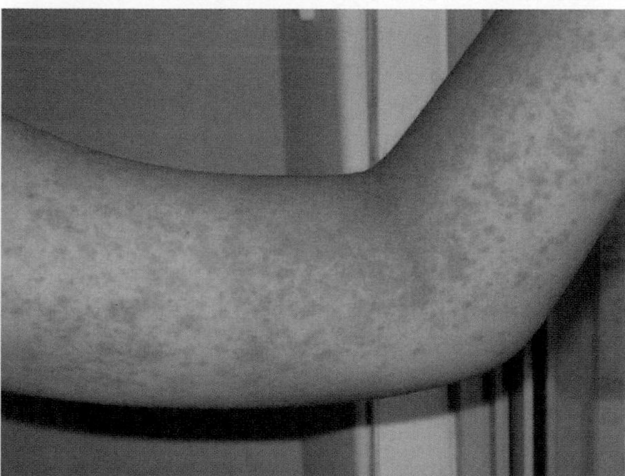

Fig. 6.15 Typical salmon-pink macular rash of systemic onset form of juvenile idiopathic arthritis in a 10-year-old boy. (Source: David Isaacs, Mike South. *Practical Paediatrics*, Seventh Edition. 2012, Elsevier Ltd.)

Therefore, transient temperature spikes with an associated pink macular rash which comes and goes with the temperature is important to recognise and may indicate systemic JIA.

These children do not develop joint symptoms until later.

Erythema Nodosum

Typically, this rash consists of erythematous painful nodules (Fig. 6.16) which are distributed over the lower

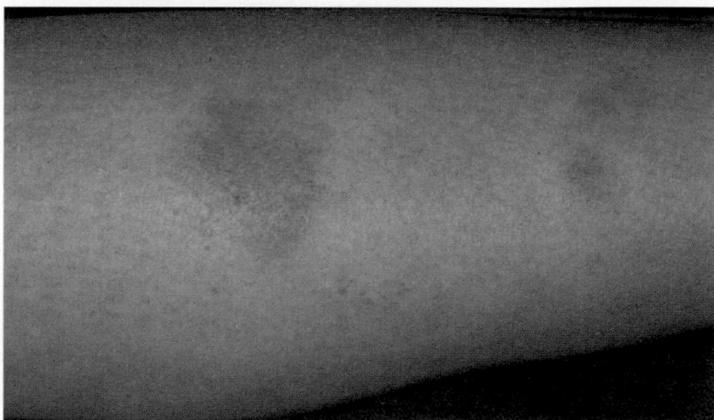

Fig. 6.16 Erythema nodosum. Tender, red, oval nodules on the extensor aspect of the legs. Note that several have darkened and resemble bruises. (Source: From Paller AS, Mancini AJ. *Hurwitz Clinical Pediatric Dermatology: A Textbook of Skin Disorders of Childhood and Adolescence*. 5th ed. Elsevier; 2016.)

limbs, often over the anterior tibial surfaces. There are a myriad of causes including group A Streptococcus, drugs, sarcoidosis and inflammatory bowel disease.

SKIN MARKERS OF NEUROLOGICAL CONDITIONS

Ash leaf macules (Fig. 6.17) are hypopigmented areas seen in tuberous sclerosis (TS). They may require a Wood lamp examination in a darkened room to detect them. TS is an important condition to pick up and may present early in infancy with developmental delay and infantile spasms. Other cutaneous features include forehead fibrous plaques, Shagreen patches and facial angiofibromas.

> In tuberous sclerosis ash leaf macules are often evident in the first few months of life.

Café au lait macules (Fig. 6.18) are very common in children, but if more than six café au lait macules over 0.5 cm in diameter are seen, then neurofibromatosis 1 (NF1) should be considered. Other features of NF1 include axillary and inguinal freckling (Fig. 6.19) with Lisch nodules (Fig. 6.20) and neurofibromas presenting later.

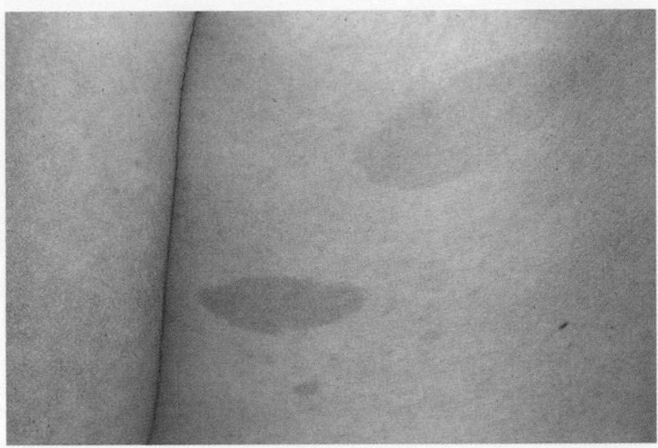

Fig. 6.18 Multiple café-au-lait macules >5 mm in diameter. (Source: James E. Fitzpatrick, Joseph G. Morelli. *Dermatology Secrets Plus*. 4th edition, Mosby, Elsevier Inc.)

IMPORTANT NEONATAL RASHES

Neonatal Lupus

Neonatal lupus results from the passage of anti-Ro and/or anti-La antibodies from affected mothers. The rash of neonatal lupus presents at, or shortly after, birth. It has a distinctive periorbital distribution. The rash is raised, red, annular and scaly (Fig. 6.21). The skin eruption will clear as maternal antibodies clear but all

Fig. 6.17 Tuberous sclerosis. Ash leaf-shaped hypopigmented macules. (Source: *Habif's Clinical Dermatology: A Color Guide to Diagnosis and Therapy*. 7th ed. 2021.)

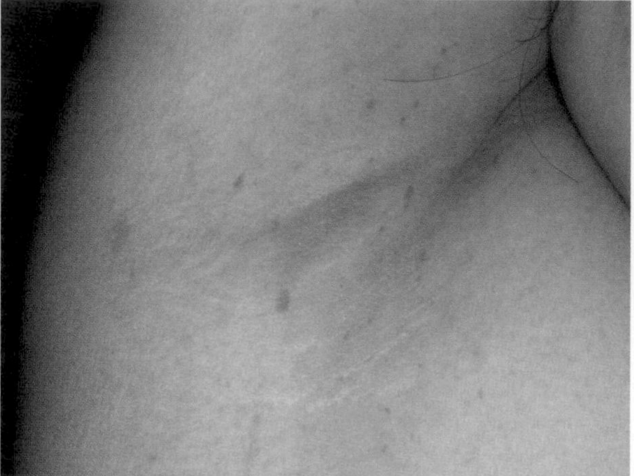

Fig. 6.19 Neurofibromatosis type 1 (NF1). Axillary freckling (Crowe sign) is present in 20% to 50% of individuals with NF1 and commonly appears between 3 and 5 years of age. Although the presence of both axillary freckling and multiple café-au-lait spots currently allows a definitive diagnosis of NF1, these features are also seen in Legius syndrome. (Source: *Paller and Mancini – Hurwitz Clinical Pediatric Dermatology: A Textbook of Skin Disorders of Childhood and Adolescence*. 6th ed. 2022.)

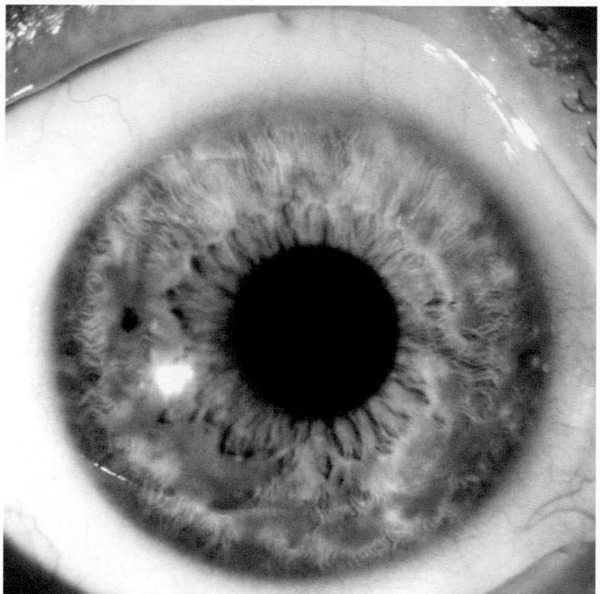

Fig. 6.20 Lisch nodules. Lisch nodules are circumferential, brown, often bilateral, hamartomatous plaques or nodules on the anterior iris. (Source: *Diagnostic Pathology: Neuropathology*. 3rd ed. 2023.)

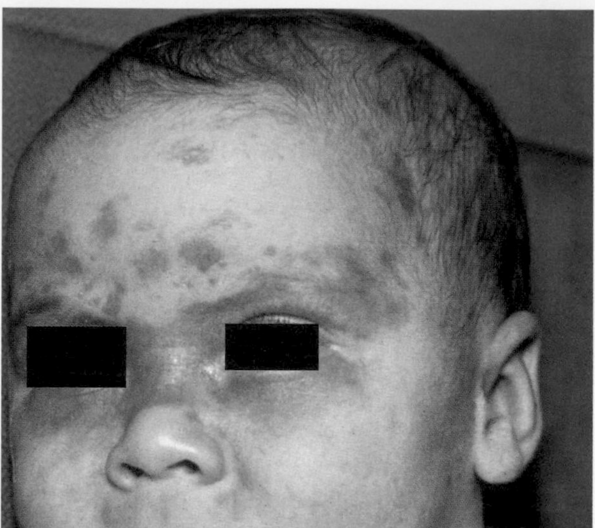

Fig. 6.21 Periocular neonatal lupus erythematosus. (Source: *Andrews' Diseases of the Skin: Clinical Dermatology*. 13th ed. 2020.)

affected infants with neonatal lupus should be screened for cardiac involvement due to the risk of complete heart block.[8] Hepatic and haematological manifestations may also be present.

About 40% to 60% of the mothers whose infants have neonatal lupus are asymptomatic. As such all mothers of affected neonates should be screened for anti-Ro/SSA antibodies in order to minimise problems in future pregnancies.

Subcutaneous Fat Necrosis

Subcutaneous fat necrosis appears as a localised red-brown indurated area over the pressure sites on neonatal skin (Fig. 6.22), often associated with therapeutic hypothermia. Fat necrosis produces 1 alpha-hydroxylase, the enzyme that converts 25-hydroxyvitamin D to 1,25 dihydroxyvitamin D, and affected infants may require treatment for subsequent hypercalcaemia.

Cutaneous Langerhans Cell Histiocytosis

Cutaneous Langerhans Cell Histiocytosis may present in a number of ways not least with crusted erosions, violaceous papules or nodules.[9] Most commonly in infants it presents as crusted papules and pustules seen over the scalp (Fig. 6.23) and skin creases of the groin that may resemble seborrheic dermatitis. A full workup

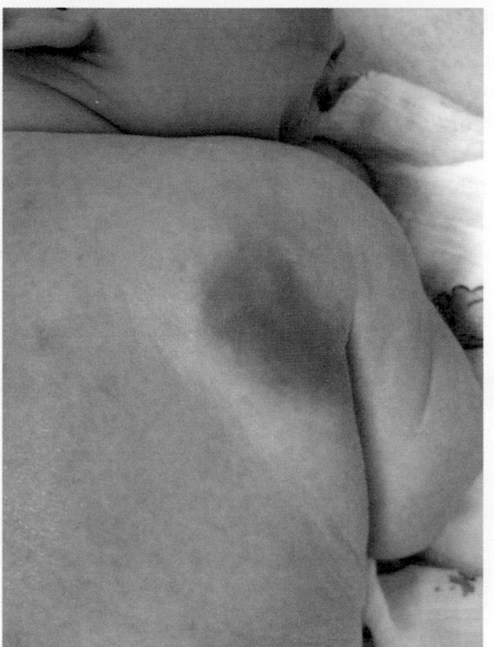

Fig. 6.22 Subcutaneous fat necrosis of the newborn. (Source: Micheletti RG, et al. *Andrews' Diseases of the Skin Clinical Atlas*. 2nd edition, 2023, Elsevier Inc.)

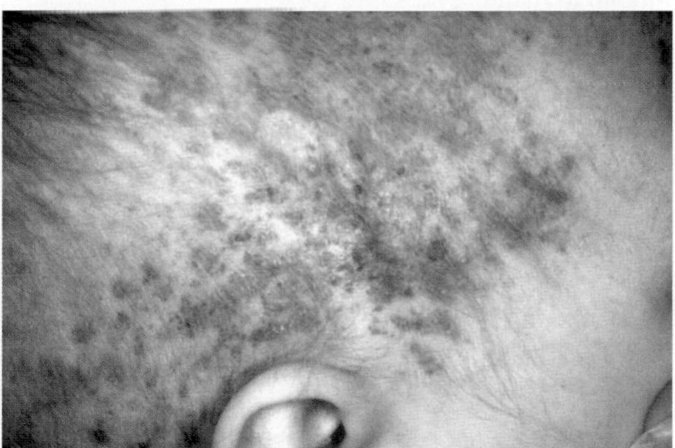

Fig. 6.23 Langerhans cell histiocytosis. (Source: Micheletti RG, et al. *Andrews' Diseases of the Skin Clinical Atlas*. 2nd edition, 2023, Elsevier Inc.)

is indicated and should include a skeletal survey, a full blood count, coagulation profile and liver function studies.[9]

Petechial Rashes in Newborns

Isolated petechiae in the superior vena cava distribution are not uncommon, but petechiae on the trunk and limbs increases the likelihood that they are clinically significant. The key blood test is the full blood count which may show low platelets. A platelet count under 10 is linked to a presumptive diagnosis of neonatal alloimmune thrombocytopenic purpura (NAIT) (Fig. 6.24).

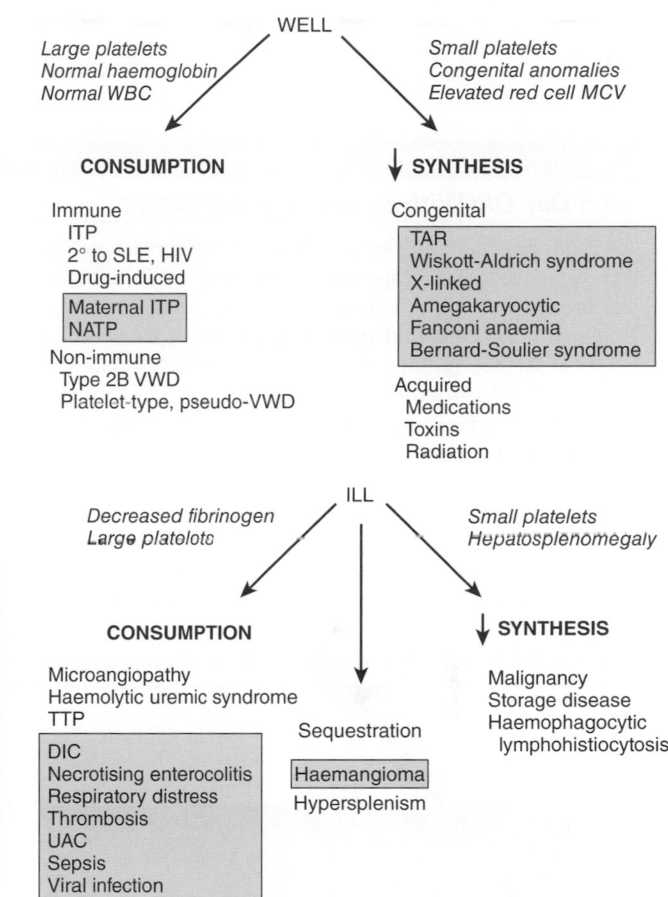

Fig. 6.24 Differential diagnosis of childhood thrombocytopenic syndromes. The syndromes are initially separated by their clinical appearance. Clues leading to the diagnosis are presented in italics. The mechanisms and common disorders leading to these findings are shown in the lower part of the figure. Disorders that commonly affect neonates are listed in the shaded boxes. *DIC*, Disseminated intravascular coagulation; *ITP*, idiopathic immune thrombocytopenic purpura; *MCV*, mean corpuscular volume; *NATP*, neonatal alloimmune thrombocytopenic purpura; *SLE*, systemic lupus erythematosus; *TAR*, thrombocytopenia – absent radius (syndrome); *TTP*, thrombotic thrombocytopenic purpura; *UAC*, umbilical artery catheter; *VWD*, von Willebrand disease; *WBC*, white blood cell; *2°*, secondary. (Source: Bordini BJ, et al. *Nelson Pediatric Symptom-Based Diagnosis: Common Diseases and Their Mimics*. 2nd ed. Elsevier; 2023.)

Treatment is with a platelet transfusion or, if suitably matched platelets are not readily available, give intravenous gammaglobulin which takes up to 24 to 36 hours to work.

Neonatal alloimmune thrombocytopenia can cause profound thrombocytopenia and is the commonest cause of intraventricular haemorrhage in term newborns.

Blistering Rashes in Newborns

Neonatal herpes simplex virus (HSV) infection needs to be considered if grouping of the vesicles is seen especially on the face and head (Box 6.6; Fig. 6.25).

Neonatal varicella (Fig. 6.26) is important to recognise and treat promptly. If varicella is seen in a pregnant

BOX 6.6 CLINICAL HISTORY

A 5 Day Old With Several Facial Blisters

A 5-day-old infant presents with a group of small vesicles on her cheek. Her temperature is normal, she is alert and is feeding well. She is reviewed by the out-of-hours service with a decision to observe and review in 24 hours.

After 24 hours, her parents note that she is now irritable, and the mother observes an episode of twitching of the infant's right hand. The infant is promptly brought to the paediatric emergency department where widespread vesicles of the face and scalp are noted. A clinical diagnosis of herpes simplex infection is made. Fluid from the skin vesicles is PCR positive for herpes simplex virus type 1 (HSV-1). The CSF protein was raised. The CSF showed a lymphocytosis and HSV-1 was found on PCR. The EEG reported a slow wave pattern in the left frontal lobe. The MRI demonstrated an area of haemorrhagic necrosis in the left frontal and parietal regions.

She was treated with intravenous aciclovir. She had developmental follow-up and showed evidence of a mild right hemiparesis.

Clinical Pearls

The presence of vesicles on the skin of a newborn infant should always raise the possibility of HSV infection.

Pitfalls to Avoid

Newborns with HSV skin lesions have a 30% risk of developing HSV encephalitis.

Prompt recognition and treatment given intravenously is required.

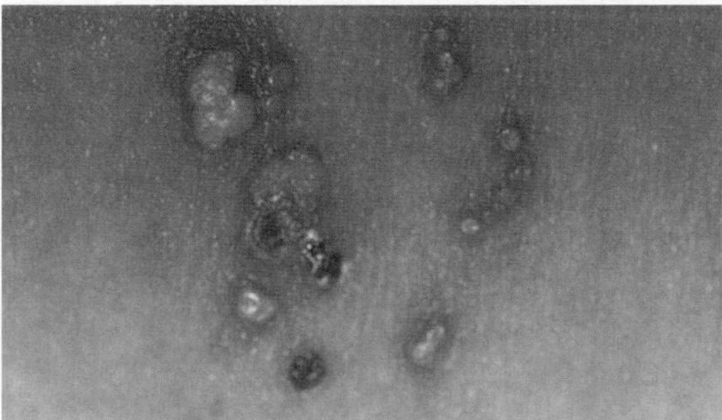

Fig. 6.25 Clustered vesicles on an erythematous base, several of which are coalescing on the skin of a neonate with herpes simplex virus infection. Three of these vesicles have ruptured, leaving shallow erosions and overlying haemorrhagic crusting. (Source: Kimberlin D, et al. *Principles and Practice of Pediatric Infectious Diseases.* 6th edition, 2022, Elsevier Inc.)

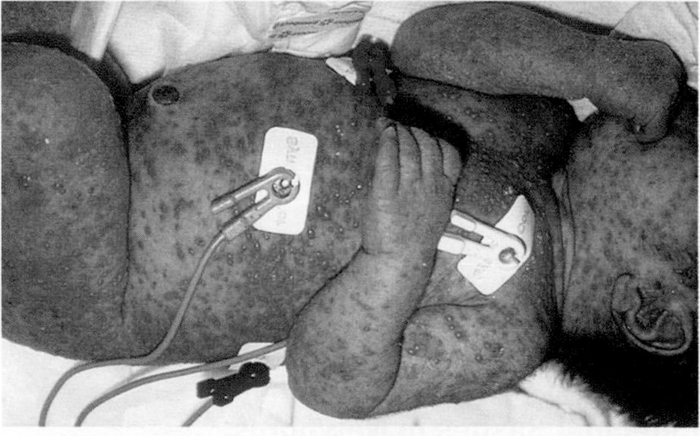

Fig. 6.26 Neonatal varicella. Disseminated, erythematous papules, vesicles and erosions. (Source: *Paller and Mancini – Hurwitz Clinical Pediatric Dermatology: A Textbook of Skin Disorders of Childhood and Adolescence.* 6th ed. 2022.)

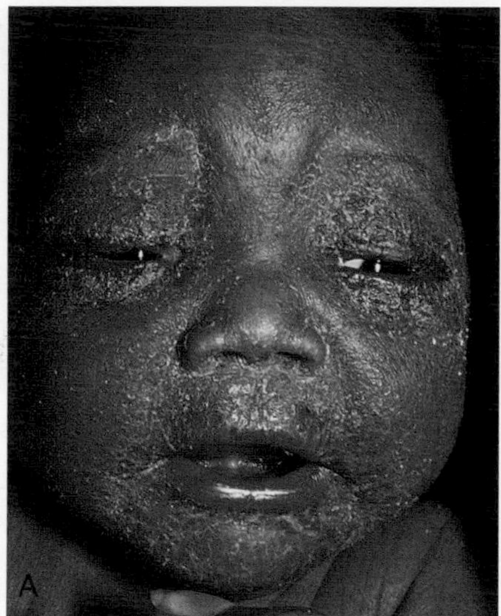

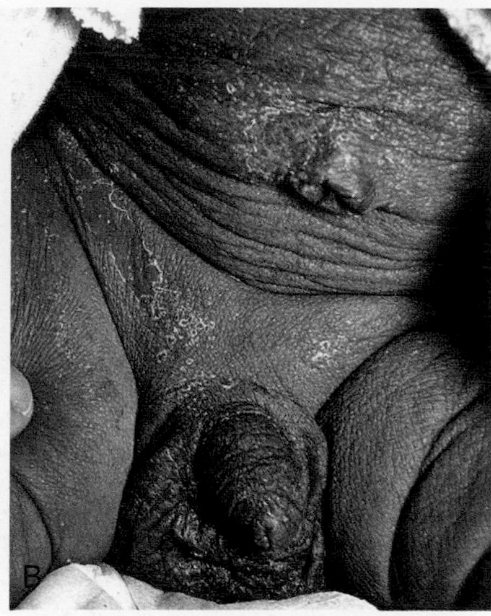

Fig. 6.27 Staph scalded skin syndrome. Staphylococcal scalded skin syndrome developed in this neonate a few days after his brother was diagnosed with impetigo. Erosive patches were most marked on the (A) face and (B) diaper areas. (Source: From Puttgen K, Cohen BA. Neonatal dermatology. In: Cohen, BA, ed. *Pediatric Dermatology*. 4th ed. Philadelphia: Elsevier; 2013:38, Fig. 2.47.)

woman within 5 days prior to delivery to 2 days post-delivery, then the infant should receive intravenous gammaglobulin prophylaxis.[10]

In newborns with staphylococcal scalded skin syndrome, a tender erythematous rash tends to start in the flexures with later circumoral erythema with crusting around the nose and mouth being characteristic (Fig. 6.27).

In dystrophic EB the presentation is with blisters that heal with scarring and nail dystrophy. Severe interdigital scarring can be seen (Fig. 6.28).

Incontinentia pigmenti (IP) is a rare X-linked skin condition caused by a defect of the *IKBKG* gene which is usually lethal in males.[11–13] Skin manifestations tend to follow Blaschko lines and divide into four stages (Fig. 6.29). The vesicular phase starts generally in the first few weeks of life (Box 6.7). These vesicles tend to be superficial on an erythematous base. Most experience the hyperpigmented stage between 3 and 6 months of age, and this phase may last for years before becoming atrophic and hypopigmented.

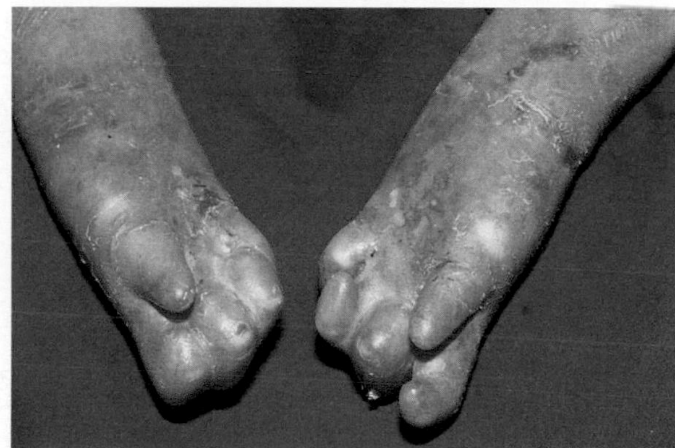

Fig. 6.28 Epidermolysis bullosa, recessive dystrophic type. (Source: *Andrews' Diseases of the Skin: Clinical Dermatology*, 13th ed. 2020.)

Alopecia, nail dystrophy and delayed eruption of teeth with an abnormal or peg shape may occur in IP.

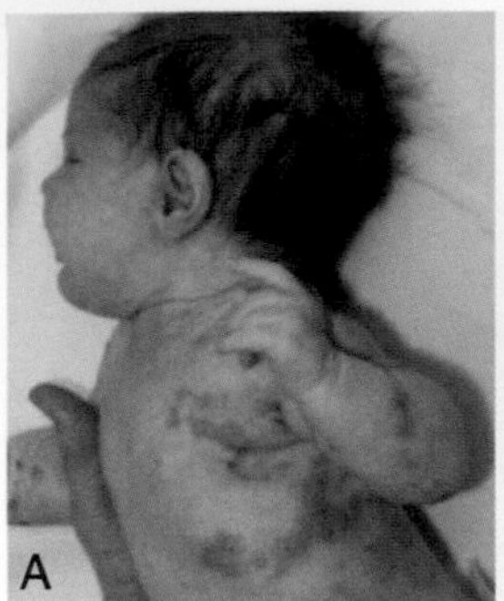

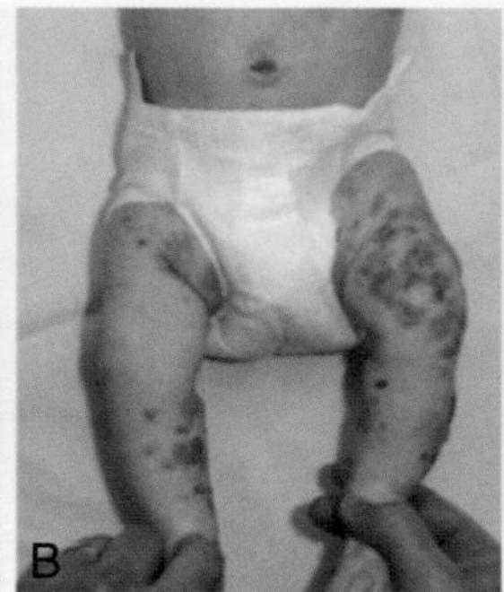

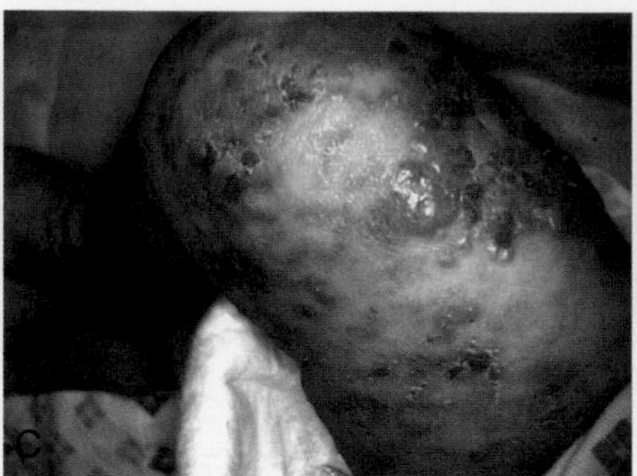

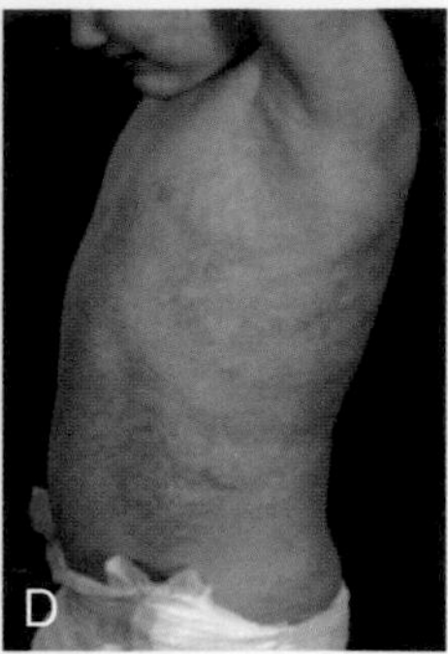

Fig. 6.29 Cutaneous features of incontinentia pigmenti. (A) Stage 1 – red, blister-like vesicular lesions affecting the trunk. (B) Stage 1 – red, blister-like vesicular lesions affecting the lower limbs. (C) Stage 2 – lesions on the right lower limb including papules and keratotic patches with some healing residual stage 1 blisters. (D) Stage 3 – marbled hyperpigmentation along the lines of Blaschko on the trunk. (Source: Graeme CM, Black et al. *Clinical Ophthalmic Genetics and Genomics*. 1st edition, Academic Press, 2022, Elsevier Inc.)

BOX 6.7 CLINICAL HISTORY

A 4-Week-Old Infant With an Unusual Rash

A 4-week-old female infant presented with an unusual rash over her right anterior thigh which had been present from birth. The rash was described as both vesicular and crusted. The infant was otherwise well with a normal feeding pattern. Birth and pregnancy history were normal with no history of perinatal varicella in the mother. The infant was referred to a paediatric dermatology service where a diagnosis of incontinentia pigmenti was made by means of genetic studies.

Clinical Pearls

Incontinentia pigmenti (IP) is very rare and usually lethal in males. The condition may be quite mild or severe. The manifestations of IP are in four separate phases. The initial stage is of a linear pattern of vesicles and pustules. This presents within 2 weeks of birth and may last up to 4 months. Stage two is the verrucous stage and tends to develop between 2 and 6 weeks of age. Stage three involves whorled skin lesions with brown pigmentation, and in stage four hypopigmentation develops. Stage four develops in adolescence, and there is a characteristic absence of hair especially of the legs. About one in four cases are inherited.

Pitfalls to Avoid

Up to 20% have ocular involvement including retinal vascularisation and risk of retinal detachment. Regular eye screening (especially under 6 months of age) by an ophthalmologist is required. Early referral with laser treatment may prevent retinal detachment.

Neurological manifestations occur in up to 30% and include microcephaly, motor delay, ataxia and seizures. Seizures are most likely in the neonatal period. Baseline MRI scan of the brain is recommended preferably in the neonatal period.

KEY LEARNING POINTS

Paediatric dermatological emergencies are relatively uncommon but important to recognise.

In assessing a rash, always estimate the body surface area involvement of the rash.

Tinea capitis is very common and presents with both scaling and a well-defined area of alopecia with broken hair follicles.

In tinea corporis, the characteristic lesion is a red annular patch with a raised border and central clearing and some scaling along the border.

Preseptal or periorbital cellulitis is important to pick up with typically redness around the eye with associated fever, and the red skin is warm to touch. The child needs to be referred to hospital if preseptal cellulitis is suspected.

Perianal infection due to *Streptococcus pyogenes* is typified by a bright red rash in the perianal area with frequent fissuring, itching and associated reluctance to pass bowel motions.

Scabies and atopic dermatitis are the most common rashes causing itch in infancy and early childhood. In infants, scabies often involves the head and neck region and the soles of the feet.

Scabies may be missed in younger children where the diagnosis of atopic dermatitis is assumed.

All close contacts of the index case should also be treated at the same time.

Be wary of an infant with atopic dermatitis with a sudden flare of the rash. Bacterial infection is suggested by weeping and crusted skin lesions or, in herpes simplex, a rapid deterioration of the rash with numerous vesicles and pustules.

The palpable purpura of Henoch-Schonlein purpura is distributed symmetrically and occurs mainly over the legs and buttocks and usually subsides after 14 days but may evolve into a bullous rash with later necrosis.

Establishing the diagnosis of Lyme disease can be challenging and recognition of the classical erythema migrans rash is important. This rash is red or bluish-red and expands over a period of days or weeks. Less than 50% can recall a prior tick bite. The most common neurological manifestation of Lyme disease in children is a facial nerve palsy.

In systemic JIA, in tandem with the fever spike, a pink macular rash appears, and this rash disappears again once the temperature settles. Recognition of this classical rash is important.

The rash of erythema nodosum consists of erythematous painful nodules which are distributed over the lower limbs, often over the anterior tibial surfaces.

Ash leaf macules are typical of tuberous sclerosis (TS) and may require a Wood lamp examination in a darkened room to pick them up.

Café au lait spots are very common, but if more than six café au lait spots over 0.5 cm in diameter are seen then neurofibromatosis 1 (NF1) should be considered.

SJS and TEN are both type IV hypersensitivity reactions which may be due to drugs (in particular antiepileptic drugs) or following *Mycoplasma* infection. They are both serious illnesses often requiring paediatric intensive care admission.

Bullous impetigo is relatively common and initially presents with transparent flaccid bullae and honey-coloured crusting.

Staphylococcal scalded skin syndrome is most often seen in preschool children and infants. There may be a generalised red rash with fever and irritability. Flaccid bullae may be seen. The mucosal surfaces are not affected. Prompt referral to hospital is indicated.

Epidermolysis bullosa (EB) is rare and may either be localised (usually hands and feet blisters with minimal trauma) or generalised.

The newborn with a blistered rash may have varicella, congenital herpes simplex, incontinentia pigmenti or epidermolysis bullosa.

Incontinentia pigmenti (IP) is a rare X-linked skin condition caused by a defect of the *IKBKG* gene which is usually lethal in males.

REFERENCES

1. Reynolds S, Matteus S, Ajay M, et al. When is a rash not 'just' a rash? A guide to recognition and treatment of paediatric dermatological emergencies. *Paediatrics and Child Health*. 2021 Jan;31(1):46–54. doi:10.1016/j.paed.2020.10.006.
2. Kullberg BJ, Vrijmoeth HD, van de Schoor F, Hovius JW. Lyme borreliosis: diagnosis and management. *BMJ*. 2020;369:m1041. doi:10.1136/bmj.m1041. Published 2020 May 26.
3. Santos JC, Pinto S, Ferreira S, Maia C, Alves S, da Silva V. Pediatric preseptal and orbital cellulitis: A 10-year experience. *Int J Pediatr Otorhinolaryngol*. 2019;120:82–88. doi:10.1016/j.ijporl.2019.02.003.
4. Baiu I, Melendez E. Periorbital and Orbital Cellulitis. *JAMA*. 2020;323(2):196. doi:10.1001/jama.2019.18211.
5. Weidinger S, Novak N. Atopic dermatitis. *Lancet*. 2016;387(10023):1109–1122. doi:10.1016/S0140-6736(15)00149-X.
6. Robinson SK, Jefferson IS, Agidi A, Moy L, Lake E, Kim W. Pediatric dermatology emergencies. *Cutis*. 2020;105(3):132–136.
7. Lee JJY, Schneider R. Systemic Juvenile Idiopathic Arthritis. *Pediatr Clin North Am*. 2018;65(4):691–709. doi:10.1016/j.pcl.2018.04.005.
8. Derdulska JM, Rudnicka L, Szykut-Badaczewska A, et al. Neonatal lupus erythematosus – practical guidelines. *J Perinat Med*. 2021;49(5):529–538. doi:10.1515/jpm-2020-0543. Published 2021 Jan 18.

9. Krooks J, Minkov M, Weatherall AG. Langerhans cell histiocytosis in children: History, classification, pathobiology, clinical manifestations, and prognosis. *J Am Acad Dermatol.* 2018;78(6):1035–1044. doi:10.1016/j.jaad.2017.05.059.
10. Sauerbrei A, Wutzler P. Neonatal varicella. *J Perinatol.* 2001;21(8):545–549. doi:10.1038/sj.jp.7210599.
11. Greene-Roethke C. Incontinentia Pigmenti: A Summary Review of This Rare Ectodermal Dysplasia With Neurologic Manifestations, Including Treatment Protocols. *J Pediatr Health Care.* 2017;31(6):e45–e52. doi:10.1016/j.pedhc.2017.07.003.
12. Thorsness S, Eyler J, Mudaliar K, Speiser J, Kim W. Asymptomatic Rash in a Male Infant with Incontinentia Pigmenti. *J Pediatr.* 2019;215:278. e1. doi:10.1016/j.jpeds.2019.07.005 .
13. Kim HY, Song HB, Kim KH, et al. Importance of extracutaneous organ involvement in determining the clinical severity and prognosis of incontinentia pigmenti caused by mutations in the IKBKG gene. *Exp Dermatol.* 2021;30(5):676–683. doi:10.1111/exd.14313.

ADDITIONAL READING

Allmon A, Deane K, Martin KL. Common Skin Rashes in Children. *Am Fam Physician.* 2015;92(3):211–216.

Gubbin J, Malbon K. Fifteen-minute consultation: The overweight teenage girl with acne. *Arch Dis Child Educ Pract Ed.* 2021;106(4):194–199. doi:10.1136/archdischild-2019-316846.

Lavery MJ, Woodcock D, Simmons W, Al-Sharqi A. A baby with a widespread itchy rash. *BMJ.* 2019;367:l5675. doi:10.1136/bmj.l5675. Published 2019 Oct 17.

Sayers DR, Clark LL. Images in health surveillance: Skin rashes in children due to infectious causes. *MSMR.* 2020;27(2):30–31.

Song Y, Zhou Q, Qiao J, Chen J. A boy with purpura on the legs. *BMJ.* 2021;372:n329. doi:10.1136/bmj.n329. Published 2021 Mar 4.

7

Diagnosing Cancer in Childhood

Michael Capra, Sarah Taaffe

CHAPTER OUTLINE

BACKGROUND

In this chapter, we will introduce a number of case scenarios and explore ways by which a diagnosis of cancer might be made in children and adolescents. Cancer in childhood is not all that rare, in fact one older child in every 450 will develop cancer by the age of 15 in the UK. Childhood cancer requires vigilance to detect and adherence to a number of golden rules. Foremost amongst these is 'three strikes and you are in' whereby if parents present three times with their child with the same symptoms, then referral and consideration of serious underlying diagnosis is recommended.[1]

The main types of childhood cancers are represented in the following diagram (Fig. 7.1). We will focus on the cancers that are most likely to be encountered.

Making the Diagnosis of Childhood Cancer

It has been estimated that a child's risk of developing cancer is low in the first year of life (1 in 4700), rising to 1 in 1000 in the preschool years and rising further from 5 to 15 years of age. Cancer risks are higher in children with specific cancer predisposition syndromes such as neurofibromatosis types 1 and 2, Down syndrome and tissue overgrowth syndromes.[1]

In our view, therefore, family doctors need support to increase awareness with guidelines that are relevant to current practice. Red flags and symptoms to consider from the NICE guidelines 2020: *Childhood cancers – recognition and referral*[2] are as summarised in Fig. 7.2.

Increasing Awareness Works

A good example has been the success of the *HeadSmart* campaign in the UK with widespread dissemination to the public and healthcare professionals with a helpful decision support website. This type of awareness campaign has therefore the potential to change practice in terms of earlier pick up of brain tumours. This campaign has been successful in reducing the total diagnostic interval (TDI) from a median of 14.5 weeks to 6.4 weeks over a period of 4 years.

Child Cancer Smart has been established in the UK to raise awareness of childhood cancers.

A **diagnostic support tool** (Fig. 7.3) by the Grace Kelly Childhood Cancer Trust has been developed with a useful pneumonic:

Concern – always respond to ongoing concern of parents
Anorexia – a poor appetite is a worrisome symptom in a young child and can be distinguished readily from food refusal which is seen almost exclusively in toddlers

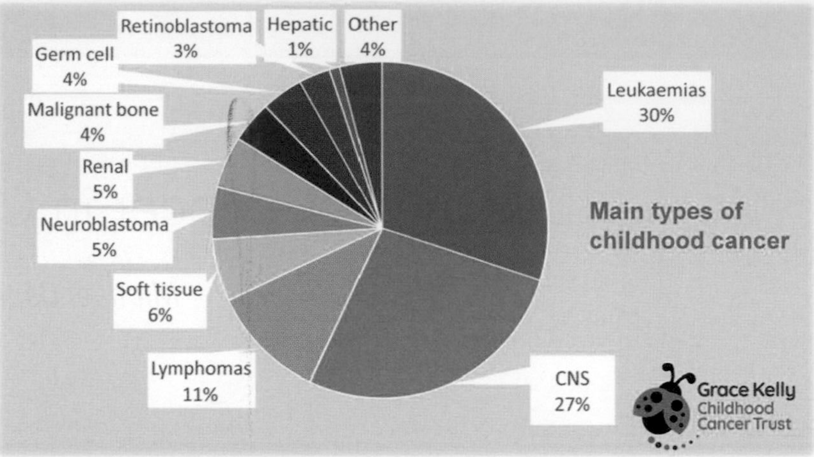

Fig. 7.1 Main types of childhood cancer. (Reproduced with permission from the Grace Kelly Childhood Cancer Trust.)

Symptoms of Concern (esp. if 2 or more)	Other Symptoms
Weight loss	Refractory constipation
Headache, worse in morning	Swollen abdomen
Constant tiredness	Palpable lumps on limbs or anywhere on body
Pallor	Haematuria
Petechiae or excessive bruising	Bleeding or swollen gums
Sudden vision change, true diplopia, new onset squint, loss of red reflex	Anorexia or nausea
Recurrent or persistent fevers of unknown origin	Non-resolving limp or leg pain Pain that is present at night or on waking
Unexplained hepatosplenomegaly	

Fig. 7.2 Symptoms of concern with cancer. (Reproduced with permission from the Grace Kelly Childhood Cancer Trust.)

Number of attendances – the general rule of 'three strikes and you are in' is apt in that repeated attendance should prompt a change in approach

Complexion – a child with cancer is often very pale and gaunt in terms of complexion

Exhaustion – a complete loss of energy or anergia is typically seen and of concern

Recurrent pyrexia – a recurrent unexplained fever is of concern and may indicate a lymphoma

Early detection and reduction in the time from first symptom to diagnosis (TDI) will support the avoidance of life-threatening presentations such as bone marrow failure, tumour lysis syndrome, raised intracranial pressure or spinal cord compression.[1] We also need to see the lowering of the staging distribution at presentation and consequently the reduction in the rates of lifelong disability.

> If a child has three visits to their family doctor within 3 months, the risk of a cancer diagnosis is increased ten-fold.

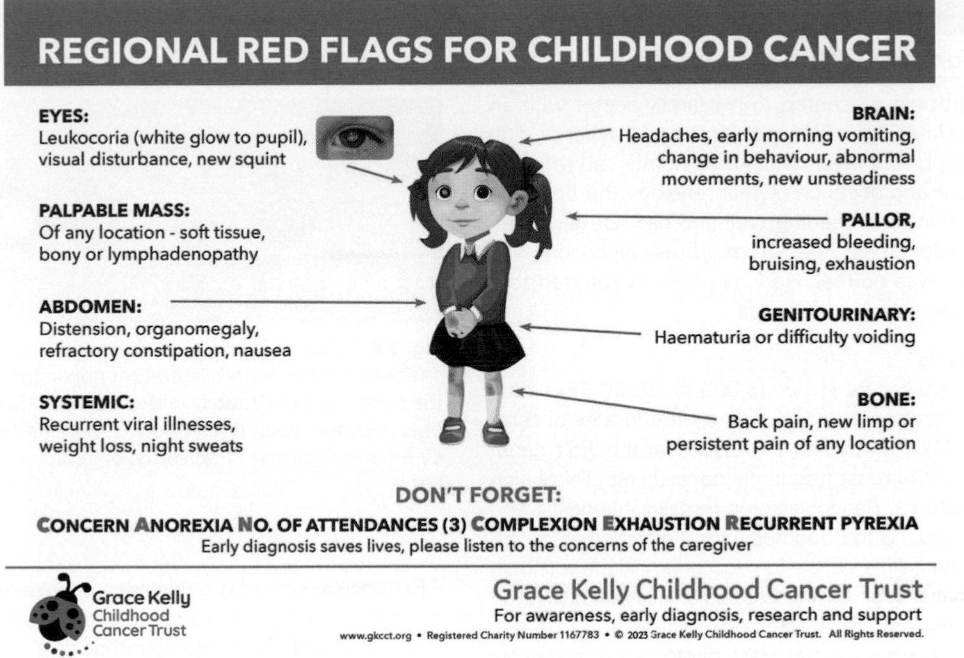

Fig. 7.3 Regional red flags for childhood cancer. (Reproduced with permission from the Grace Kelly Childhood Cancer Trust.)

AVOIDING DIAGNOSTIC DELAY

Delays in diagnosis are reported regularly and are a cause of great distress to families and a leading cause of malpractice claims.[3] Factors leading to a lengthy diagnostic delay include older age, the level of paediatric training of the first responder, the presence of non-specific symptoms, the histology of the tumour and its location. Parental profession, whether urban or rural resident and distance from a paediatric oncology centre did not alter the time to diagnosis.

Long delays in diagnosis may be expected in low-grade astrocytoma and localised Ewing's sarcoma. Conversely, fast-growing tumours such as nephroblastoma, leukaemia and non-Hodgkin's lymphoma will be diagnosed quicker. Therefore, the time to diagnosis depends in large part on the tumour's biology.

Contrary to the popular view, expert opinions in malpractice claims assert that no adverse association exists between delayed diagnosis and prognosis for most CNS tumours, osteosarcoma and Ewing's sarcoma. On the other hand, initial invasion, survival and the risk of blindness are increased if the diagnosis of retinoblastoma is delayed (Box 7.1).[3]

There is no doubt that *delays in diagnosis matter to families,* as early referral does significantly reduce the suffering they experience. Data from abdominal malignancies from the UK and Europe suggests that they tend to present to hospital later in the UK with a consequent need for a more prolonged and intensive treatment process and less favourable clinical outcomes. The NICE *Suspected Cancer* guidelines[4] are used extensively in adults with suspected cancer but rarely for children and young people. The key measure of success is the total diagnostic interval (TDI).

BOX 7.1 CLINICAL HISTORY

An 18 Month Old With a White Pupil

An 18 month old presented to his family doctor with an apparent 'white' pupil. This was first noted when a digital photograph was taken showing a normal red reflex of the right eye and absence of this reflex on the opposite side. The infant was feeding well and had normal developmental milestones. Apart from left eye leucocoria, his examination was normal. He was promptly referred to a specialist ophthalmology service.

Clinical Pearls

Retinoblastoma is rare (1 per 15,000 to 20,000 live births) but is the most frequently seen intraocular tumour of childhood (Fig. 7.4). It is due to a mutation of the *RB1* gene. Leucocoria is the most frequently noticed first clinical sign of retinoblastoma. Retinoblastoma remains intraocular and curable for about 3 to 6 months after the first signs of leucocoria appear.[5] Differentials for leucocoria include retinopathy of prematurity, ocular toxocariasis and cataract. Delayed diagnosis enables retinoblastoma to spread from the eye and thereby reduces survival. Flash photography can enable the earlier detection of leucocoria (as in this instance). All bilateral retinoblastoma cases are inherited.

Pitfalls to Avoid

Retinoblastoma is certainly a cancer where early diagnosis significantly improves prognosis, as once the tumour spreads outside of the eye, survival rates fall.

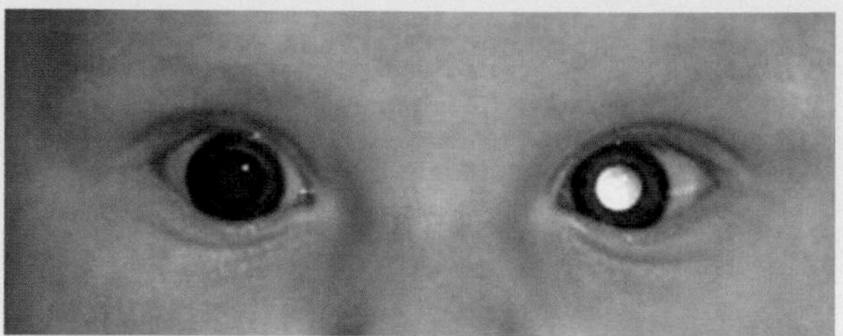

Fig. 7.4 Leucocoria and mild esotropia in the left eye of a 4-month-old boy with bilateral retinoblastoma (Group A in the right eye and Group D in the left eye). (Source: Christopher J. Lyons, Scott R. Lambert. *Taylor and Hoyt's Pediatric Ophthalmology and Strabismus*. 6th edition, 2023, Elsevier Ltd.)

Extraocular spread is rarely seen in developed countries due to the earlier diagnosis, but sadly, it is quite common in low- and middle-income countries as a result in delayed presentation/detection.

Retinoblastoma is best managed by a multidisciplinary team. Multicentre clinical trials are currently looking at treatment options – recently more conservative treatment modalities including intraarterial chemotherapy, cryotherapy, laser therapy and intravitreal chemotherapy are proving effective while sparing the eye.

SYMPTOMS ASSOCIATED WITH COMMON CANCERS

Acute Lymphoblastic Leukaemia

Acute leukaemia is the most common form of childhood cancer. In the UK, about 1 in 2000 children develop leukaemia, and most family doctors will see a case of childhood leukaemia just once or twice in their careers.

There are **two** key presenting features in acute leukaemia:

- Bone marrow failure – leading to anaemia, neutropenia and thrombocytopenia
- Tissue infiltration – leading to bone pain, lymphadenopathy (Fig. 7.5) and hepatosplenomegaly (Box 7.2)

About 80% of childhood leukaemia is acute lymphoblastic (ALL) with the remainder being acute myeloid (AML). There are a number of differential diagnoses for leukaemia to be considered not least infections (in particular Ebstein-Barr virus (EBV) or parvovirus), aplastic anaemia, idiopathic thrombocytopenic purpura and juvenile idiopathic arthritis.

Standardised treatment protocols have been agreed internationally and have led to an overall excellent prognosis. Adverse prognostic factors include those aged over 10 or with a white cell count over 50. Chemotherapy is the mainstay of treatment. Rarely bone marrow transplantation is required for children who do not enter remission or who later relapse.

Brain Tumours

Despite the fact that 70% of children and adolescents now survive a brain tumour, it is still the leading cause of death due to cancer in childhood. The diagnosis of a brain tumour poses unique challenges. Low-grade gliomas tend to be associated with prolonged symptoms and consequent delayed diagnosis, whereas high-grade gliomas tend to have a rapid onset of symptoms. Tumours located in the cerebellum (such as medulloblastoma

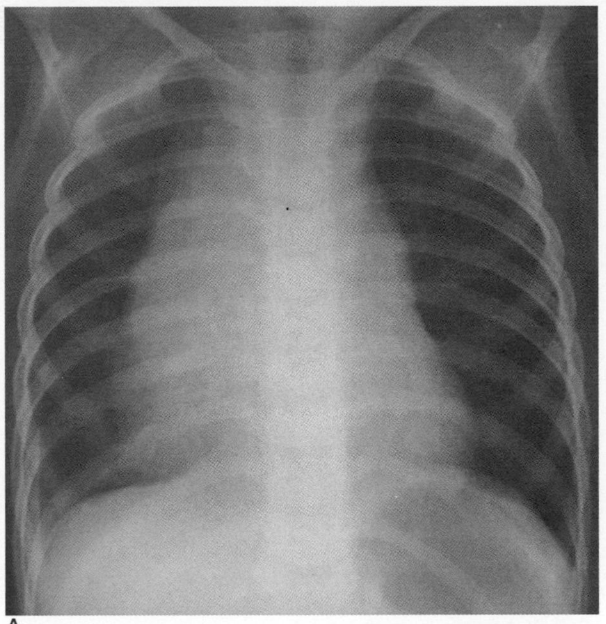

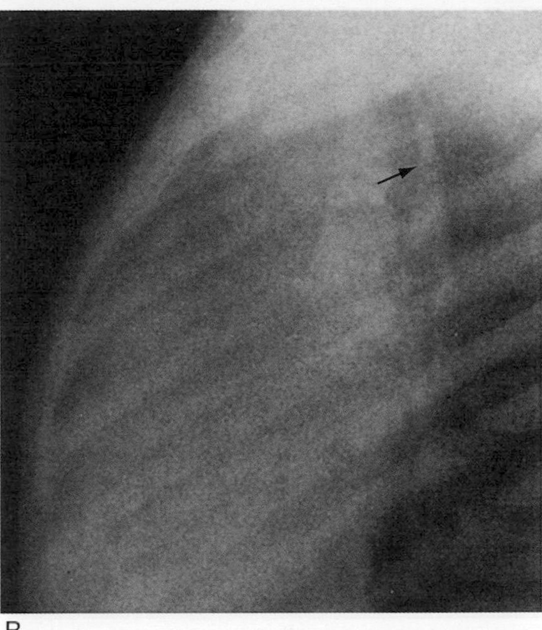

Fig. 7.5 Anterior mediastinal mass. Chest radiograph (A) PA and (B) lateral. Large anterior mediastinal mass displacing the trachea posteriorly (*arrow*) due to T-cell acute lymphoblastic leukaemia. Similar appearances may be seen with lymphoma. (Source: *Grainger & Allison's Diagnostic Radiology: A Textbook of Medical Imaging*. 5th ed. 2008.)

BOX 7.2 CLINICAL HISTORY

Just Another Child With Dietary Iron Deficiency Anaemia

A 4-year-old girl is referred by her family doctor to the paediatric outpatients with a history of pallor, angular cheilitis and reduced energy noted over a period of 6 weeks. Her energy levels were low and her exercise tolerance had significantly reduced. Her diet was poor in that she consumed up to 1 litre of cow's milk per day, and the working diagnosis was of dietary iron deficiency anaemia. She had no bruising but did have a low-grade pyrexia for a number of days. Her examination revealed a very pale girl with shotty cervical nodes and significant hepatosplenomegaly. She had an urgent full blood count performed which showed a low white cell count of 1.8 with neutropenia and a haemoglobin of 7.4 g %. The blood film was reviewed by a haematologist and blast cells were seen. She went on to have a bone marrow biopsy, and a diagnosis of ALL was made. She was transferred to a paediatric oncology service.

Clinical Pearls

Common presenting features of acute leukaemia include pallor, petechiae and unexplained bruising, tiredness, lethargy and bone pain or a limp, lymphadenopathy, hepatosplenomegaly or enlarged testes.

Definitive diagnosis is via the detection of leukaemic blast cells on either blood film or bone marrow aspirate. Bone marrow aspirate or biopsy is the definitive test, and one looks for morphology (presence of blast cells), immunophenotyping and cytogenetic analysis. The majority of children with ALL will have precursor B cell type with just 15% having the T cell phenotype.

Pitfalls to Avoid

The presenting features of acute leukaemia may be nonspecific and mimic self-limiting childhood illnesses. The act of balancing parental anxiety around self-limiting illnesses versus the detection of serious illness within this group can be extremely challenging.

Listening to the parental instinct, taking note of the number of presentations to healthcare and focusing on examination can aid in defining the difference.

If in doubt, take a full blood count.

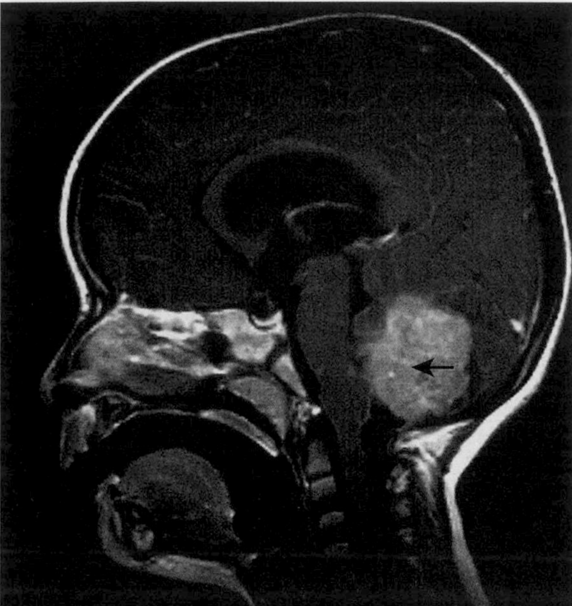

Fig. 7.6 Sagittal magnetic resonance image of a medulloblastoma. The tumour (arrow) can be seen filling the fourth ventricle between the pons anteriorly and the cerebellum posteriorly. There is associated obstructive hydrocephalus due to blockage of cerebrospinal fluid flow through the fourth ventricle. (Source: *Principles and Practice of Surgery*. 8th ed. 2023.)

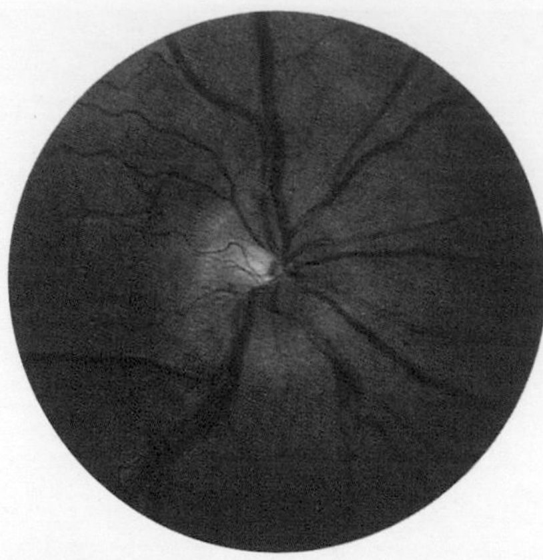

Fig. 7.7 Papilloedema: optic disc swelling caused by raised intracranial pressure. (Source: Glynn, M., Drake, W.M. (eds). *Hutchison's Clinical Methods: An Integrated Approach to Clinical Practice*. 25th edn. Elsevier; 2023.)

[Fig. 7.6]) and brain stem, tend to have a shorter duration of symptoms as opposed to supratentorial tumours which may present with seizures, papilloedema (Fig. 7.7) and other features of raised intracranial pressure. Symptoms at presentation relate primarily to the location of the tumour. Craniopharyngioma, low-grade optic nerve glioma and germ cell tumours often have a delayed presentation.

Posterior fossa tumours, such as cerebellar astrocytoma, medulloblastoma and ependymoma, may present with hydrocephalus due to outlet obstruction of the fourth ventricle.

Preschool children with a brain tumour may present with persistent or recurrent vomiting, abnormal eye movements, significant behavioural change with lethargy in particular, problems with balance and walking, seizures, head tilt or a progressively increasing head circumference. In school-going children and adolescents, a crescendo pattern of headaches is a key symptom that should prompt a request for neuroimaging (Box 7.3). In the adolescent, delayed or arrested puberty, in addition to precocious puberty may also indicate the presence of a brain tumour and must prompt investigation.

BOX 7.3 CLINICAL HISTORY

Always Beware the Second Diagnosis

A 10-year-old girl presents with a 12-month history of headaches occurring once every 4 weeks. She experiences bifrontal headaches which may last a few hours and are felt to represent tension headaches. Paracetamol is helpful in alleviating the headaches. The headaches were not associated with nausea or vomiting. Clinical examination is normal.

Her parents have become more concerned, as over the past 8 weeks the headaches have changed considerably. They are worse immediately after wakening but improve as the day progresses. She feels nauseous in the mornings and has vomited the last four mornings. Coughing makes the pain worse. Her parents report that she is more irritable, and her teacher has noted her school performance has worsened significantly. She also appears to be somewhat unsteady on her feet.

Clinical Pearls

Tension headaches and migraine are by far the commonest reasons for frequent headaches in childhood and adolescence. By contrast brain tumours are rare but, as in this instance, both can coexist. Tension headaches was the correct initial diagnosis in this case, but the pattern of headaches did change quite dramatically, and this should always prompt a re-think for an alternative diagnosis.

The headache description, frequency and pattern are key, and one should ask the family to keep a headache diary and review this diary and re-examine the child after 6 to 8 weeks.

Pitfalls to Avoid

Looking for this *crescendo pattern* of headaches with an ever-increasing frequency and severity of headaches should prompt consideration of raised intracranial pressure and the urgent requirement for neuroimaging.

Children between 5 and 12 years old may also present with recurrent vomiting, abnormal eye movements, blurred vision or diplopia, behavioural change or seizures.[6]

HeadSmart UK[7] have developed some visual prompts to support awareness of symptoms in various age ranges, including babies, children and teens. Presenting symptoms differ within these groups, and it is important that the general practitioner is aware of this spectrum of presentation (Fig. 7.8).

If a brain tumour is suspected, neuroimaging (either an MRI or CT scan) should be promptly coordinated.

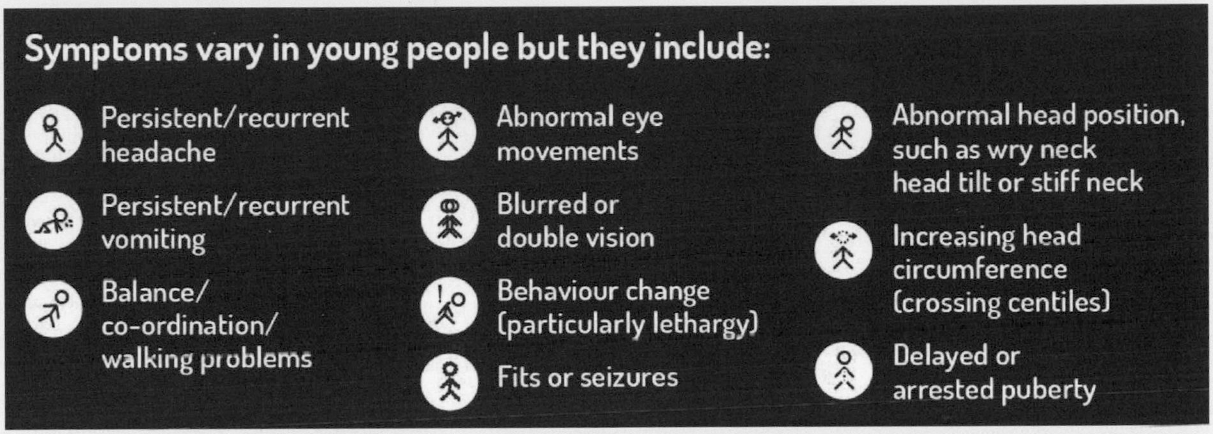

Fig. 7.8 Symptoms of brain tumour in young people. (Source: Reproduced with permission from HeadSmart. HeadSmart is funded and promoted by The Brain Tumour Charity and run in partnership with the Children's Brain Tumour Research Centre (CBTRC) and the Royal College of Paediatrics and Child Health (RCPCH). The Brain Tumour Charity Registered Charity No. 1150054 (England and Wales) SC045081 (Scotland), CBTRC Charitable Status Inland Revenue No. X15294, RCPCH Registered Charity No. 1057744 (England and Wales) SC038299 (Scotland).)

Neuroblastoma

Neuroblastoma affects primarily children under 8 years of age, and over 50% to 75% of cases are in children under 2 years of age. Neuroblastoma arises in primitive cells of the sympathetic nervous system, with the majority of primary tumours (75%) being abdominal mainly originating in the adrenal medulla or lumbar sympathetic ganglia. Neuroblastoma is a very challenging diagnosis to make, as the presenting signs and symptoms often masquerade as other entities, hence a high index of suspicion is required. Generally the symptoms include abdominal pain, vomiting, loss of appetite with weight loss, fatigue, bone pain and unexplained fevers (Box 7.4).

Nephroblastoma

Nephroblastoma is the commonest cause of a large abdominal mass picked up incidentally in a child (Box 7.5). Clues on examination of the abdomen are the size, location and consistency of the mass, whether the mass extends across the midline or into the pelvis and whether there are systemic signs (tachycardia, hypertension or tachypnoea) or signs of cachexia. An abdominal ultrasound is the most appropriate initial imaging to be requested.

BOX 7.4 CLINICAL HISTORY

Repeated Attendances to the Practice

A 2-year-old boy presented to his family doctor on four occasions over a six-month period with vague symptoms of abdominal cramps and bloating, marked irritability, excess sweating and weight loss. Prior to this period of time, he had been a cheery and energetic toddler who was very active. He was noted by his mother to be lacking in energy and to be constantly in some discomfort with frequent loose bowel motions. Finally she brought him to the emergency department and he was assessed by the team on duty.

His examination showed him to be quite pale, underweight and he had some degree of abdominal distension without organomegaly. He was admitted in view of his sick appearance and his mother's concerns.

He had a full work up and his abdominal ultrasound showed a large left adrenal mass. His MRI confirmed this mass, and his spot urinary catecholamines were markedly elevated. Thus a diagnosis of neuroblastoma was made, and he went on to have cross-sectional imaging, together with a metaiodobenzylguanidine (MIBG) scan and a bone marrow aspirate and biopsy to detect metastatic disease (Fig. 7.9).

Clinical Pearls

Time and time again it is proven that parental instincts are invariably correct. Neuroblastoma accounts for just over 5% of all childhood cancers and can be challenging in terms of diagnosis. Some cases regress spontaneously (especially in neonates) and others progress inexorably despite therapy.

The most common site of neuroblastoma is the abdomen, hence presentation with progressive abdominal distension or abdominal discomfort, including loss of appetite and weight, is common. Presenting signs and symptoms may include bone pain, limp, pallor, bruising (including periorbital ecchymoses known as raccoon eyes) (Fig. 7.10), proptosis and skin lesions. Catecholamine production by the tumour may result in vague symptoms such as flushing, sweating and irritability.[7]

Vasoactive intestinal polypeptide may cause secretory diarrhoea. Rarely, opsoclonus myoclonus or 'dancing eye syndrome' may be a further neurological presentation.

Surgical resection is the primary treatment for localised neuroblastoma. Two exceptions to this rule are neonates with stage 4S disease (primary lesion with cutaneous, hepatic and or bone marrow metastases) and infants under 6 months of age with stage 1 small adrenal tumours. In these cases, careful observation may be employed with intervention for those with disease progression. Adjuvant chemotherapy, radiotherapy and immunotherapy may complete treatment relative to the stage and biological characteristics of the disease.[8]

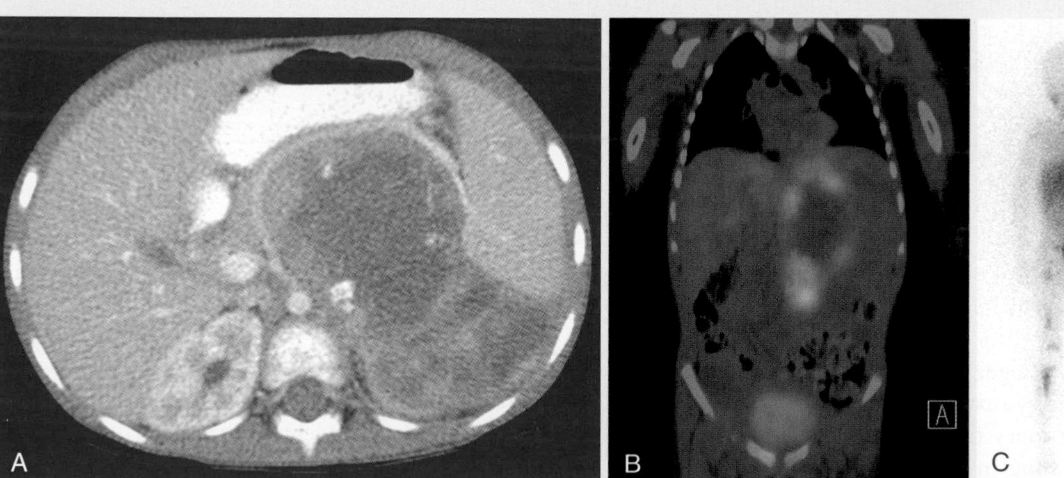

Fig. 7.9 (A) CT scan of an abdominal neuroblastoma with central necrosis at diagnosis. (B) Coronal fused CT and metaiodobenzylguanidine (MIBG) image of the same child with extensive retroperitoneal mass and central necrosis, probably an adrenal primary with extensive lymph node involvement. (C) MIBG avid neuroblastoma with increased uptake of radiolabelled tracer can be detected in multiple sites of disease, including bone and soft tissue. (Source: *Nelson Textbook of Pediatrics*. Copyright © 2020 Elsevier Inc.)

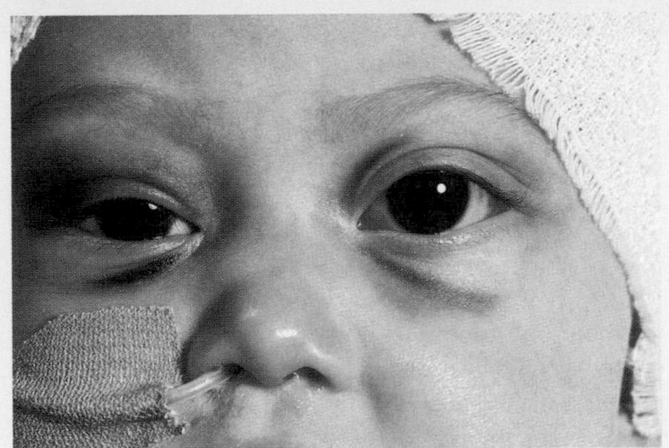

Fig. 7.10 Periorbital ecchymoses in a patient with orbital neuroblastoma. (Source: Christopher J. Lyons, Scott R. Lambert. *Taylor and Hoyt's Pediatric Ophthalmology and Strabismus.* 6th edition, 2023, Elsevier Ltd.)

Infants and children with localised stage 1 and 2 disease and favourable biology have survival rates over 90%. Overall outcomes are determined by the child's age, tumour stage and biology.

Pitfalls to Avoid

Symptoms are often relatively nonspecific and may include irritability, pain, limp, diarrhoea, poor weight gain or weight loss and excessive flushing or sweating. Always consider neuroblastoma in a younger child who looks very unwell and has other symptoms as listed above.

In 90% of cases, catecholamines and their detectable metabolites namely homovanillic acid (HMA) and vanillylmandelic acid (VMA) are found in spot urine samples, so a spot urine for HMA and VMA is a very useful test if the diagnosis is being considered.

BOX 7.5 CLINICAL HISTORY

A 4 Year Old With an Abdominal Mass

A previously well 4 year old is found to have a mass noted by his parents following a bedtime bath. He is not unwell and has no relevant past or perinatal history. His very concerned parents made an urgent appointment to see their family doctor, and the child is brought early the following morning. The family doctor is not certain that she can feel a mass but, in view of the parent's concern, refers the child into hospital for review.

Clinical Pearls

Nephroblastoma (Wilms tumour) tends to present with a painless and enlarging abdominal mass that does not cross the midline (Fig. 7.11). About 25% of children with Wilms tumour have hypertension and less than 10% have frank haematuria.

Extremely preterm infants, children with Beckwith-Wiedeman syndrome and those with familial polyposis have heightened risk of developing hepatoblastoma where an elevated alpha-fetoprotein is a recognised tumour marker.

In older children (usually over 10 years of age) non-Hodgkins lymphoma may present with abdominal distension, constipation and ascites. Ovarian tumours in girls are seen in over 5 year olds and may present with a palpable abdominal mass and perhaps pain if there is ovarian torsion.

Pitfalls to Avoid

Incidental finding of an abdominal mass in a young child at bath time is most likely due to Wilms tumour. Other presentations include a swollen abdomen, macroscopic or microscopic haematuria, an alteration in bowel habit or intermittent fevers. For older girls consider ovarian tumours and adolescents, non-Hodgkins lymphoma.

Prompt referral is required with ultrasound being the imaging modality of choice.

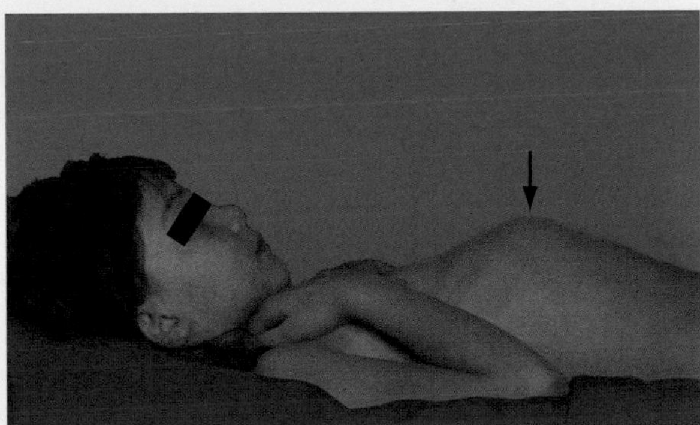

Fig. 7.11 Nephroblastoma. This 9-year-old girl presented with a large unilateral mass (*arrowed*), which was later confirmed to be arising from the left kidney (Wilms tumour or nephroblastoma). (Source: Quick CRG, Biers SM, Arulampalam, THA, eds. *Essential Surgery: Problems, Diagnosis and Management.* 6th ed. Elsevier.)

KEY LEARNING POINTS

Reducing the TDI (time from first symptoms to diagnosis) as noted above can impact the outcome for the child and family with ideally the avoidance of life-threatening presentations such as bone marrow failure, tumour lysis syndrome, raised intracranial pressure or spinal cord compression. Earlier detection and therefore the lowering of the staging distribution at presentation, will no doubt see the rates of lifelong disability fall.

'Three strikes and you are in' is a useful mantra for family doctors to consider.[1] Ask the caregiver how many times they have presented to healthcare with this issue.

Be aware of parental instincts, as so often they are proven to be correct.

Always examine the child carefully, symptoms may overlap with other childhood illnesses, but the examination may assist in clarifying the diagnosis. If you have concerns, but not enough to refer, prebook or encourage a follow-up appointment.

Safety net, with clear advice on where, when and why to return. As a family doctor, if concerned, it is best to contact your local paediatric service and talk to one of the paediatricians to see what the next best steps are.

REFERENCES

1. Walker DA. Helping GPs to diagnose children's cancer. *Br J Gen Pract*. 2021;71(705):151–152. doi:10.3399/bjgp21X715241. Published 2021 Mar 26.
2. *Childhood cancers — recognition and referral: symptoms suggestive of childhood cancers*. London: NICE; 2020. Available at https://cks.nice.org.uk/topics/childhood-cancers-recognition-referral/.
3. Brasme JF, Morfouace M, Grill J, et al. Delays in diagnosis of paediatric cancers: a systematic review and comparison with expert testimony in lawsuits. *Lancet Oncol*. 2012;13(10):e445–e459. doi:10.1016/S1470-2045(12)70361-3.
4. Suspected cancer: recognition and referral. NICE Guideline, 2015. Available at https://www.nice.org.uk/guidance/ng12/evidence/full-guideline-pdf-2676000277.
5. Weaver MS, Heminger CL, Lam CG. Integrating stages of change models to cast new vision on interventions to improve global retinoblastoma and childhood cancer outcomes. *BMC Public Health*. 2014;14:944. doi:10.1186/1471-2458-14-944. Published 2014 Sep 11.
6. Wilne SH, Dineen RA, Dommett RM, Chu TP, Walker DA. Identifying brain tumours in children and young adults. *BMJ*. 2013;347:f5844. doi:10.1136/bmj.f5844. Published 2013 Oct 9.
7. Headsmart website. Accessed at www.headsmart.org.uk.
8. Densmore JC, Densmore EM. Abdominal Masses. In: Kleigman RM, Lye PS, Bordini B, Toth H, Basel D, eds. *Nelson Pediatric Symptom-Based Diagnosis*. Philadelphia: Elsevier; 2018:283–301.

ADDITIONAL READING

Coleman MP, Forman D, Bryant H, et al. Cancer survival in Australia, Canada, Denmark, Norway, Sweden, and the UK, 1995-2007 (the International Cancer Benchmarking Partnership): an analysis of population-based cancer registry data. *Lancet*. 2011;377(9760):127–138. doi:10.1016/S0140-6736(10)62231-3.

Dimaras H, Kimani K, Dimba EA, et al. Retinoblastoma. *Lancet*. 2012;379(9824):1436–1446. doi:10.1016/S0140-6736(11)61137-9.

Dommet R, Redaniel T, Stevens M, Martin R, Hamilton W. Risk of childhood cancer with symptoms in primary care: A population-based case-control study. *British Journal of General Practice*. 2013;63(606):e22–e29. doi:10.3399/bjgp13X660742.

Dommett RM, Redaniel T, Stevens MCG, et al. Risk of childhood cancer with symptoms in primary care: a population-based case-control study. *Br J Gen Pract*. 2013. doi:10.3399/bjgp13X660742.

Grace Kelly Childhood Cancer Trust. Accessed at https://www.gkcct.org/

Leslie SW, Sajjad H, Murphy PB. Wilms Tumor. In: *StatPearls*. Treasure Island (FL): StatPearls Publishing; September 17, 2021.

National Cancer Registration and Analysis Service. Retrieved from http://www.ncin.org.uk/publications/routes_to_diagnosis.

Price SJ. Advances in imaging low-grade gliomas. *Adv Tech Stand Neurosurg*. 2010;35:1–34. doi:10.1007/978-3-211-99481-8_1.

Ripperger T, Bielack SS, Borkhardt A, et al. Childhood cancer predisposition syndromes – A concise review and recommendations by the Cancer Predisposition Working

Group of the Society for Pediatric Oncology and Hematology. *Am J Med Genet A*. 2017;173(4):1017–1037. doi:10.1002/ajmg.a.38142.

Scotting PJ, Walker DA, Perilongo G. Childhood solid tumours: a developmental disorder. *Nat Rev Cancer*. 2005;5(6):481–488. doi:10.1038/nrc1633.

Shanmugavadivel D, Liu JF, Murphy L, Wilne S, Walker D; HeadSmart. Accelerating diagnosis for childhood brain tumours: an analysis of the HeadSmart UK population data. *Arch Dis Child*. 2020;105(4):355–362. doi:10.1136/archdischild-2018-315962.

Smith CF, Drew S, Ziebland S, Nicholson BD. Understanding the role of GPs' gut feelings in diagnosing cancer in primary care: a systematic review and meta-analysis of existing evidence. *Br J Gen Pract*. 2020. doi:10.3399/bjgp20X712301.

Thorbinson C, Calton E, Brennan B. An approach to oncological abdominal masses in children. *Paediatrics and Child Health*. 2021;31(7):295–299. Available at https://www.sciencegate.app/app/redirect#aHR0cHM6Ly9keC5kb2kub3JnLzEwLjEwMTYvai5wYWVkLjIwMjEuMDQuMDA2.

Uzunova L, Bailie H, Murray MJ. Fifteen-minute consultation: A general paediatrician's guide to oncological abdominal masses. *Arch Dis Child Educ Pract Ed*. 2019;104(3):129–134. doi:10.1136/archdischild-2018-315270.

8

The Child With a Limp

Carol Blackburn

CHAPTER OUTLINE

Limping in children is relatively common and is most often due to trauma resulting in either a fracture or a soft tissue injury in the older child. There is usually a clear history of trauma and a clear temporal relationship between the injury and the symptom of limping in the child.

Limping is often quite straightforward, but there are some serious underlying potential causes of limp that a primary care doctor or trainee in the emergency department needs to consider. The correct differential diagnosis is important, as some conditions are time-critical and therefore important to detect and replace in a timely manner. The conditions that are especially important to diagnose include septic arthritis, osteomyelitis, slipped capital femoral epiphysis (SCFE) and occasionally malignancies arising from bone.

APPROACHING THE CHILD WITH A LIMP

> The approach to a child with a painful limp is relatively straightforward and is based around the maxim that the child should continue to be kept under review until the symptoms resolve or a clear diagnosis is evident.

For a painless limp, an expectant approach prior to referral is reasonable whereas for a painful limp, prompt referral to the emergency department is advisable.

The history, as always, is key. Age is important, as certain conditions are age-related. Common differentials in toddlers include transient synovitis or a toddler's fracture. In older children transient synovitis can also occur, but reactive arthritis and juvenile idiopathic arthritis (JIA) are also important differentials. In adolescence (especially if obese) the key differential is SCFE.

A clear description of the pain experienced is required including whether or not pain is present daily. Seek a detailed description of the pain in terms of its site, duration, frequency and precipitating or relieving factors. Stiffness (over 15 minutes) especially in the morning is noteworthy, as significant stiffness may point to an inflammatory cause. Pain related to activity and improved by rest is more likely to relate to overuse injury or joint hypermobility.

Enquire whether there are any systemic symptoms such as fever (try to establish if a pattern is evident), fatigue, poor appetite or weight loss.

If the onset of joint pain is sudden and severe, consider septic arthritis, osteomyelitis or trauma.

Limping, especially in the mornings, and difficulty in running and jumping may indicate trauma or an arthritis affecting joints of the lower limbs. Young children with transient synovitis may have an early morning limp which is improved by the time they attend the emergency department.

The examination should focus on whether or not the child looks unwell, measuring the temperature and conducting a full examination with a focus on assessing the child's gait. Be aware that hip pain may be referred to the knee and examine the hips of children presenting with atraumatic knee pain. Check both the active and passive movement of the affected joint.

Dealing With Uncertainty

> It is reasonable to manage children with a history of an atraumatic limp of less than 72 hours duration and no 'red flag' features in an expectant way.

It is essential to provide safety netting advice and arrange a follow-up.[1] Ensure there are no 'red flags' such as a fever above 38.5°C, inability to weight bear or a markedly reduced range of movement. Those with significant symptoms and signs require onward referral and further investigations in hospital.

In an under 10 year old with a limp, apart from minor trauma, the most common diagnosis is transient synovitis of the hip. With transient synovitis there will often be a history of a recent or concurrent viral illness.

In most cases a self-limiting cause for the limp will be identified, but a small number are due to conditions such as septic arthritis or SCFE which require prompt recognition and treatment. The key is a careful assessment to identify the small number that require further investigation.

The great majority will have minor injuries. Also be aware that a significant number of young children have joint hypermobility and are more likely to have joint pains intermittently. These pains are typically at night and may follow a busy day of significant activity.

Joint Hypermobility Syndrome

> Joint hypermobility is very common (occurs in 10%–20% of children) and is a quite frequent cause of noninflammatory joint pain in children.

Joint hypermobility syndrome is a frequent cause of pain associated with sporting activities and always improves with rest (Fig. 8.1).

Common clues suggesting the possibility of joint hypermobility, as per the Beighton score,[2] include a prior history of developmental dysplasia of the hip, a history of delayed walking with bottom shuffling, recurrent ankle sprains, tiring easily when compared to peers, joint dislocations, poor catching and handwriting skills and so-called 'growing pains' with leg pains associated with nocturnal awakening.

Transient Synovitis

Transient synovitis generally affects the hip, occurs most commonly in the 4- to 8-year-old age group and is seen more often in boys. Typical features are hip pain and mild restriction of hip movement, in particular, hip abduction and internal rotation. Hip ultrasound will confirm the presence of hip effusion (see Chapter 18 interpreting commonly requested radiological investigations). Laboratory tests and X-rays are generally normal. If the history supports a diagnosis of transient synovitis, the authors recommend analgesia and gentle mobilisation with recourse to investigations (X-ray and bloods) only if the symptoms do not resolve within 14 days.

In some paediatric emergency departments, point-of-care ultrasound is used to confirm the presence of a hip effusion, otherwise formal radiological ultrasound

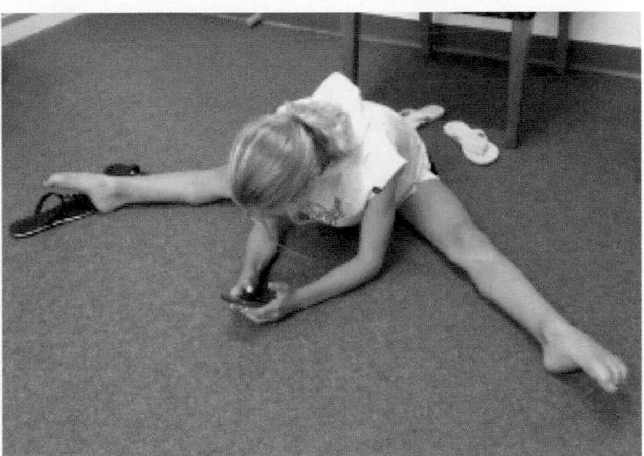

Fig. 8.1 Casual posturing seen with joint hypermobility. (Source: J. Gordon Burrow, Keith Rome, Nat Padhiar. *Neale's Disorders of the Foot and Ankle.* 9th edition, 2020, Elsevier Ltd.)

may also be used to confirm the diagnosis if there is uncertainty.

> If transient synovitis is suspected but fails to resolve within 2 weeks, then plain film imaging of the hips looking for Perthes disease should be requested.

Perthes Disease

Perthes disease typically affects boys aged 4 to 8 years. In Perthes, avascular necrosis of the femoral head is typically seen. Generally, it is a self-limiting condition, and revascularisation occurs over a 3-year period, but a late diagnosis or Perthes occurring over age 8 carries a poorer prognosis with surgery sometimes required.

A non-resolving apparent transient synovitis (2 weeks on) requires further investigation for Perthes disease initially via plain film imaging of both hips (condition can also be bilateral), then either by MRI (the preferred modality) or technetium bone scan in conjunction with referral for specialist orthopaedic follow-up. A typical evolution of radiological changes may be noted on serial X-ray from initial sclerosis to fragmentation with later flattening of the femoral epiphysis (Fig. 8.2). The treatment of Perthes aims to contain the femoral head within the acetabulum and may be surgical or nonsurgical. In general, Perthes has an excellent long-term prognosis.[1]

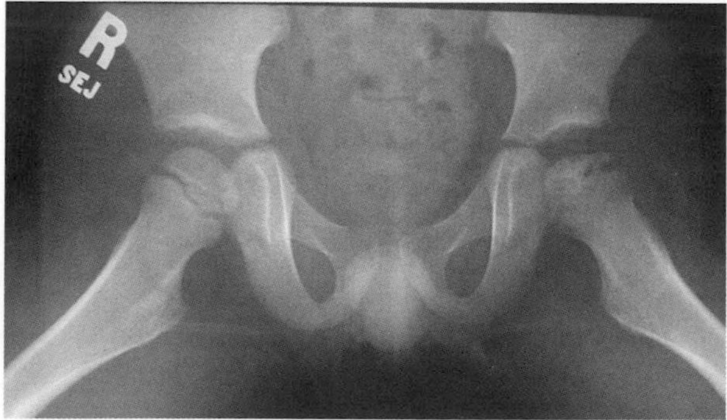

Fig. 8.2 Legg-Calvé-Perthes disease of the left hip. (Source: From Cummings NH, Stanley-Green S, Higgs P. *Perspectives in Athletic Training*. Mosby; 2009.)

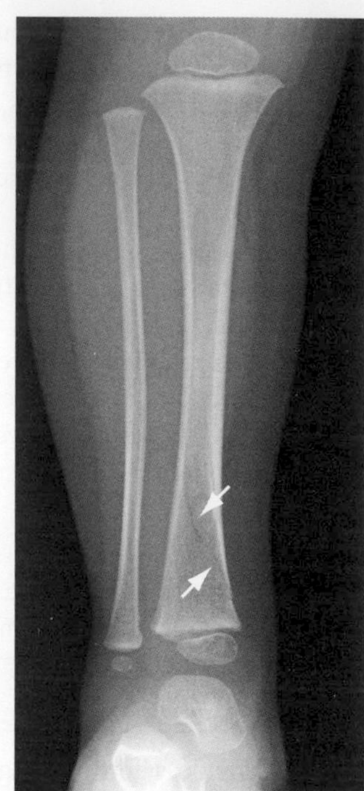

Fig. 8.3 Toddler's fracture. AP radiograph shows an oblique fracture of the distal tibia (*arrows*). These nondisplaced fractures of the lower extremities of toddlers are always subtle and are often only detected on follow-up radiographs by the development of tell-tale periosteal reaction. Most toddler's fractures occur in the tibia. (Source: May DA, et al. *Musculoskeletal Imaging*. 5th edition, 2022, Elsevier Inc.)

Toddler's Fracture

A toddler's fracture is an undisplaced spiral fracture of the tibia.[3] These occur typically between the ages of 9 months and 4 years with a peak incidence around 20 months. Tenderness over the tibial shaft is generally absent. Diagnosis is by X-ray (Fig. 8.3) or, in some instances, bone scan. The history may be vague and there may be a history of seemingly innocuous trauma such as tripping while walking, catching a leg while going down a slide or falling from a low height such as a couch. Toddler's fractures are commonly referred for orthopaedic trauma clinic follow-up.

Reactive Arthritis

Reactive arthritis is a sterile synovitis associated with infection elsewhere in the body and is the commonest cause of acute arthritis in childhood. Reactive arthritis most often follows a viral upper respiratory tract infection. *Shigella*, *Salmonella*, *Campylobacter* and *Yersinia enterocolitica* infections can all be associated with reactive arthritis. Many viruses are also implicated as causes of reactive arthritis not least rubella (typically affects small joints of the hand), herpes simplex, cytomegalovirus, varicella (usually pauci-articular) and mumps (large joint arthritis).

IMPORTANT CONDITIONS TO ALWAYS CONSIDER

Septic Arthritis and Osteomyelitis

> Septic arthritis and osteomyelitis should always be considered in any child with a painful limp and a history of fever.[1]

The typical presentation of septic arthritis is with fever, a limp and refusal to weight bear. In infancy, septic arthritis may present as reduced movement of the affected limb. Septic arthritis is most frequently seen in infants, toddlers and preschool children. The most affected joints are the hip, knee and ankle. *Staphylococcus aureus* is the commonest causative organism, but *Kingella kingae* is increasingly recognised in younger children under 3 years old. High fever is typical of septic arthritis due to methicillin-resistant *Staphylococcus aureus* (MRSA), and *Kingella kingae* infection is associated with mild fever. Diagnosis is confirmed by joint fluid aspiration prior to commencement of intravenous antibiotics (Fig. 8.4).

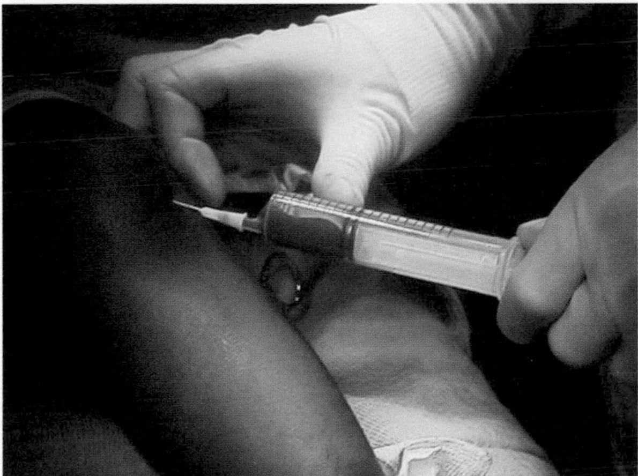

Fig. 8.4 Aspiration of blood-stained pus from the knee of a child with septic arthritis. (Source: *Textbook of Orthopaedics, Trauma and Rheumatology*. 2nd ed.)

Prompt referral to an orthopaedic team for joint aspiration, a surgical washout and intravenous antibiotics is important and necessary to avoid joint destruction. Local infectious diseases or antimicrobial guidance should be sought.[4] Children with a delay in diagnosis or MRSA infection have a worse prognosis, as delay in diagnosis and treatment can lead to damage to the growth plate or avascular necrosis.

The stakes are therefore very high and early diagnosis is essential. In any child with a fever who is refusing to weight bear, septic arthritis must be considered, and the child should be referred for prompt investigation (Box 8.1). In the emergency department setting septic arthritis is an example of an occasion where Erythrocyte Sedimentation Rate (ESR) is of diagnostic relevance. Using Kocher's criteria, if a child has a

BOX 8.1 CLINICAL HISTORY

A 3 Year Old With a Painful Hip

A 3-year-old active boy had a minor fall while out playing and 24 hours later was noticed to have a limp and complained of pain. He had an associated fever but no other symptoms of note. Over the next 10 days he was seen by his family doctor on three occasions and was then referred to the emergency department for further assessment. On arrival he looked unwell, was feverish and his left hip was held in flexion and external rotation. An orthopaedic opinion was sought and a joint aspiration performed. His joint aspirate grew *Kingella kingae,* and he was commenced on intravenous antibiotics. Six months after admission his left hip X-ray still showed striking changes, and he had some residual limping.

Clinical Pearls

In a febrile child with a limp, septic arthritis is the diagnosis not to miss.

Septic arthritis presents with fever, painful limp and refusal to weight bear.

Pitfalls to Avoid

Delayed diagnosis and treatment can lead to damage to the growth plate or avascular necrosis.

Antibiotic choices may vary, but cefazolin is recommended for under 5-year-olds and cefazolin or flucloxacillin for children over 5 years of age. Always refer to local antimicrobial guidance.

temperature above 38.5°C, is unable to weight bear and has an ESR above 40 mm/hr and a white cell count above 12 × 10^9/L, evidence from some studies suggests this conveys a 99% likelihood of septic arthritis.[4] More recently CRP has been evaluated as part of the decision tool, and a CRP >20 mg/L may be applied in place of ESR.

Slipped Capital Femoral Epiphysis

SCFE is a frequently seen hip disorder in adolescence (Fig. 8.5). While classically described in adolescents who are overweight, it can also occur in active adolescents with normal BMI who have had a recent growth spurt. Therefore, maintaining an index of suspicion for SCFE in adolescents with new limp is important, as late

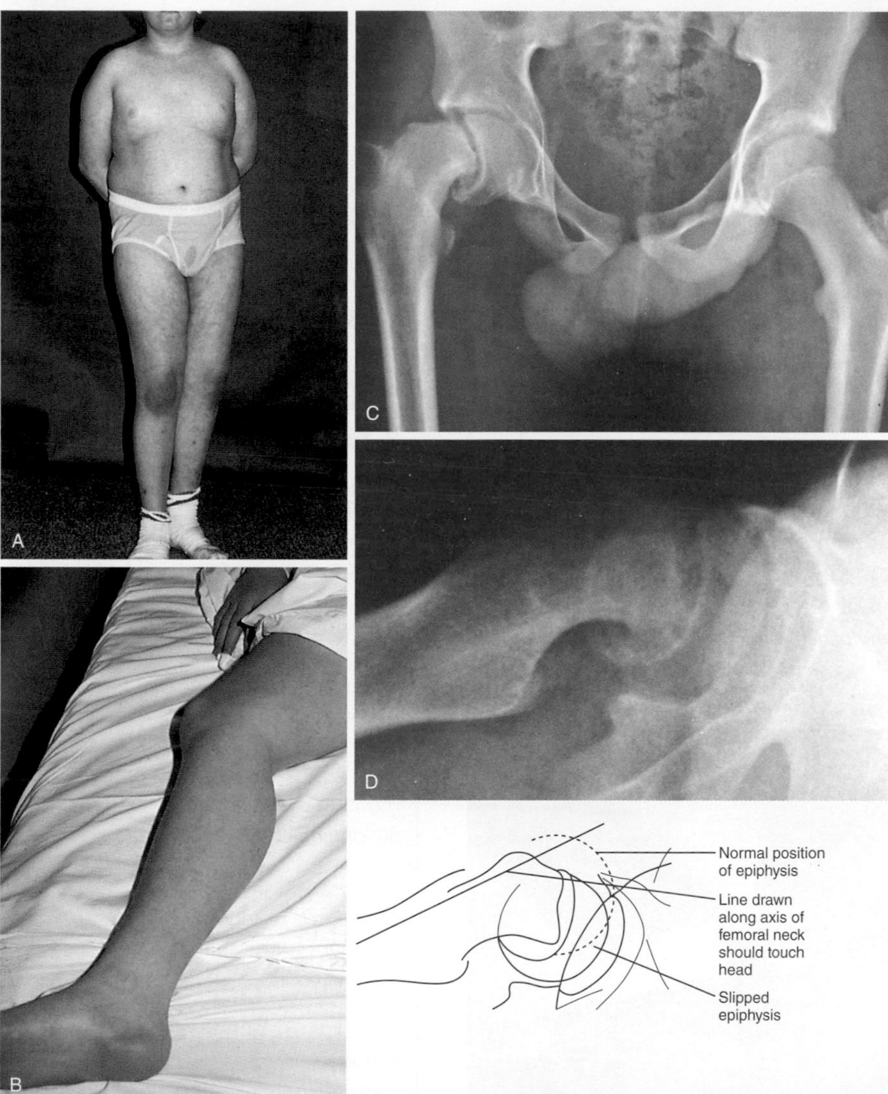

Fig. 8.5 Slipped capital femoral epiphysis. (A) This obese boy presented with a painful limp during early puberty. Note his reluctance to bear weight on the involved right leg. (B) When he lies supine, the affected leg is positioned in external rotation because this minimises discomfort. Attempts at motion produce pain in the acutely slipped epiphysis. (C) In the anteroposterior radiograph, the right femoral head is displaced medially in relation to the femoral neck as a result of epiphyseal separation. (D) In the lateral view, the femoral head is seen to be displaced posteriorly in relation to the femoral neck. A line drawn along the axis of the femoral neck should normally touch the head. (Source: *Zitelli and Davis' Atlas of Pediatric Physical Diagnosis*. 7th ed. 2018.)

diagnosis affects long-term outcome for the affected hip with the risk of avascular necrosis or chondrolysis.[5]

Onset of symptoms may be acute or insidious (Box 8.2). Often there is a history of minor trauma, and this may confound the differential diagnosis.

Stress on the growth plate may relate to obesity, conditions such as hypopituitarism or hypothyroidism and chronic renal failure. A period of rapid growth in adolescence may also weaken the epiphyseal plate. The peak age of diagnosis of SCFE is 11 to 12 years in girls and 12 to 13 years in boys.

> Typical presenting features of SCFE include medial knee, hip, groin and thigh pain.

The child may present with knee pain in up to 15% of cases, and this can be misleading. If no history of trauma, knee pain in an adolescent may be due to SCFE. On examination there is typically a limitation of internal rotation and abduction of the affected hip.

BOX 8.2 CLINICAL HISTORY

A 12 Year Old With a 4-Week History of Groin Pain

A 12-year-old boy presents with a 4-week history of groin pain and difficulty walking. He has pain on passive rotation of the hip and pain on exercise. There is no history of trauma or fever. Clinical examination shows that the right leg is held in external rotation. Bloods are normal, and a hip X-ray, frog lateral views, are requested which confirm SCFE on the right hip. Surgical fixation of the unstable right hip was performed.

Clinical Pearls

Do not miss SCFE in an afebrile older child (over 10 years of age) with hip or knee pain without a history of trauma and restricted movement of the hip on examination.

SCFE is more common in boys, is bilateral in 20% and requires a high index of suspicion in an adolescent presenting with hip, groin, thigh or knee pain, as *early diagnosis is critical*.

Pitfalls to Avoid

Not all SCFE adolescents are obese as actively growing adolescents may present with a severe slip, regardless of age or sex.

Bilateral X-ray films should always be requested, as SCFE is bilateral in up to 60% of cases. Frog lateral X-rays provide the best view for identifying SCFE on X-ray, using the 'line of Klein' and looking for asymmetry between left and right femoral neck to detect early or subtle cases of SCFE.

> SCFE should be managed surgically as soon as it is recognised, and urgent referral to an orthopaedic surgeon is advised.

The child should avoid weight bearing on the affected hip. Place the child on bed rest in order to avoid acute displacement of a chronic slip. The key aim of orthopaedic intervention is to halt progression of the slip. The mainstay of treatment of a stable SCFE is fixation of the epiphysis with a single screw. Those with an unstable slip require urgent orthopaedic repair (reposition the slip and fix with two screws) and fixation of the opposite hip. Osteonecrosis is much more likely in unstable SCFE. Surgical treatment of an early slip leads to a near-normal outcome.

Benign and Malignant Bone Tumours

Nocturnal pain may be seen in benign bone tumours such as osteoid osteoma or in leukaemia but is more often related to joint hypermobility and is sometimes described as 'growing pains'.

Both a simple bone cyst and osteoid osteoma can present with a limp. For bone cysts, symptoms may relate to a pathological fracture. These cysts tend to be in either the proximal humerus or femur but can occur in any bone.

Osteoid osteoma presents with pain which is typically much worse at night and is relieved by non-steroidal anti-inflammatory agents such as ibuprofen. Most benign bone cysts are picked up on plain X-ray where they are seen as well-circumscribed lesions (Fig. 8.6). A bone scan is helpful in the diagnosis of osteoid osteoma.

For malignant bone tumours, such as Ewing's sarcoma, chondrosarcoma or osteogenic sarcoma, pathological fractures, weight loss, fever and persistent pain are presenting features that should arouse concern (Fig. 8.7). Tumours of the spine may lead to muscle weakness with consequent limping.

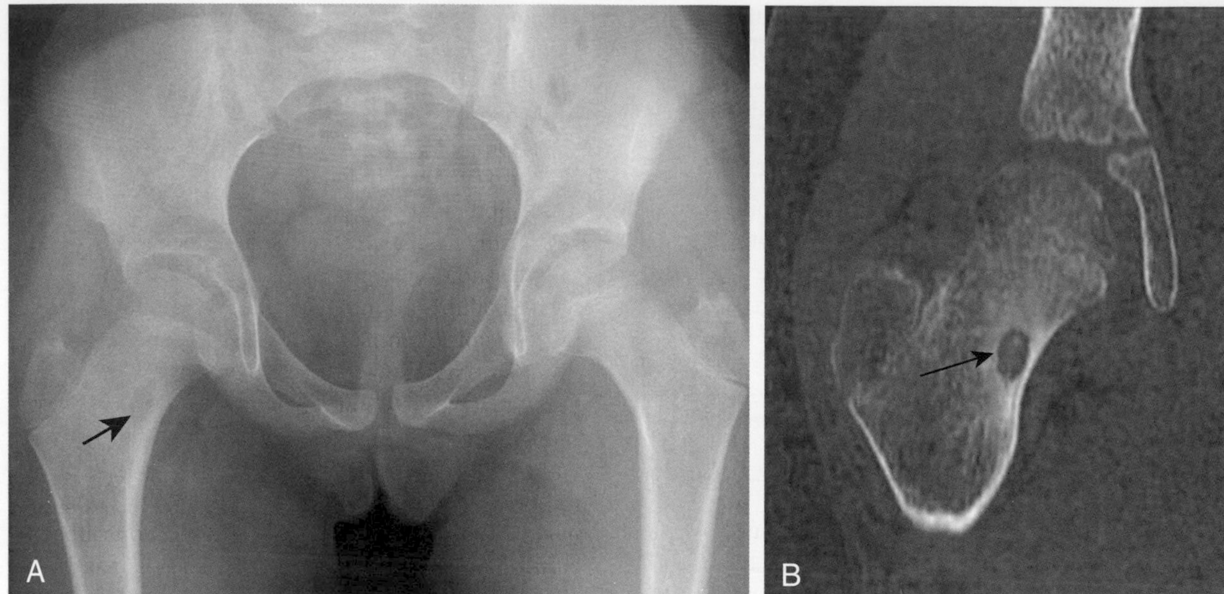

Fig. 8.6 (A) Anteroposterior radiograph of the pelvis in an 8-year-old girl with right hip pain and limp for 1 year demonstrates a focal lucent lesion at the inferior aspect of the right femoral neck (*arrow*). (B) Coronal reformatted image of a computed tomography scan of the pelvis in an 8-year-old girl with right hip pain and limp for 1 year demonstrates the osteoid osteoma at the inferior aspect of the right femoral neck (*arrow*). (Source: Sarah Sarvis Milla, Shailee Lala. *Problem Solving in Pediatric Imaging*. 1st edition, 2023, Elsevier Inc.)

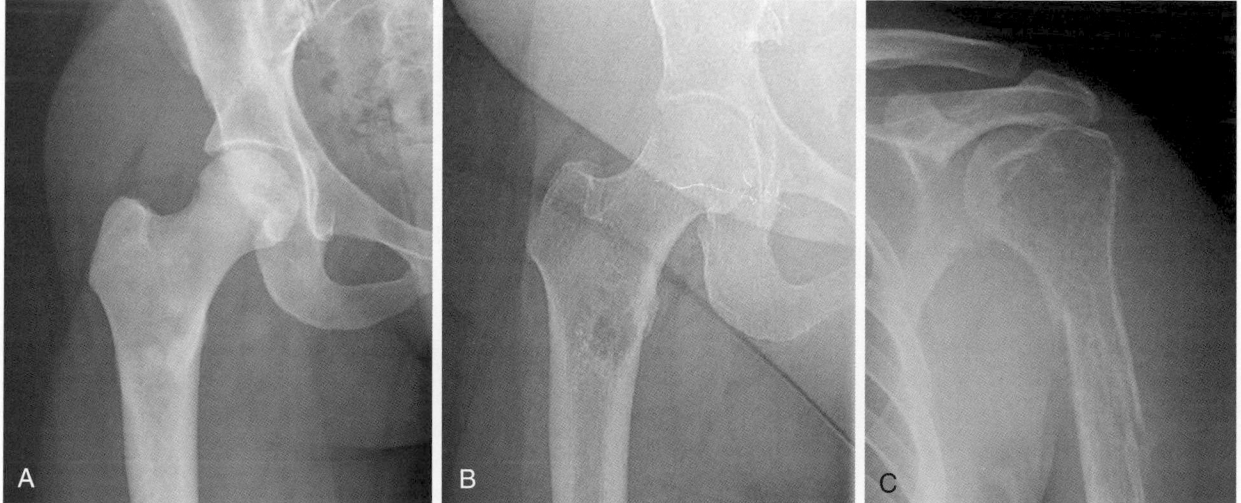

Fig. 8.7 High-grade primary malignancy. (A) Osteosarcoma proximal femur. (B) Chondrosarcoma proximal femur. (C) Ewing's sarcoma – late progression with pathological fracture. (Source: Paul Jenkins, David W. Shields, Timothy O White. *McRae's Elective Orthopaedics*. 7th edition, 2023, Elsevier Ltd.)

KEY LEARNING POINTS

A limping child is always of concern until a diagnosis is made or the symptom resolves. Septic arthritis may be difficult to distinguish from more common conditions such as minor trauma or transient synovitis.

Definitive diagnosis of transient synovitis is based on a confirmed hip effusion (picked up by hip ultrasound), and the exclusion of other potential causes.

In all children presenting with a painful limp and associated fever, septic arthritis should be suspected. For septic arthritis, timely orthopaedic input is required and treatment is joint aspiration to confirm diagnosis and intravenous antibiotics. In septic arthritis, early antibiotic treatment has significantly improved the prognosis, but complications may occur if the treatment is delayed beyond 5 days.

Perthes disease typically presents in boys aged 4 to 8 years, and slipped capital femoral epiphysis tends to occur in obese or overweight adolescents or in those with a recent growth spurt. Early orthopaedic referral is essential.

Osteoid osteoma presents with pain which is typically much worse at night and is relieved by non-steroidal anti-inflammatory agents such as ibuprofen.

For malignant bone tumours, such as Ewing's sarcoma or osteogenic sarcoma, pathological fractures, weight loss, fever and persistent pain are presenting features that should arouse concern.

REFERENCES

1. Adamson J, Waterfield T. Fifteen-minute consultation: The limping child. *Arch Dis Child Educ Pract Ed.* 2020;105(3):137–141. doi:10.1136/archdischild-2018-315905.
2. Malek S, Reinhold EJ, Pearce GS. The Beighton Score as a measure of generalised joint hypermobility. *Rheumatol Int.* 2021;41(10):1707–1716. doi:10.1007/s00296-021-04832-4.
3. Perry DC, Bruce C. Evaluating the child who presents with an acute limp. *BMJ.* 2010;341:c4250. doi:10.1136/bmj.c4250. Published 2010 Aug 20.
4. Pääkkönen M. Septic arthritis in children: diagnosis and treatment. *Pediatric Health Med Ther.* 2017;8:65–68. doi:10.2147/PHMT.S115429. Published 2017 May 18.
5. Perry DC, Arch B, Appelbe D, et al. The British Orthopaedic Surgery Surveillance study: slipped capital femoral epiphysis: the epidemiology and two-year outcomes from a prospective cohort in Great Britain. *Bone Joint J.* 2022;104-B(4):519–528. doi:10.1302/0301-620X.104B4.BJJ-2021-1709.R1.

ADDITIONAL READING

Ali AM, Hani A, Zaw H. A child with a painful limp. *BMJ.* 2019;365:l1349. doi:10.1136/bmj.l1349. Published 2019 May 8.

Allen MM, Rosenfeld SB. Treatment for Post-Slipped Capital Femoral Epiphysis Deformity. *Orthop Clin North Am.* 2020;51(1):37–53. doi:10.1016/j.ocl.2019.08.008.

Loder RT, Gunderson ZJ, Sun S, Liu RW, Novais EV. Slipped Capital Femoral Epiphysis Associated With Athletic Activity [published online ahead of print, 2022 May 2]. *Sports Health.* 2022. doi:10.1177/19417381221093045.

Mooney JF, 3rd Murphy RF. Septic arthritis of the pediatric hip: update on diagnosis and treatment. *Curr Opin Pediatr.* 2019;31(1):79–85. doi:10.1097/MOP.0000000000000703.

Obana KK, Siddiqui AA, Broom AM, et al. Slipped capital femoral epiphysis in children without obesity. *J Pediatr.* 2020;218:192–197e1. doi:10.1016/j.jpeds.2019.11.037.

Wright J, Ramachandran M. Slipped capital femoral epiphysis: the european perspective. *J Pediatr Orthop.* 2018;38(Suppl 1):S1–S4. doi:10.1097/BPO.0000000000001161.

9

Child Protection and Safeguarding Concerns

Sabine Maguire

CHAPTER OUTLINE

Child physical abuse is a recognised global issue with very significant long-term negative effects for affected children. Even in countries with mandatory reporting, child physical abuse is both under-recognised and under-reported.[1] A core duty and responsibility as a healthcare professional is to both recognise and report suspected abuse to safeguard the child from further abuse.

All healthcare professionals have a duty to protect children from harm.[1] Not identifying an inflicted injury may lead to the child or a sibling presenting with further serious or fatal injury. On the other hand, an incorrect call suggesting inflicted injury may have major negative implications for the family including needless separation of the child from the family. So, the stakes could not be higher.

As in most acute situations, first responders such as family doctors and emergency department staff need to have the ability to recognise various forms of child abuse and refer to appropriate services. This is a difficult issue emotionally and does put healthcare professionals under pressure to make the right call.

RECOGNISING CHILD ABUSE

The desired approach involves careful, open-minded questions that enable the professionals to explore any concerns in a gentle and safe way. A failure to listen, or to consider, the voice of the child are frequent findings in reviews of professional practice and can lead to the diagnosis of abuse being delayed. Ask short, nonleading questions. Adopt the '*Opening doors*' approach using the following principles (see Table 9.1).[2]

Family doctors (or primary care providers) may suspect maltreatment where they have a serious level of concern but not confirmation of abuse. In this instance, consultation with a senior colleague within the practice or with a paediatrician is advisable.

TABLE 9.1 Opening Doors' Approach in Taking the History

Listen attentively to the child, and give the child enough time
Adapt your communication style to meet the child's needs
Ask questions one at a time, and pause between questions to enable the child to respond in his/her own words
Keep a careful written record of the questions asked and the child's responses to these questions
Reflect back using the child's own words if needed
Let the child know what you plan to do next

Remember that physical injuries tend to escalate in severity over time if abuse is not diagnosed. Always follow local child protection guidelines and statutory processes.

> Never be judgmental or be tempted to adopt a role as a quasi-investigator or police officer. The younger the infant, the greater the risk of serious physical injury, and so unexplained bruising or injuries in infancy deserve additional attention and thought.

Important considerations are whether the injuries sustained are consistent with the history given and the child's developmental stage. A delay in seeking medical advice, aggressive responses when delicate questions are posed, a negative attitude towards the child and inconsistencies in the story are all causes for concern.

IMMEDIATE ACTIONS

If a healthcare professional suspects child maltreatment, a referral to the local child protection team is required, and local safeguarding pathways should be followed. If there is an immediate risk to the child or other children in the household, an emergency protection order is sought, and the child should be moved to a place of safety (in some countries admission to hospital). A child protection case conference or multidisciplinary review is then convened and involves all the relevant professionals and the family (not routine in the United States or Canada but occurs in the UK) where information is shared, risks are identified, and a child protection plan is developed. The decisions of this multidisciplinary group are heavily dependent on the reports and input from healthcare professionals. In North America, the Suspected Child Abuse and Neglect team convene a multidisciplinary assessment with law enforcement if required.

The key priority is that appropriate investigations to identify occult injury are conducted as soon as possible. If under 24 months of age, request a full skeletal survey which includes oblique views of the ribs with a follow-up skeletal survey, excluding the skull and pelvis, 11 to 14 days later. If under 12 months old, the infant should also have neuroimaging (ideally MRI) and a formal ophthalmological examination, preferably with RedCam imaging. Investigations such as a full blood count and clotting screen are also necessary if unexplained bruising.

TAKING THE HISTORY

The role of the doctor is to ascertain whether the history provided is in keeping with the clinical findings. A detailed medical and social history, full examination with appropriate investigations, helps to identify any potential occult injuries.

> The clinician must determine if the injuries sustained and the history provided are consistent or not.

In particular, the mechanism of injury, the force required to cause the injury and the developmental age of the child should be in keeping with the findings. For instance, a young infant rolling off a couch would not be expected to sustain a significant head injury or present to hospital unconscious or with seizures.

Consider the events leading up to the injury and the parental or caregiver responses post injury. With respect to suspected immersion burns, ask open-ended questions in relation to the child's alleged position at the time of scalding, who was there at the time and the exact timings involved if known. Vague, changing or inconsistent mechanisms of injury should always lead to additional concern. Likewise, if investigating patterned contact burns, consider potential causative agents and the plausibility of the child sustaining those injuries by themselves. Performing an investigation of the scene of the injury is very helpful, including determination of hot water temperature, the location of taps for scalds and is usually coordinated by the community social work team.

Documentation of prior injuries or emergency department attendances is important as is a detailed review of prior contact with social services. Be sure to contact the family doctor (primary care provider) and health visitor (or public health nurse) with parental consent, seeking a detailed background of professional input prior to this presentation.

Birth and perinatal history should focus on whether single or multiple birth (maltreatment is increased in multiple births), whether preterm and admitted to neonatal intensive care and whether ongoing neurodevelopmental concerns (again a higher risk of maltreatment).

A detailed social history is critical looking for family and other stressors.

PHYSICAL EXAMINATION

Examine the child in an area with good lighting. Pay close attention to how the child and parents interact. Ensure the child is examined fully.

> Document injuries on a body map with measurements, and ensure the paperwork is correctly signed and dated.

Bruises

Bruising is a normal process and is very common amongst active and adventurous toddlers. It is key for family doctors to be aware of suspicious bruising that might indicate physical abuse, and there are clear 'rules of thumb' that should be followed.

> Any bruises in infants under 9 months of age or who have not started walking should be considered suspicious.

The motor development of the infant or child is key in the interpretation of bruises.

Accidental bruises are typically anterior and over bony prominences, such as shins and forehead and relate to simple falls especially in toddlers.

The Cardiff group have been able to demonstrate a strong relationship between the presence, number and location of 'everyday' bruises in infants and children at different stages of development and have also shown the expected pattern of bruising in inherited bleeding disorders.[3]

The neck region, ears and genitalia seldom get bruised during normal childhood activities at any age, and bruising at these sites should cause concern. Bruising, if associated with petechiae in a child without a bleeding disorder, is of concern. Be aware that bruises are often hidden in areas typically covered by clothing, so you must undress the child to visualise all the skin especially for bruising (Box 9.1; Fig. 9.1).

BOX 9.1 CLINICAL HISTORY

Unexplained Bruising in a 3 Year Old

A 3-year-old girl and her mother attend their family doctor with classic symptoms of impetigo with yellow-crusted lesions around the mouth. She is sitting in her buggy quietly, and her lesions are visible around her mouth. She is prescribed oral antibiotics by her family doctor.

Her mother returns 1 week later. She brings her daughter into the consultation again in the buggy. The doctor notices that the child is extremely quiet, and the impetigo has not improved. A full examination is requested by the family doctor.

The girl is noted to be very withdrawn. Upon undressing, it is noted that the child is covered in bruises. These bruises are over both anterior tibial surfaces, the buttocks and the lower back, and they are felt to be bruises of concern. The family doctor states her dual concern that the impetigo has progressed and the worrisome nature of the bruises.

Clinical Pearls

When clinical progress is not as expected, always review the diagnosis, and carefully examine the child. There is no substitute for clinical examination and, without undressing the child, valuable clinical signs can be missed.

A calm nonaccusatory approach with a focus on getting the child assessed in hospital is required. A detailed assessment confirmed that concerns about child abuse were valid, and a child protection plan was drawn up.

Pitfalls to Avoid

Always be aware of the differential diagnoses of physical abuse

Seek a second opinion if concerned about a skeletal survey result

Never jump to conclusions until all the facts are available

Consider Differential Diagnoses

Sometimes bruising may be difficult to the inexperienced eye to differentiate from Mongolian blue spots, café au lait spots or other pigmented birthmarks. Bruising may also relate to coagulopathy such as due to idiopathic thrombocytopenic purpura, Von Willebrand's disease, haemophilia (Fig. 9.2), other inherited bleeding disorders or acute leukaemia, and these differentials should always be considered.

It may be tempting to date the bruises seen, but as bruises cannot be dated with any degree of accuracy, it is best simply to document if there is a pattern or clustering of bruises, and measure such bruises with an appropriate tape measure.

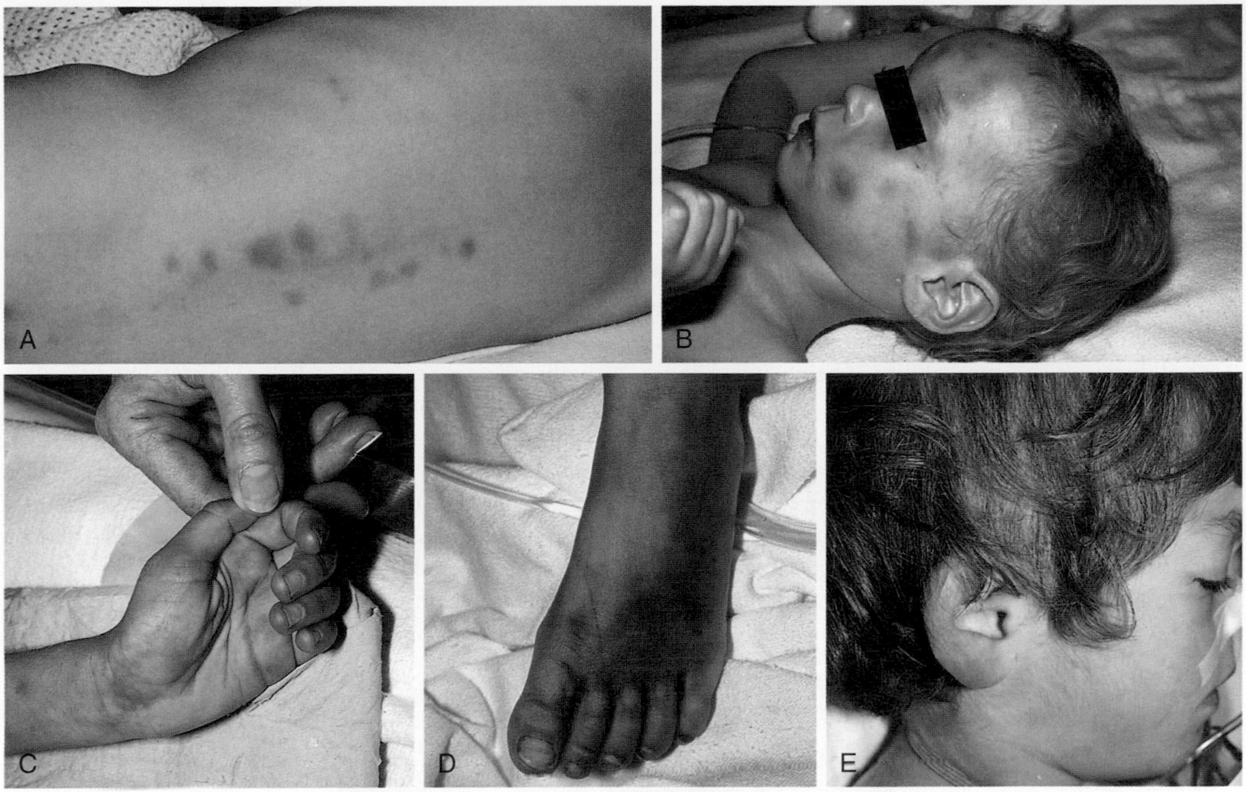

Fig. 9.1 Inflicted bruises found in unusual locations. (A) Multiple ecchymoses are evident over the back and upper chest of this child who presented in a poorly nourished condition. (B) The same patient with multiple bruises involving differing planes of the face and forehead. Note the fingerprint bruise on the cheek. (C, D) This child had severe contusions over the hands and feet, which were inflicted with a ruler. (E) He also had a markedly swollen and contused ear and patches of hair loss where the perpetrator had pulled out hanks of hair. (Source: *Zitelli and Davis' Atlas of Pediatric Physical Diagnosis*, 7th ed. 2018.)

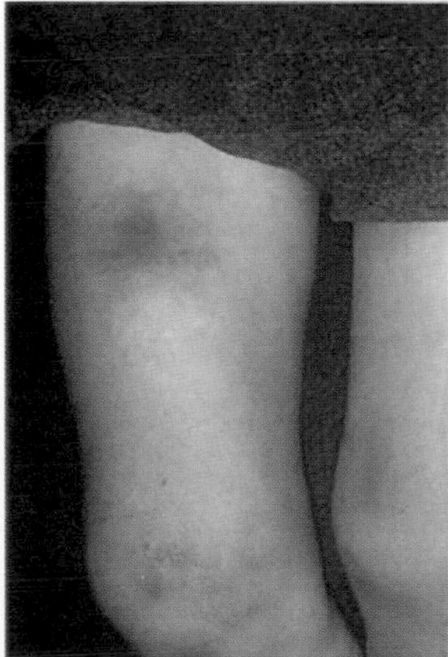

Fig. 9.2 Deep haematoma in haemophilia A factor VIII deficiency. (Source: Declan Millett, Richard Welbury. *Orthodontics and Paediatric Dentistry*. 1st edition, Churchill Livingstone, 2000, Elsevier Ltd.)

It is vital to obtain high-quality images of any bruises of concern. Correct imaging should involve a minimum quality entry-level digital single lens reflex (DSLR) camera and lens at least 60 mm (wide angle lens distorts image), a right-angled rigid ruler next to the bruise and the use of cross-polarised imaging, which helps to improve the definition of the bruise boundary.[3]

FRACTURES

Bone fractures are the second most common presentation of physical abuse after soft tissue injuries. Fractures other than skull in a child under 12 months of age are always suspicious of child abuse. Spiral or oblique fractures have, however, been described in infants playing in static activity centres, and hairline tibial fractures can occur in toddlers who have just started to walk.

To reduce the likelihood of errors in terms of radiological interpretation, double reporting of skeletal surveys by two radiologists with at least 6 months paediatric radiology training is the recommendation of the Royal College of Radiologists.[4] Improved digital communication of radiology images between centres enables second opinions to be sought by smaller centres.

Fractures With Higher Risk Profiles

Nonsupracondylar fractures of the humerus, femoral shaft fractures and metaphyseal fractures of any long bone all have a higher probability of being due to abuse in nonambulatory children (Fig. 9.3).

> Any rib fractures are highly specific for abuse.

Rib fractures are uncommon in accidental trauma (even in road traffic accidents and high falls) and very rarely follow in paediatric cardiopulmonary resuscitation.

BURNS

Burns are a relatively common injury in children, and it is estimated that about 1 in 10 are due to maltreatment.[5]

Key points in the history include a changing story about the mechanism of injury or indeed no mechanism proposed. Prior attendances for injuries or burns may add concern.

Be aware that full-thickness and caustic burns are often nonpainful and may evolve from a superficial to a deeper burn over time. Abuse is more likely if a scald is bilateral in distribution, involves the groin and lower limbs, affecting more than 10% of the total body surface area and if full thickness.

In a so-called forced immersion, there is a symmetrical burn to both sides of the body with clear margins, a so-called 'glove and stocking' pattern and apparent sparing of skin folds with a uniform burn depth (Fig. 9.4). The distribution of intentional scalds may be over the lower limbs, buttocks or perineal region and may be either unilateral or bilateral.

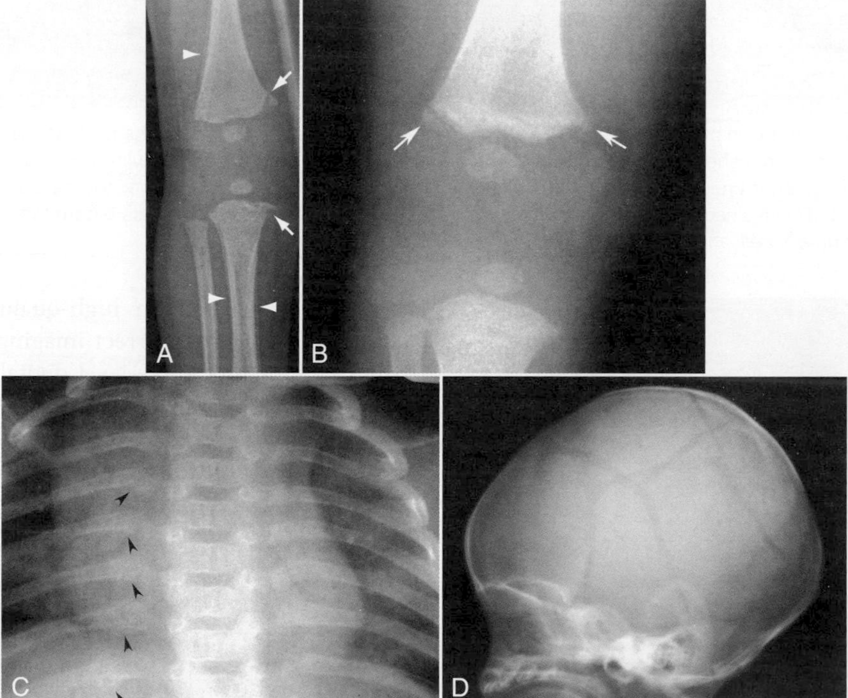

Fig. 9.3 Child abuse, skeletal findings. (A, B). Classic metaphyseal lesions (*arrows*). Also note the periosteal new bone formation in (A) (*arrowheads*). (C) Posterior rib fractures. The fracture lines are not visible, but the callus formation indicates their presence (*arrowheads*). These can be undetectable at the time of injury, illustrating the usefulness of follow-up radiographs. Even on delayed radiographs, subtle fractures of child abuse may remain nearly occult and must be carefully sought. (D) Multiple skull fractures. This finding is less specific for child abuse than the classic metaphyseal lesion and posterior rib fracture. (Source: May DA, et al. *Musculoskeletal Imaging*. 5th edition, 2022, Elsevier Inc.)

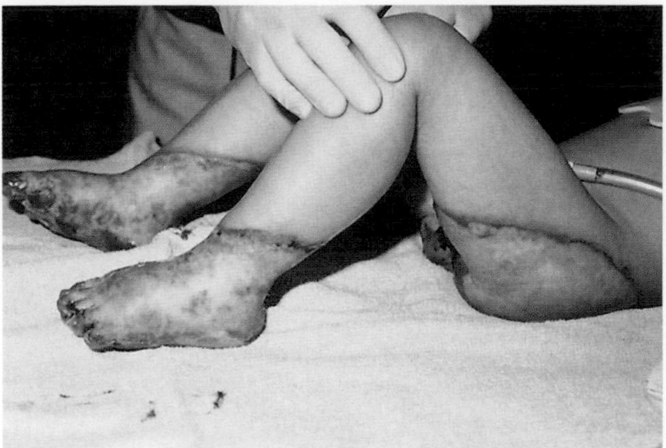

Fig. 9.4 Burn pattern typically seen after forced immersion in hot water. (K. L. McCance, S. E. Huether, V. Brashers & N. Rote (Eds), *Pathophysiology: The Biologic Basis for Disease in Adults and Children.* 8th edition, 2019, Elsevier Inc.)

Accidental scalds are most often due to spillages of hot drinks or liquids and are typically seen on the head, neck and upper body and mostly result from pulldown injuries.

The burn pattern is of irregular margins, irregular burn depth and asymmetrical involvement, with the deepest burn at the site of initial contact (e.g. the face, neck, shoulder or upper limb).

Contact burns may be due to hair straighteners, cigarettes, irons, domestic heaters or hairdryers. Accidental contact burns from irons, hair straighteners, oven hobs, solid fuel fires and oven doors are not infrequent. Accidental contact burns typically occur on the fingers or palm of the child's hand. Phototoxic dermatitis occurs when a plant psoralen or citric juice comes in contact with the child's skin and is exposed to sunlight leading to a sudden onset of blister formation with erythema around the base. Similarly cultural remedies such as cupping may cause confusion.

ABUSIVE HEAD TRAUMA

Abusive head trauma (AHT) is characterised by repetitive acceleration/deceleration forces, with or without blunt head impact, occurring in infants and resulting in intracranial, ocular and sometimes other injuries such as fractures or bruising. It has a variable presentation, with initial inconsolable crying, seizures, apnoea, vomiting, drowsiness, irritability and brief resolved unexplained events (BRUE) (Box 9.2).

Up to one-third of children presenting with AHT have abuse missed on first presentation.

BOX 9.2 CLINICAL HISTORY

A 3-Month-Old Infant Presenting With a Seizure

A male infant was born by lower segment caesarean section at 34 weeks gestation weighing 1.8 kg at birth. The infant stayed for 12 days in hospital for mild physiological jaundice and some minor feeding issues. His mother and her new partner were both living in rented accommodation. After discharge home, he presented on two occasions to the local emergency department with irritability, excess crying and an episode of brief apnoea felt to be a BRUE. He was observed on one occasion for 4 hours and discharged home. No communication with either the health visitor or primary care doctor ensued.

At 3 months of age, the infant had a sudden episode of collapse with a short, generalised seizure and was rushed to hospital via ambulance. On assessment he had a depressed level of consciousness and was therefore admitted to paediatric intensive care. Subsequent MRI brain scan showed bilateral subdural bleeds. Indirect ophthalmoscopy showed multiple bilateral retinal haemorrhages, and skeletal survey confirmed old rib fractures.

A case conference was convened, and a diagnosis of abusive head trauma was made, and the infant was subsequently taken into care.

Clinical Pearls

This case highlights the classical presentation of AHT with subdural bleeding, retinal haemorrhages and multiple rib fractures. Presentations are not always clear-cut if all these characteristics are not present.

Good communication with both the family, fellow professionals and the social work team is essential, and it is important to always keep an open mind and to conduct all family interviews in a professional and nonaccusatory way.

Pitfalls to Avoid

From the perspective of a primary care doctor, supporting families in the care of newborns, understanding their needs and providing support for stressed parents whose infants have significant crying reduce the risk of shaking injuries.

Your role as a paediatrician is to document the facts and inform others of your professional opinion in terms of likely cause. It is not to solve the mystery or to evolve into being an amateur detective.

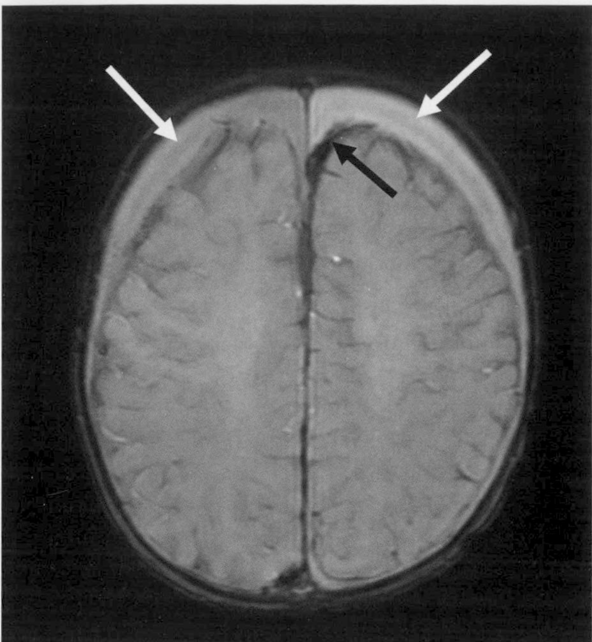

Fig. 9.5 Nonaccidental injury. A pale and difficult to rouse 3 month old. Gradient echo sequence MRI shows bilateral frontal subdural collections (*white arrows*), each with slightly different signals and each extending into the interhemispheric fissure. The left subdural also extends around to the posterior aspect of the parietal lobe and into the posterior aspect of the interhemispheric fissure. The dark signal (*black arrow*) adjacent to the medial frontal lobe is consistent with blood products in the subarachnoid space. Collections in at least three different spaces, right and left subdural and left subarachnoid spaces, each with different signal characteristics and in the absence of a history of trauma, are highly suggestive of nonaccidental injury. (Courtesy Prof Stephanie Ryan.)

In considering AHT, questions needing to be asked include whether the history is consistent with the injuries seen, whether there was an immediate onset of symptoms, where there is evidence of both subdural bleeding (Fig. 9.5), with or without hypoxic ischaemic injury and retinal haemorrhages (Fig. 9.6), whether there are potential home stressors and lastly (and most importantly) whether other differential diagnoses have been ruled out (Box 9.3).

CHILD SEXUAL ABUSE

The definition of child sexual abuse (CSA) is the involvement of a child in sexual activity that he or she does not fully comprehend, is unable to give informed consent to

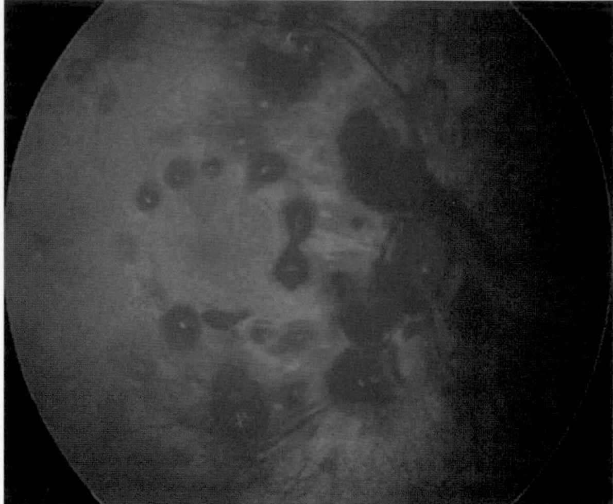

Fig. 9.6 Retinal haemorrhages in abusive head trauma (AHT). (Source: *Building Blocks in Paediatrics*, 2023.)

and is unprepared developmentally for and that violates the laws or social taboos of society. Worldwide the prevalence of CSA is anywhere from 3% to 30% with girls being twice as likely to be abused as boys. It is estimated that a small minority (sadly just 1 in 8) come to the attention of statutory authorities.

Taking the History

Best practice is to interview the parents separately from the child to prevent the child being unduly influenced by what they say.[6] Ensure that you have a chaperone when interviewing the child without their carer.

Careful documentation is required clearly outlining the concerns of the parents, disclosure by the child and the source of disclosure. Take a full general, developmental and psychosocial history, and speak to the family doctor for further details about the family.

Mild sexual play may occur innocently between children of the same age and does not warrant child protection referral. Of greater concern, however, is sexual behaviour between children who are 4 or more years apart in age, where a variety of behaviours occur on a daily basis or if the behaviour is linked to emotional distress or coercion. These children may display these behaviours persistently and become angry when someone tries to stop the behaviour.

The Brook Traffic Light Tool is a useful resource to distinguish developmentally appropriate from concerning sexual behaviour in each age group.[7]

BOX 9.3 CLINICAL HISTORY

Not What It Seemed at First

A 12-month-old male infant fell from his cot and cried immediately. The day after his fall he was noted to have a boggy swelling of the scalp but was otherwise in good form.

Five days after his fall, he collapsed with marked pallor and a reduced level of consciousness. He was rushed to the local hospital and was noted to have unequal pupils, therefore urgent neurosurgical transfer was coordinated. On examination he was noted to have a persistent boggy swelling of the scalp and bruising over the anterior chest, legs, wrists and forearms. He was intubated and had an urgent CT brain scan which demonstrated a 6 cm intracerebral bleed with midline shift.

His urgent transfer for neurosurgical intervention was expedited and prior to surgery, he had a coagulation profile performed which showed that the APTT was markedly prolonged. An urgent haematology review was sought, and his factor VIII level was found to be less than 1% of normal. He was given factor VIII prior to surgery and made an excellent recovery. He subsequently developed posthaemorrhagic hydrocephalus requiring a ventriculo-peritoneal shunt. He is currently well and has regular haematology and neurosurgical reviews.

Clinical Pearls

The key learning point in this case was, of course, that the history of the injury was very clear and consistent and the gap of 5 days before symptoms is in no way typical of AHT.

Pitfalls to Avoid

The bruising was of significant concern and was, accounted for by the coagulation disorder (haemophilia A). The administration of factor VIII prior to urgent neurosurgery was critical in this case.

In one in three children with haemophilia A there is no family history, and it results from a new (de novo) genetic mutation.[5]

If severe haemophilia, presentations during the first year of life include bleeding following circumcision, intramuscular immunisations or rarely (as in this instance) with intracranial bleeding.

Some only present as they start to mobilise around 12 to 24 months when 'pea-sized' lumpy bruises are commonly seen. These 'pea-sized' bruises were evident in this case (see Fig. 9.2).

Measurement of factor VIII or IX clotting activity both confirms the diagnosis and establishes the severity.

Interviewing the Child

A very skilled and sensitive interview technique is required. Approach the child at his or her own level in terms of development and readiness to disclose. Free recall questions are preferred, and using anatomical dolls can assist with the history especially in younger children. Video recordings of the interview are often helpful.[8]

The Examination

The appearance of the rim of the hymen may change with position and therefore the child should be examined in both knee-chest and supine positions.[8] Conducting a physical examination for alleged CSA requires special training. Videography using a colposcope is the preferred method for documenting examination findings.

> It is important to remember that 95% of cases of CSA display NO PHYSICAL FINDINGS if examined 48 hours or more after the alleged abuse.

If there are explicit or specific concerns about possible CSA, it is best to refer for a specialist examination at a multiagency safeguarding hub.

Physical findings in CSA may include bruising or laceration of the labia (in the absence of a straddle history), penile or perineal bruising, an acute laceration of the posterior fourchette or vestibule (without involving the hymen), an acute hymenal laceration either partial or complete and laceration of the perineum.

> If injuries are found on examination, differential diagnoses of CSA such as accidental injuries, normal anatomical variations, lichen sclerosis (Fig. 9.7) and urethral prolapse should be considered.

You should be aware of female genital mutilation (FGM) which is a common practice in many countries. FGM can be associated with a risk of haemorrhage or infection. FGM can lead to significant psychological issues and long-term urological and gynaecological complications. Safeguarding issues may arise if there is

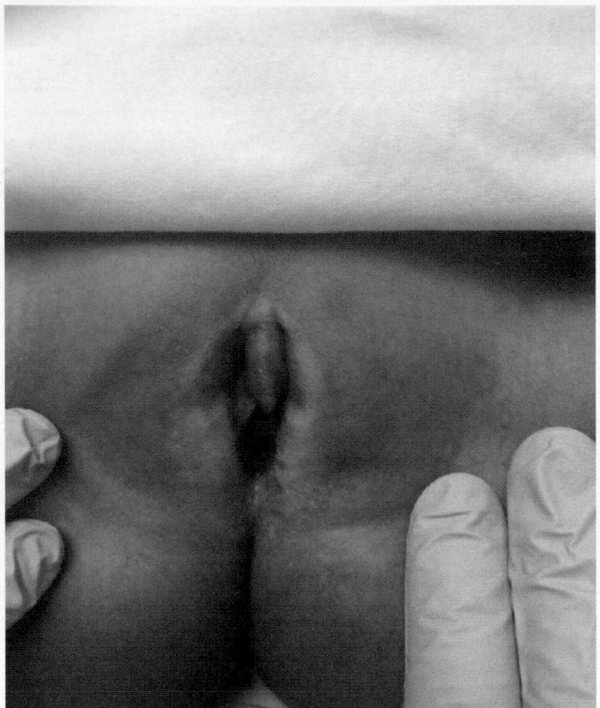

Fig. 9.7 Lichen sclerosis diagnosed in a 5-year-old child. A sharp demarcation of hypopigmented, thin epithelium is seen with characteristic 'parchment paper' changes in the affected area. (Source: *Holcomb and Ashcraft's Pediatric Surgery*. 7th ed. 2020.)

a suspicion that a young girl may be due to travel to their country of origin for the purposes of this procedure.

> In the emergency department setting, it is important that staff are able to recognise a classical straddle injury, excessive self-gratification behaviour in a preschool child, genital itch due to threadworms and lichen sclerosis.

Laboratory Testing

Indications for testing for sexually transmitted (STI) infections include a history of penetration of the genitalia or anus, abuse by a stranger, abuse by someone known to have an STI or at high risk due to intravenous drug use or multiple sexual partners. Children who are prepubertal require a second confirmatory test.

Lack of Disclosure

It is uncommon for children to disclose CSA spontaneously, and this disclosure may only occur at a much later age, quite often in adulthood. Feelings of shame and guilt often preclude disclosure by the child. CSA can be linked to many symptoms including depression, posttraumatic stress, anxiety and behavioural problems. Deliberate self-harm and an increased risk of suicide are seen. Some have nonspecific symptoms such as constipation with overflow or dysuria and daytime wetting.

Sadly, 7 years is the average time interval from the start of CSA to disclosure.[9]

Key Issues to be Addressed in Assessment

The key issues are the child's safety and communication with relevant professionals with expertise in CSA assessment. Always consider the child's mental health and whether a physical or forensic examination is required.

Always reassure the child that they are doing the right thing in giving you a history of what has taken place thereby navigating the child through 'secrets'.

The need for a forensic evaluation depends on the time interval between the alleged episode and presentation. This was in the past 72 hours but has now been extended to 7 days. Acute presentations of alleged CSA are uncommon in children.

FACTITIOUS INDUCED ILLNESS

Factitious induced illness (FII) is defined as occurring when someone persistently fabricates symptoms on behalf of another, usually a child, causing that person to be regarded as ill, or induces illness in another person, usually a child. FII is, perhaps, not the rare 'enigma' that many believe it to be and can be managed with a multidisciplinary approach.[10]

> Clues to a possibility of FII include an unusual, bizarre and recurrent illness with inconsistent histories, observations and tests.

The child experiences physical harm because of unnecessary investigations and emotional harm relating to fulfilling the sick role, social isolation, confusion and anxiety. Almost all (98%) of perpetrators are women and the mother of the child. The mother may have a background in healthcare. The father is typically either emotionally or geographically absent.

The illness begins only when the perpetrator is present and the child is inexplicably better away from the perpetrator. The perpetrator tends to be happy in hospital and always appears knowledgeable and calm.

Treatment of the presenting symptoms is ineffective and there may be a history of previous unusual illness or deaths in the family. Admission to hospital and extensive investigations are required (Box 9.4).

BOX 9.4 CLINICAL HISTORY

Frequent GP Attendance

A 2-year-old boy attends his GP on a regular basis with his mother. He has attended five times over the last 4 months. He is an only child.

He presents with repeated episodes of fresh blood in his nappy. His last episodes were 2 days ago. His Mum describes his nappy as soaked through, very red in colour, with no obvious source seen. It was described as alarming. He is lethargic and slightly off his food but otherwise looks well. His examination is normal apart from a slightly tight foreskin.

His mother is extremely anxious and is increasingly worried as to why he is recurrently unwell. She is fearful that he may have a serious underlying condition.

He is referred to the local paediatric service for further review based on parental concerns. An extensive series of investigations including renal ultrasound and cystoscopy are normal. His bloods investigations including renal and coagulation profiles were normal. He remains in hospital for over 3 weeks and is seen by several specialists who are increasingly baffled by his presentation. His mother is on first-name terms with both the nursing and medical team and, in desperation, he is referred to a tertiary paediatric hospital. A detailed assessment there showed normal observations and investigations. A case conference is convened with input from a host of professionals, and a diagnosis of factitious induced illness (FII) is made.

Clinical Pearls

FII needs to be considered before it can be recognised and should always be considered in the differential diagnosis of medically unexplained or perplexing symptoms.

The calm attitude and behaviour of the mother despite very worrying symptoms are quite characteristic.

Pitfalls to Avoid

Avoid, if possible, a series of never-ending and increasingly invasive investigations. Identify a multiprofessional and multiagency team which will formulate a consensus as to what the appropriate next steps should be. Admission to hospital is often required as is the monitoring of the child's condition when the chief caregiver (usually the mother) is not present. Referral to child protection services is warranted, and the behaviour of the mother may escalate further once she has been confronted with allegations regarding FII. A plan for rehabilitation should be agreed. Psychiatric evaluation of the parents is recommended.

KEY LEARNING POINTS

First responders such as family doctors and emergency department staff need to be able to recognise various forms of child abuse, and refer to services as appropriate.

Unexplained bruising or injuries in infancy deserve additional attention and thought.

Important considerations are whether the injuries sustained are consistent with the child's developmental stage and whether the injuries could readily be explained by the story given by the carers.

The clinician must not jump to conclusions or be judgemental, rather they should calmly determine if the injuries sustained and the history provided are consistent or not.

Ensure the child is examined fully. Document injuries on a body map with measurements, and ensure the paperwork is correctly signed and dated.

A naked eye assessment will not be able to determine the age of a bruise.

Abusive bruises are found mainly on the head and neck (ear, neck and cheeks in particular), soft tissue areas such as inner thigh, upper arm or in genital areas.

Rib fractures (especially if multiple) have a high predictive value for abuse.

All children under 24 months where physical abuse is suspected should have a full skeletal survey, with repeat limited survey 11 to 14 days later.[10]

Abusive burns account for 1 in 10 children admitted to burns units and are more frequent in infancy.

Accidental scalds are most often due to spillages of hot drinks or liquids.

AHT has a variable presentation, not least at first inconsolable crying, seizures, apnoea, vomiting, drowsiness, apparent sepsis and apparent life-threatening events.

Child sexual abuse is common (1 in 20), many do not disclose, and a specialist examination is required when a child makes an allegation or disclosure.

There are specific competencies and professional standards defined by the RCPCH for doctors conducting specialist examinations.

95% of cases of child sexual abuse display NO PHYSICAL FINDINGS on examination.

The absence of physical findings never excludes CSA. Videography using a colposcope is the preferred method to document examination findings.

REFERENCES

1. Flaherty EG, Sege RD, Griffith J, et al. From suspicion of physical child abuse to reporting: primary care clinician decision-making. *Pediatrics*. 2008;122(3):611–619. doi:10.1542/peds.2007-2311.
2. Marchant R, Carter J, Fairhurst C. Opening doors: suggested practice for medical professionals for when a child might be close to telling about abuse. *Arch Dis Child*. 2021;106(2):108–110. doi:10.1136/archdischild-2020-320093.
3. Johnson EL, Jones AL, Maguire S. Bruising: the most common injury in physical child abuse. *J. Paediatrics*. September 3, 2021. doi:10.1016/j.paed.2021.08.001.
4. Halstead S, Scott G, Thust S, Hann G. Review of the new RCR guidelines (2017): The radiological investigation of suspected physical abuse in children. *Arch Dis Child Educ Pract Ed*. 2019;104(6):309–312. doi:10.1136/archdischild-2017-314591.
5. Mullen S, Begley R, Roberts Z, Kemp AM. Fifteen-minute consultation: Childhood burns: inflicted, neglect or accidental. *Arch Dis Child Educ Pract Ed*. 2019;104(2):74–78. doi:10.1136/archdischild-2018-315167.
6. Vrolijk-Bosschaart TF, Brilleslijper-Kater SN, Benninga MA, Lindauer RJL, Teeuw AH. Clinical practice: recognizing child sexual abuse – what makes it so difficult? *Eur J Pediatr*. 2018;177(9):1343–1350. doi:10.1007/s00431-018-3193-z.
7. Brook Organisation: Sexual Behaviours Traffic Light Tool. Accessed online at https://www.brook.org.uk/education/sexual-behaviours-traffic-light-tool/.
8. Gifford J. A practical guide to conducting a child sexual abuse examination. *J. Paediatrics*. July 31, 2019. doi:10.1016/j.paed.2019.07.006.
9. Bosschaart TF. *Recognizing child sexual abuse: An unrelenting challenge*. University of Amsterdam. UvA-DARE (Digital Academic Repository); 2018. Accessed online at. https://pure.uva.nl/ws/files/28237276/Chapter_9.pdf.
10. Tully J, Hopkins O, Smith A, Williams K. Fabricated or induced illness in children: A guide for Australian health-care practitioners. *J Paediatr Child Health*. 2021;57(12):1847–1852. doi:10.1111/jpc.15663.

ADDITIONAL READING

Abusive head trauma in infants. *BMJ Best Practice*. 2018. Accessed online at. https://bestpractice.bmj.com/topics/en-us/688/references.

Ali S, Patel R, Armitage AJ, Learner HI, Creighton SM, Hodes D. Female genital mutilation (FGM) in UK children: a review of a dedicated paediatric service for FGM. *Arch Dis Child*. 2020;105(11):1075–1078. doi:10.1136/archdischild-2019-31833.

Arthurs OJ, Williams D, Steele A. Safeguarding children: are we getting it right? *Arch Dis Child*. 2022;107(9):780–781. doi:10.1136/archdischild-2021-32321.

Child Protection Evidence Systematic review on Bruising (March 2020). Royal College of Paediatrics and Child Health. Accessed online at https://childprotection.rcpch.ac.uk/wp-content/uploads/sites/6/2021/02/Child-Protection-Evidence-Chapter-Bruising_Update_final.pdf

Child Protection Evidence Systematic review on Burns (July 2017). Royal College of Paediatrics and Child Health. Accessed online at https://childprotection.rcpch.ac.uk/child-protection-evidence/burns-systematic-review/

Child Protection Evidence Systematic review on Head and Spinal Injuries (August 2019). Royal College of Paediatrics and Child Health. Accessed online at https://childprotection.rcpch.ac.uk/child-protection-evidence/head-and-spinal-injuries-systematic-review/

Child Protection Evidence Systematic review on Retinal Findings (September 2020). Royal College of Paediatrics and Child Health. Accessed online at https://childprotection.rcpch.ac.uk/child-protection-evidence/retinal-findings-systematic-review/

Debelle G, Oates A. Making the case for greater certainty in child protection. *Arch Dis Child*. 2022;107(9):777–778. doi:10.1136/archdischild-2021-323703.

Dubowitz H, Bennett S. Physical abuse and neglect of children. *Lancet*. 2007;369(9576):1891–1899. doi:10.1016/S0140-6736(07)60856-3.

Gifford Jo. A practical guide to conducting a child sexual abuse examination. *Paediatrics and Child Health*. 2019;29(10)):448–454.

Glenn K, Nickerson E, Bennett CV, et al. Head computed tomography in suspected physical abuse: time to rethink? [published online ahead of print, 2020 Oct 29]. *Arch Dis Child*. 2020. doi:10.1136/archdischild-2020-320192 archdischild-2020-320192.

Hodes D, Ayadi O'Donnell N, Pall K, et al. Epidemiological surveillance study of female genital mutilation in the UK. *Arch Dis Child*. 2021;106(4):372–376. doi:10.1136/archdischild-2020-319569.

Lindauer RJ, Brilleslijper-Kater SN, Diehle J, et al. The Amsterdam Sexual Abuse Case (ASAC)-study in day care centers: longitudinal effects of sexual abuse on infants and very young children and their parents, and the consequences of the persistence of abusive images on the internet. *BMC Psychiatry*. 2014;14:295. doi:10.1186/s12888-014-0295-7. Published 2014 Nov 8.

10

Important Cardiac Diagnoses in Children

Terence Prendiville

CHAPTER OUTLINE

Just under 1% of children have a congenital heart lesion, but up to 40% of healthy school-aged children will have a vibratory innocent heart murmur if examined by a healthcare professional.[1] These murmurs can often come and go throughout childhood, either with normal growth or during times of physiological stress (e.g., fever). The findings of a murmur, be that innocent or not, and the subsequent referral for evaluation by a paediatric cardiologist, results in a significant degree of parental anxiety with almost half of the parents believing this represented heart disease in their child and an anxiety about their ongoing participation in exercise prior to formal evaluation.[2]

In this chapter we will explore the approach to the child with a murmur, when cardiology referral is indicated, pitfalls in diagnosis and when to be concerned when a child presents with syncope, chest pain or a tachycardia.

Complicating this often-benign physical finding of a murmur in a child is that distinguishing between an innocent and a pathologic murmur can be challenging. However, there are several associated clinical findings and a certain degree of 'pretest probability' factors based on past medical history and the family history that help inform the healthcare professional on whether to refer for further evaluation or not.

On referral of a child for assessment of a murmur, echocardiography clearly has a role to play in confirming the diagnosis in a child with what is thought to be a pathological murmur on exam. Arguably, there is also a role for echocardiography in reassuring an anxious family[3] and in making sure that the evaluating paediatric cardiologist does not miss a rare and clinically subtle finding.[4] It is worth noting that under the 2014 'Appropriate Use Criteria for Initial Transthoracic Echocardiography in Out-patient Pediatric Cardiology' published by the American Academy of Pediatrics and the American Heart Association, an echocardiogram for a presumptively innocent murmur with an otherwise normal exam and a benign family history is classified as 'rarely appropriate'.[5] Nonetheless, in current clinical practice, a substantial majority of children being evaluated by paediatric cardiologists will undergo echocardiography for a combination of validation of clinical suspicion, reassurance and both parental and referring physician expectation. Given the fact that echocardiography is a finite resource and that most of the efforts of paediatric cardiology should be focused on the cohort of children with clinically significant heart disease, there is a burden of responsibility on the referring physician to 'filter' those healthy children with innocent murmurs from those with a higher degree of clinical suspicion, erring on the side of caution. This necessitates a thoughtful and calculated risk assessment in each child over a defensive practice policy in referral practice.[6]

OPPORTUNITIES TO PICK UP CONGENITAL HEART DISEASE

Antenatal Screening

It is now a recommendation that all fetuses are screened for congenital heart disease at 20 weeks gestation, and those with a concern for congenital heart disease (CHD) and take out CHD raised on ultrasound will be seen promptly by a paediatric cardiologist. Nonsyndromic parents who themselves have congenital heart disease or have a previous child with congenital heart disease (first-degree relative) have an increased risk (4.2%) of a subsequent child being born with any form of CHD in a future pregnancy.[7] Of all those infants requiring a procedure to treat a congenital heart malformation in the first year of life, just over 50% were diagnosed through antenatal screening, allowing planned delivery and elective transfer to a specialist cardiology service soon after birth.[8] This is over double the pick-up rate from 10 years previously with a hope this trend will continue to improve antenatal detection going forward. Nonetheless, there will always be a significant proportion of complex congenital heart disease that is challenging to detect antenatally (e.g., total anomalous pulmonary venous drainage) or not yet manifest anatomically (e.g., coarctation of the aorta or persistent ductus arteriosus) at the time of fetal assessment.

Assessing Murmurs in Early Infancy

The identification of congenital heart disease is one of the important aspects of the newborn examination. Ideally the heart should be examined between 6 and 48 hours after birth to allow time for the patent ductus arteriosus to close following withdrawal of endogenous prostaglandin that had been secreted from the placenta and for the pulmonary vascular resistance to begin to fall to unmask left-to-right ventricular shunt lesions or valvular pulmonary stenosis. The current reality is, however, that most newborn examination is performed prior to discharge on day one of life.

To assist with screening for critical congenital heart defects in newborn infants prior to discharge, a simple pulse oximetry algorithm has been shown to be effective in detecting clinically significant disease. A threshold of 95% oxygen saturations or greater in either foot is required for discharge with further clinical assessment warranted. The sensitivity for critical CHD is reported at 75% and for major CHD at 49%.[9]

> Pulse oximetry is a simple, safe and acceptable test that adds value to existing screening and helps identify critical congenital heart disease that would otherwise go undetected.

Murmurs can be heard in 0.6 to 1.37% of newborns but up to 42.5 to 54% of these infants will subsequently have a diagnosis made of a congenital cardiac lesion.[10,11] This yield is significantly higher than in any other paediatric age cohort. Infants who have a murmur picked up in the first 6 weeks of life who otherwise appear well and with low clinical suspicion for CHD should be reviewed in 2 weeks to ascertain whether the murmur is still present and to see if the infant has developed symptoms. There is little doubt that murmurs picked up in the first 6 weeks are more likely to be significant than if picked up later, and thus referral for paediatric cardiology opinion may be indicated.

Always assess upper and lower limb pulse volumes as part of the routine clinical examination using the pads of the index and middle fingers applied gently and along the axis of the femoral vessels. Low pulse volumes in all four limbs are a feature of critical aortic stenosis or hypoplastic left heart syndrome. Decreased or absent femoral pulses are a feature of coarctation of the aorta. Note that radio-femoral delay is rarely clinically apparent in young infants with fast heart rates. A greater than 20 mmHg difference in the averaged systolic values between the upper and lower limbs is considered significant as an indicator for coarctation. A palpable thrill, either between the upper chest rib spaces or the suprasternal notch, infers a clearly pathological characteristic to an auscultated murmur.

The clinical hallmarks of congestive heart failure (CHF) from the neonatal period onwards are an active precordium, hepatomegaly and a gallop rhythm. The precordium is assessed with the examiner's hand placed across the left chest, assessing for a more forceful cardiac impulse than is otherwise normally appreciated.

A third heart sound (S3) is a low-pitched, mid-diastolic sound, best appreciated by listening for a triple rhythm. It has been likened to the galloping of a horse and is called a gallop rhythm. It is usually heard in addition to background sinus tachycardia.

BOX 10.1 CLINICAL HISTORY

A Young Infant With an Apparently Normal Cardiovascular Examination as a Newborn

A male infant is born by spontaneous vertex delivery and weighs 3.5 kg at birth. He had a normal cardiovascular examination in the newborn period and was discharged home at 48 hours of age. At 8 weeks of age, he attends his family doctor with concerns about diminished feeding over the prior 2 weeks. His weight gain has plateaued over the same time. He is irritable, upset and has sweating of the scalp, particularly with feeds. His mother also states that he is breathing quickly and looks pale. A loud pansystolic murmur is noted on examination along with an active precordium and a 3 cm liver edge.

Clinical Pearls

Ventricular septal defects (VSDs) are either muscular or perimembranous and account for 30% of all congenital heart disease.

As the peripheral vascular resistance (PVR) naturally falls during the first 6 weeks of life to approximately 20% of the systemic vascular resistance (SVR), a significant increase in left to right shunting through the ventricular septal defect will develop. This results in clinically significant pulmonary over-circulation, presenting with signs and symptoms of congestive heart failure (CHF).

Examination findings in CHF include tachypnoea, tachycardia, an S3 gallop rhythm, a left parasternal heave and hepatomegaly.

Assess the precordium for thrills (palpable murmurs) and heaves, and look especially for a left parasternal heave or a displaced apex beat.

In an infant with a large VSD (Fig. 10.1), heart failure may develop at *4 to 6 weeks* of age.

On the other hand, CHF that develops in the *first week of life* (especially the first 3 days) is usually due to a critical obstructive lesion, typically critical aortic stenosis, hypoplastic left heart syndrome or coarctation of the aorta.

Pitfalls to Avoid

VSDs usually become symptomatic at 4 to 6 weeks of age, and often a murmur is *not* evident on the newborn discharge examination.

If left untreated, a VSD can cause marked failure to thrive and progressively irreversible pulmonary hypertension. This can manifest as a prominent S2 (P2) on cardiac auscultation. Longstanding pulmonary hypertension may eventually lead to reversal of shunt flow with consequent cyanosis and secondary polycythaemia.

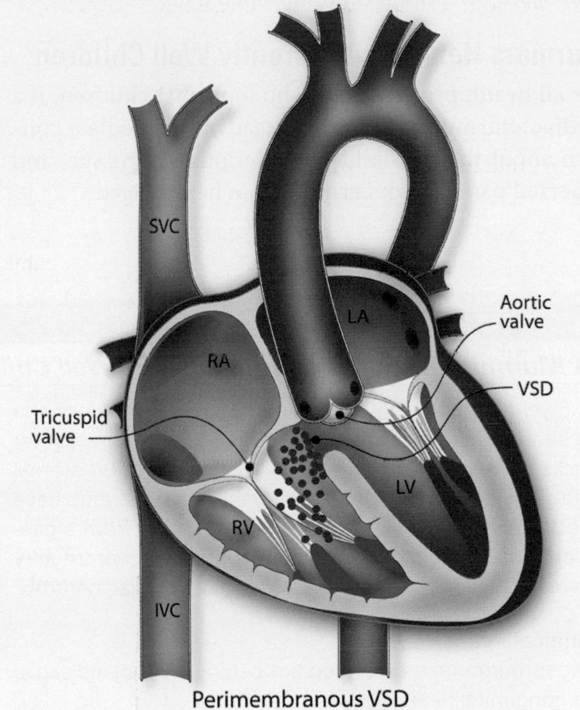

Fig. 10.1 Perimembranous VSD. (Reproduced with permission of Dr Bill Evans.)

A palpable liver edge more than 2 cm beneath the costal margin infers hepatomegaly and, if CHF is marked, may also be identified along with splenomegaly (Box 10.1).

CONGENITAL HEART DEFECTS

Congenital heart defects are strongly associated with many of the common chromosomal abnormality syndromes, and infants with a major chromosomal abnormality require cardiac screening on this basis alone, regardless of the clinical exam findings. Trisomy 21, the most common form of syndromic CHD, has a frequency of CHD of 40%; 22q11.2 deletion (Di George syndrome) is associated with CHD of 75 to 85%; Turner syndrome (45, X) is associated with CHD of 25%. In addition to chromosomal abnormalities, microdeletions (Williams Beuren syndrome) and phenotypic RASopathies (Noonan syndrome) are both also highly associated with CHD (75% and 80%, respectively).

Environmental exposures for the fetus are also of relevance in subsequent CHD. Foetal alcohol syndrome has a strong association with congenital heart defects (33–100%).[12] Maternal pregestational and, to a lesser extent, gestational diabetes is a numerically more common contributor to CHD risk with 3 to 6% of pregnancies complicated by CHD.[13] Lithium use in the first trimester of pregnancy has a relatively small impact (2.41%) on CHD risk, based on more recent published data.[14]

Murmurs Heard in Apparently Well Children

For all health professionals who look after children, if a cardiac murmur is heard, this leads to immediate concern about the possibility of a serious heart issue, and expected parental concerns need to be managed.

> There are a plethora of so-called innocent murmurs and, in amongst them, a small number of children with significant congenital heart disease.

Innocent murmurs are always systolic, soft, localised and tend to vary with either respiration or posture. Murmur variations with posture are important. A venous hum is heard in the sitting position but disappears by laying the child supine.

Conversely, a vibratory Still's murmur is maximally heard in the supine position and may disappear on standing. The description by Sir George Still over a century ago of the murmur bearing his name 'a bruit that has somewhat of a musical character with a characteristic sound like that made by twanging a piece of tense string' is truly accurate (Box 10.2).

Rarely congenital heart disease may present with apparent neurological symptoms (Box 10.3).

BOX 10.2 CLINICAL HISTORY

A Murmur Picked Up Incidentally in a Well Child

A 6-year-old active boy has an intercurrent viral illness and is seen by his family doctor. He is pyrexial, and his doctor picks up a soft systolic murmur at the upper left sternal border. Despite being reassured, the child's parents have become worried and are seeking an opinion from a paediatric cardiologist. The family live in a rural community over 100 miles from the nearest tertiary cardiac centre.

Clinical Pearls

Most murmurs in childhood are benign and *not* indicative of congenital heart disease.

Innocent murmurs are typically of low intensity (less than grade 2/6), short duration, present in systole only, located along the left sternal edge without radiation, associated with normal splitting of S2 and with no additional cardiac findings such as an active precordium, gallop rhythm or palpable liver edge.

A vibratory Still's murmur (the diagnosis in this case) is the most common innocent murmur of childhood and is typically audible between the ages of 2 and 6 years old.

The likelihood of finding significant cardiac pathology from a murmur found on examination decreases after the first year of life with up to *40%* of healthy, school-aged children having innocent murmurs on careful cardiac auscultation.

If a murmur is deemed innocent, then endocarditis prophylaxis is not required.

A chest X-ray and electrocardiogram rarely assist in the diagnosis of heart murmurs in children, and should clinical judgement indicate concern, a referral to paediatric cardiology for echocardiography is indicated.

Pitfalls to Avoid

Structural heart disease is more likely when murmurs have certain characteristics such as a holosystolic, grade 3 or higher in intensity with a harsh-sounding quality, associated with a systolic click or present in diastole.

BOX 10.3 CLINICAL HISTORY

Apparent Fits With Underlying Congenital Heart Disease

A female infant had her first presentation to her family doctor at 9 months with sweating during feeds. Her weight was between the 9th and 25th centile, and she had a normal cardiovascular examination. She was referred to her local emergency department and discharged home.

She was admitted at 12 months of age with episode of unresponsiveness, limb shaking and apnoea with a normal temperature. On this occasion a grade 2 systolic murmur was heard. She had a chest X-ray while in hospital, but the report was not filed in the chart. The working diagnosis was possible seizures.

She had a further episode of central cyanosis, limb shaking and apnoea lasting 40 seconds at 16 months of age. On this occasion no murmur was heard. Her EEG was normal, and her ECG showed evidence of left axis deviation (Fig. 10.2). Left axis deviation is not a normal finding, but this was not appreciated at the time.

At 24 months of age, there had been a history of episodes of frequent desaturation and transient loss of consciousness. She also had symptoms of excessive tiredness, breathlessness and failure to gain weight. Examination on this occasion revealed tachycardia and tachypnoea and an enlarged liver (3 cm hepatomegaly), and thus she had an urgent admission to hospital. Urgent advice and transfer to the tertiary paediatric cardiology team were sought.

Subsequent investigations demonstrated an ostium primum ASD with pulmonary hypertension.

Clinical Pearls

Atrial septal defects (ASD) are the third most common congenital heart lesion and account for 25 to 30% of congenital heart disease diagnosed in adulthood (Fig. 10.3).

Typical features of an ASD are a widely split-second heart sound that does not vary with respiration, a soft systolic murmur in the pulmonary area and a loud second heart sound (P2) if there is a degree of pulmonary hypertension.

Ostium primum ASD is associated with a haemodynamically significant shunt and thus needs surgical closure. Most ASDs are asymptomatic in childhood, and pulmonary hypertension is very rare. Left axis deviation is characteristic of an ostium primum ASD.

Pitfalls to Avoid

Most children with ASD are asymptomatic, but the rates of exercise intolerance, atrial arrythmias, right ventricular dysfunction and pulmonary hypertension all increase with age.

Ostium primum ASD is associated with the development of pulmonary hypertension, and increasing pulmonary vascular resistance can lead to a reduction in shunt flow with the murmur becoming quieter (as in this instance).

It is essential to be able to interpret correctly basic investigations or seek advice if required.

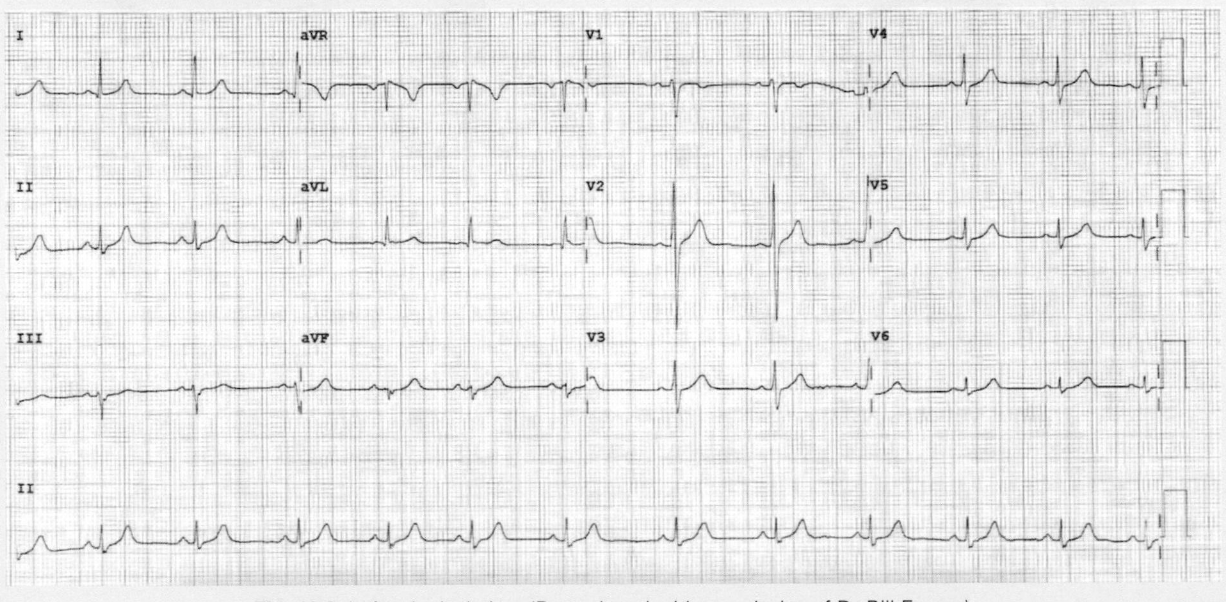

Fig. 10.2 Left axis deviation. (Reproduced with permission of Dr Bill Evans.)

Continued

BOX 10.3 **CLINICAL HISTORY—CONT'D**

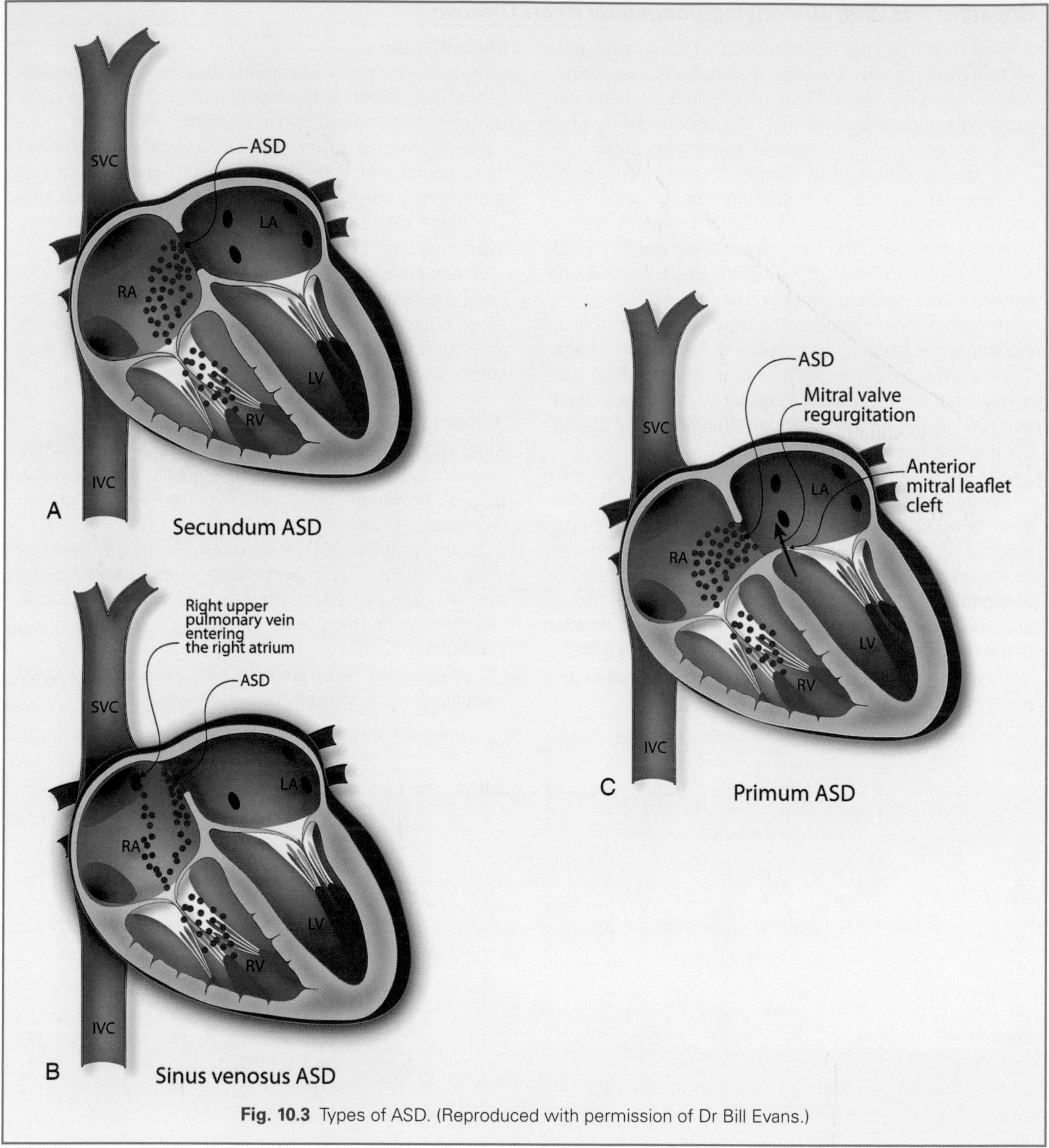

Fig. 10.3 Types of ASD. (Reproduced with permission of Dr Bill Evans.)

THREE SYMPTOMS OF CONCERN – CHEST PAIN, SYNCOPE AND PALPITATIONS

Chest Pain

Chest pain is relatively common in childhood and adolescence and is the referring complaint in a significant number of new patient referrals to paediatric cardiology outpatient clinics. It can be a source of great concern to the family given the association in later life between chest pain and ischaemic heart disease. Thankfully, in the paediatric population, only a tiny minority (1 in 100 in one large series) of all cases of chest pain in children are found to have a cardiac aetiology with the vast majority being thought to be either transiently musculoskeletal, psychogenic or idiopathic in origin.[15] There is also no evidence to suggest on longer-term follow-up that paediatric chest pain correlates in any way with future cardiac pathology. Nonetheless, the perception of chest pain is real for the patient and is important for the clinician to acknowledge. Standardised management algorithms have been developed and well validated for chest pain in the paediatric cohort.[16] The vast majority of patients are satisfied with reassurance when it is thought to be benign and don't seek long-term follow-up thereafter.

Costochondritis is often preceded by a viral illness. Very brief and sharp, stabbing pain worsened by deep inspiration is typical of precordial catch and happily usually self-resolves.[17] Exercise-induced asthma with linked bronchospasm has symptoms of chest tightness, coughing and wheeze. Herpes zoster (or shingles) can cause significant chest pain or burning before the typical vesicular rash appears.

> Chest pain or syncope brought on by exercise or exertion should be taken seriously and is considered a 'red flag', especially if there is a family history of sudden cardiac death, cardiomyopathy or inherited arrhythmia.

These patients in the above categories should always be referred for a paediatric cardiology opinion.

Hypertrophic cardiomyopathy (HCM) is characterised by hypertrophy of the basal septal wall of the left ventricle with associated obstruction of the left ventricular outflow tract in more severe cases (Fig. 10.4).

Most patients with HCM are asymptomatic but, with increasing age, chest pain in addition to exertional dyspnoea may be reported. Syncope or palpitations need urgent evaluation in this patient cohort, and there remains a small but not insignificant risk of sudden death. There are now clear guidelines on when a patient with HCM requires placement of an automatic implantable cardioverter-defibrillator.

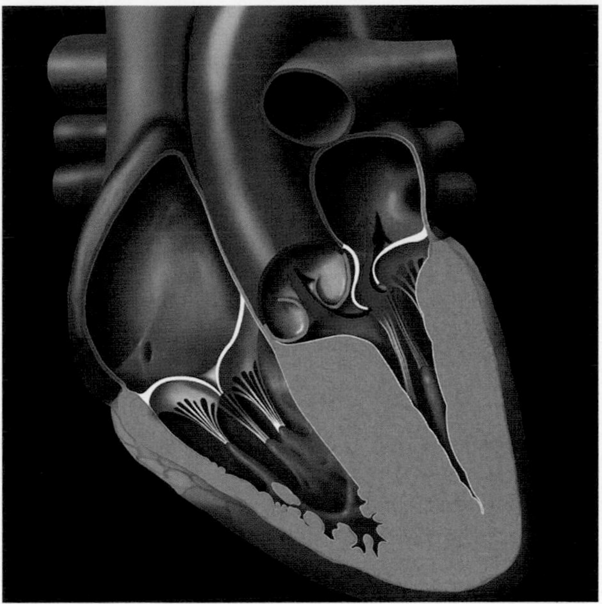

Fig. 10.4 'Five-chamber' graphic demonstrates concentric hypertrophic obstructive cardiomyopathy (HOCM). Septal hypertrophy and systolic anterior motion (SAM) of the mitral valve leaflet combine to cause left ventricular outflow tract (LVOT) obstruction and mitral regurgitation. (A. Carlson Merrow Jr., Selena Hariharan. *Imaging in Pediatrics*. 1st edition, AMIRSYS, 2018, Elsevier INC.)

HCM is inherited in an autosomal dominant pattern with often a positive family history or a family history of sudden death. Typical features of more advanced disease (left ventricular outflow tract obstruction) include the finding of a harsh ejection systolic murmur that is louder on standing up or performing the Valsalva manoeuvre.

Generally, HCM comes to light either as part of family screening or if a child or adolescent presents with symptoms such as breathlessness, angina or syncope that are related to exercise.

Diagnosis of HCM can be suggested by ECG and confirmed by echocardiography or cardiac MRI, and referral to a paediatric cardiologist for family screening should take place. HCM is diagnosed if the left ventricular wall thickness exceeds two standard deviations from normal diameter (corrected for body surface area) excluding other causes of left ventricular hypertrophy not least uncontrolled hypertension or left heart obstructive lesions (e.g., valvular aortic stenosis).

Chest pain is very rarely cardiac in nature (under 1%) with the key question being whether it is brought on by exertion or associated with syncope.

Syncope

Syncope can be a frightening experience for both the child and witnesses. Up to one in five children experience an episode of syncope before the age of 15.[18] The history is generally the key to making the diagnosis. In taking the history, details such as the child's age, the time of day (early morning is typical of simple faints), the environmental conditions, activity immediately prior to the episode and whether any injuries were evident are key pieces of information.

Autonomic dysfunction in vasovagal (or neurocardiogenic) syncope leads to bradycardia and subsequent brief hypotension resulting in transient loss of consciousness. The great majority (~75%) of childhood syncope is vasovagal in origin with breath-holding (7%), epilepsy (6%), acute anxiety (4.5%) and hypoglycaemia (1%) accounting for a small percentage of other causes. Cardiac arrhythmia is responsible for 2%.[18]

The commonest prior event in neurogenic (vasovagal) syncope is either prolonged standing or rapidly assuming an upright position, but a noxious stimulus (e.g., phlebotomy), hair grooming, swallowing something ice-cold or micturition may all act as triggers. The loss of consciousness is typically brief (under 2 minutes), incontinence is rare and myoclonic jerks may be a feature further adding to confusion and concern. A prodrome of pallor, nausea and a clammy sensation is quite frequently seen. Unprovoked syncope with a sudden onset (with or without exertion) and rapid recovery is suspicious for a possible cardiac aetiology and warrants further evaluation.

The corrected QTc interval can be assessed using Bazett's formula either manually (Fig. 10.5) or by using one of a number of multiple online calculators, for example – (https://www.qtcalculator.org/). A long QTc of > 0.45 seconds (>450 msec) is considered a threshold of significance, but the formal diagnosis of Long QT syndrome has multiple considerations including the clinical history, family history and other ECG parameters. These are summated in the Schwartz score for Long QT syndrome diagnostic confidence.[19]

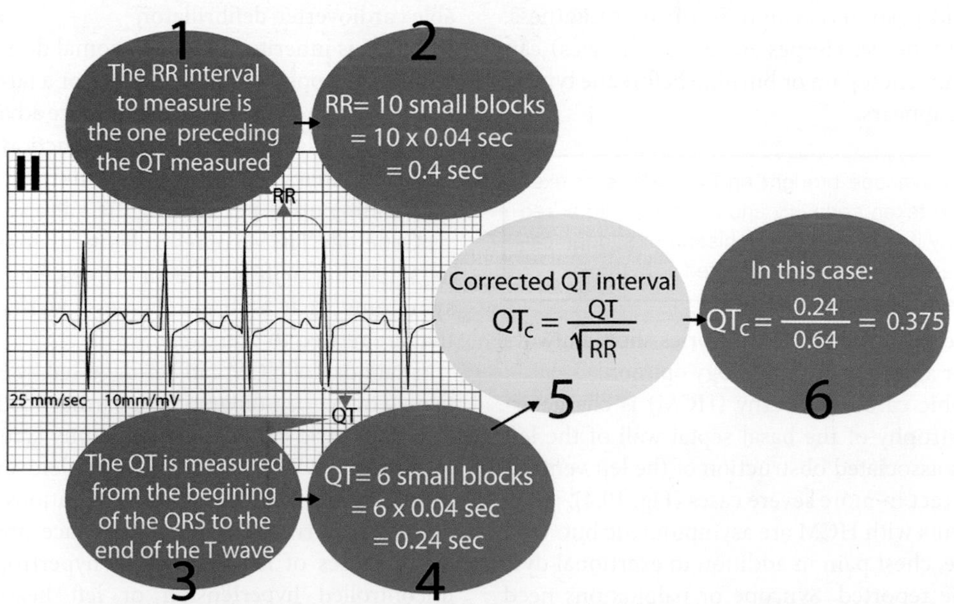

Fig. 10.5 Measuring QTc interval. (Reproduced with permission of Dr Bill Evans.)

Long QT syndromes are usually inherited in an autosomal dominant fashion, and thus there may be a family history of sudden death.

Long QT syndromes generally present with sudden onset syncope and brief seizure activity (including unexplained nocturnal incontinence) but not usually with palpitations or presyncope.[20]

If any of the above red flags or a family history of sudden cardiac death or arrhythmias, referral to a paediatric cardiologist and further evaluation is warranted.

Palpitations in Childhood

Palpitations are a very common complaint in older children and adolescents. Again, the history is all-important. Ask whether the palpitations are abrupt (more suspicious for a cardiac aetiology) or gradual in onset and offset. Asking the patient to tap out the rate can be helpful with supraventricular tachycardia typically being 'too fast to count' (Box 10.4).

Enquire how long they last (generally more benign if duration is seconds) and whether they are linked to rest or associated with exercise (supraventricular tachycardia is seen in both). Seek other associated symptoms such as chest discomfort potentially from rapid tachycardia or syncope which constitutes a red flag. Chest pain reported separate from the episode of palpitation is much less suspicious.

Supraventricular tachycardia (SVT) typically is sudden in onset, with a heart rate that is generally too fast to count (180–220 beats per minute) and terminates relatively abruptly.

BOX 10.4 CLINICAL HISTORY

A 4-Week-Old Male Infant With a Very Fast Heart Rate

A 4-week-old male infant presents to his family doctor on a number of occasions with episodes of marked pallor and is noted also to have poor weight gain from birth. His birth weight was 3.4 kg and his weight at 4 weeks was 3.48 kg. His parents brought him to his local paediatric unit for further assessment. The examining doctor noted a fast pulse rate and a sensation of 'buzzing' under the fingertips on palpation of the precordium. She requested an ECG and placed him on a cardiac monitor. His ECG showed a supraventricular tachycardia (SVT) (Fig. 10.6).

Further questioning revealed that he had episodes of marked pallor, irritability, poor feeding and lethargy over the previous 4 weeks. His peripheries were noted to be cool during these episodes. Cardiology advice was promptly sought. His SVT was managed initially with the use of crushed ice mixed with water in a sealed plastic bag held over his forehead and nose for 10 to 15 seconds. As these vagal manoeuvres were unsuccessful, a rapid bolus of intravenous adenosine followed by a 5 to 10 mL normal saline flush was given and was successful, and he reverted to sinus rhythm.

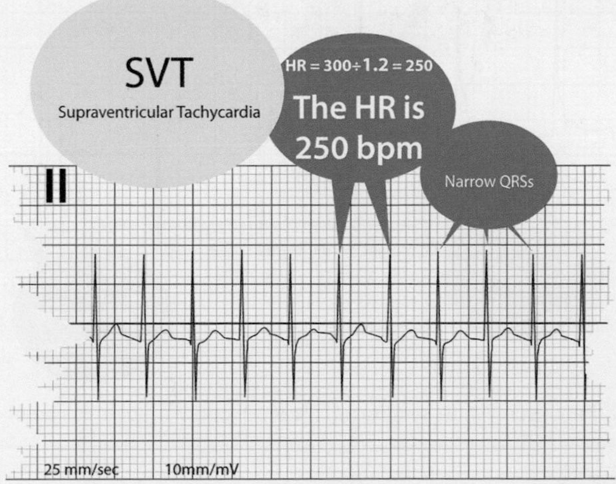

Fig. 10.6 Supraventricular tachycardia (SVT). (Reproduced with permission of Dr Bill Evans.)

Continued

BOX 10.4 CLINICAL HISTORY—CONT'D

Clinical Pearls

It is imperative to consult paediatric cardiology as soon as the diagnosis of SVT is suspected, as myocardial function can be quite significantly impaired when there are clinical signs of related cardiogenic shock. In older children, a relatively clear history of sudden onset and sudden cessation of tachycardia or palpitations is suspicious along with associated chest discomfort or acute shortness of breath. Daily symptoms lasting for a few seconds are unlikely to be due to SVT.

Most new diagnoses of SVT are in either young infants, frequently secondary to an accessory pathway or in the older child with an AV node re-entrant mechanism. In Wolff-Parkinson-White syndrome the typical ECG changes are of a short P-R interval, delta wave and a widened QRS complex (Fig. 10.7).

In older children, a Valsalva manoeuvre can be performed by asking the child to blow through an occluded straw or to do a handstand (with the assistance of a parent). Carotid or ophthalmic massage are *not* recommended.

Premature atrial contractions (PACs), premature ventricular contractions (PVCs) and extrasystoles, while commonly seen, do not cause symptoms in children or adolescents and are generally thought of as benign. If the child has no correlating symptoms, then a PAC picked up on ECG is not usually of clinical importance.

Pitfalls to Avoid

Premature ventricular contractions can result in a referral to a paediatric cardiologist, but the aetiology often is benign after initial basic assessment (ECG, Holter study and echocardiography) with no pharmacotherapy indicated.

Ventricular tachycardia (VT) (Fig. 10.8) is always considered pathological in childhood and can be due to a particular ventricular myocardial focus (e.g., right ventricular outflow tract VT), acute myocarditis, hypertrophic or dilated cardiomyopathy, congenital heart disease or cardiac ion channelopathies such as long Q-T syndrome or catecholaminergic polymorphic VT.

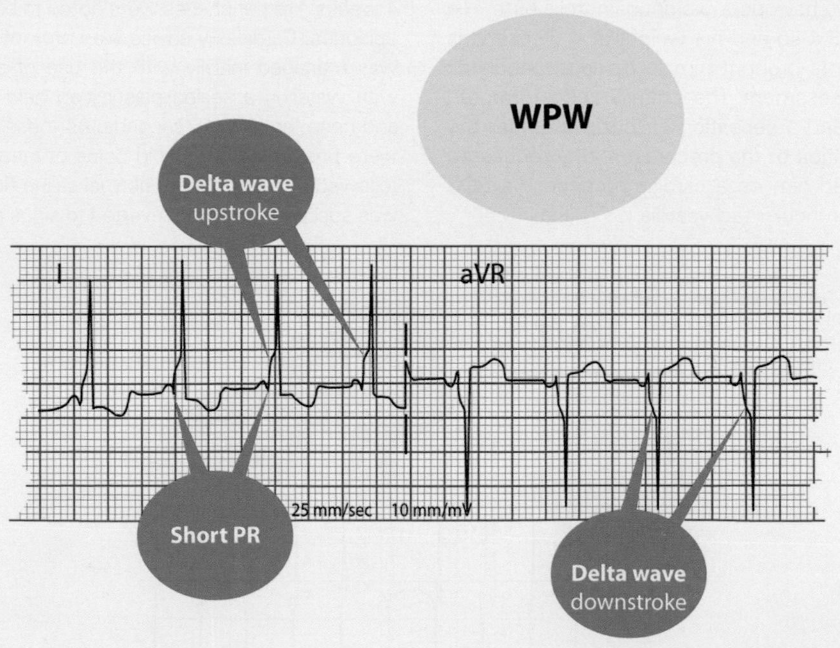

Fig. 10.7 Wolff-Parkinson-White syndrome. (Reproduced with permission of Dr Bill Evans.)

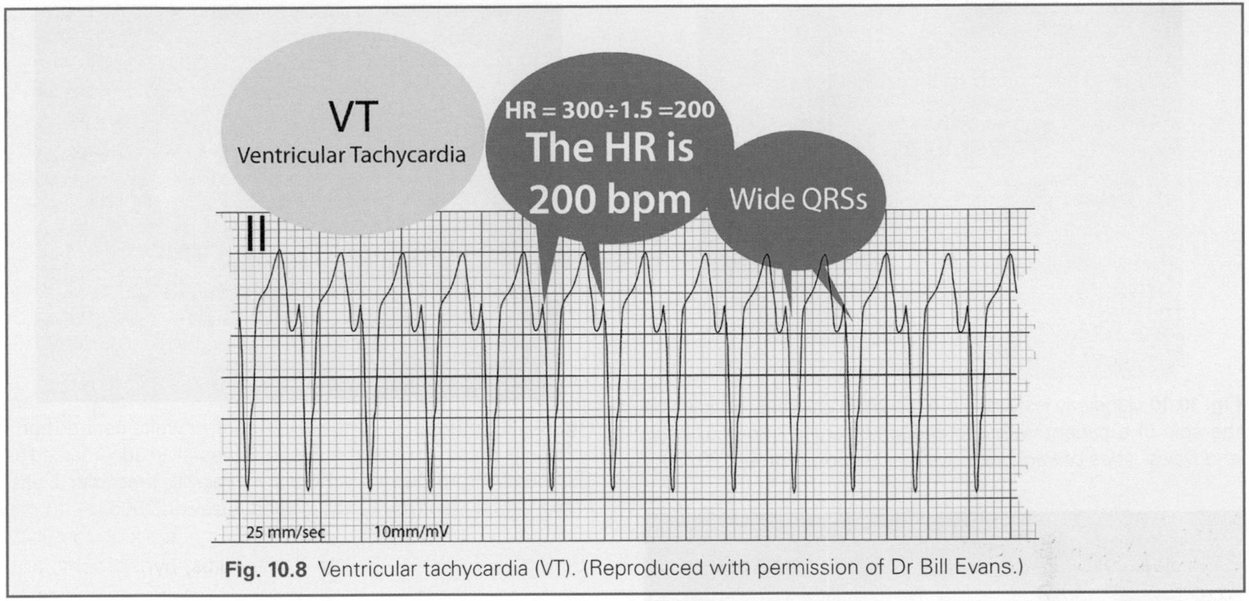

Fig. 10.8 Ventricular tachycardia (VT). (Reproduced with permission of Dr Bill Evans.)

PROLONGED FEVER AND THE HEART

Kawasaki disease, acute myocarditis, acute or subacute endocarditis and rheumatic fever are important but rare conditions to consider when faced with a child with prolonged fever.

Clearly the recognition of Kawasaki disease (see Chapter 4, Approaching the febrile infant or child) and treatment with intravenous gammaglobulin has been proven to significantly reduce the prevalence of coronary artery dilatation and aneurysms.

Endocarditis can be quite a challenging diagnosis to make. In many cases, the child may have a mild congenital heart malformation such as mitral valve prolapse (MVP), a bicuspid aortic valve or a small patent ductus arteriosus and, of course, endocarditis may also occur in structurally normal hearts.

> Chief presenting symptoms of endocarditis are a persistent fever, malaise, arthralgias, splenomegaly and new or changing murmurs.

Look out for classical features such as petechiae, splinter haemorrhages (Fig. 10.9), Janeway lesions (flat painless ecchymoses of the palms and soles) (Fig. 10.10) and Osler nodes (painful, erythematous lesions of the fingertips or toe pads) (Fig. 10.11), Roth spots of the retina (Fig. 10.12) or glomerulonephritis. Endocarditis is most often due to infection with *Streptococcus viridans* or *Staphylococcus aureus*.

Diagnosis is by fulfilling two major Duke criteria (positive blood culture on two occasions with the same organism or echocardiographic findings of vegetations, an abscess or new or worsening valvular regurgitation)

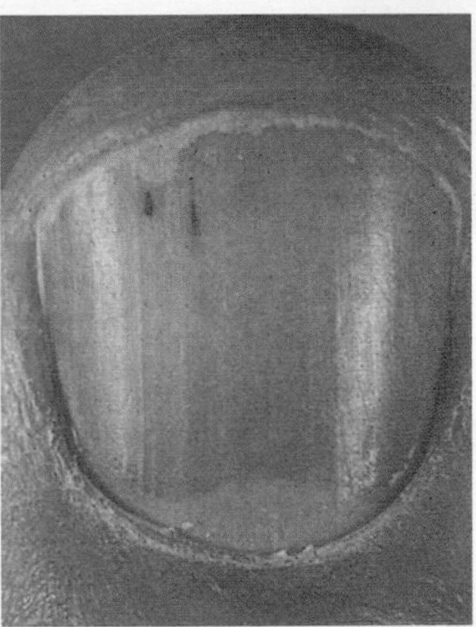

Fig. 10.9 Splinter haemorrhages. (Source: From Forbes CD, Jackson WF. *Color Atlas and Text of Clinical Medicine*. 3rd ed. Mosby; 2002. Reproduced by kind permission.)

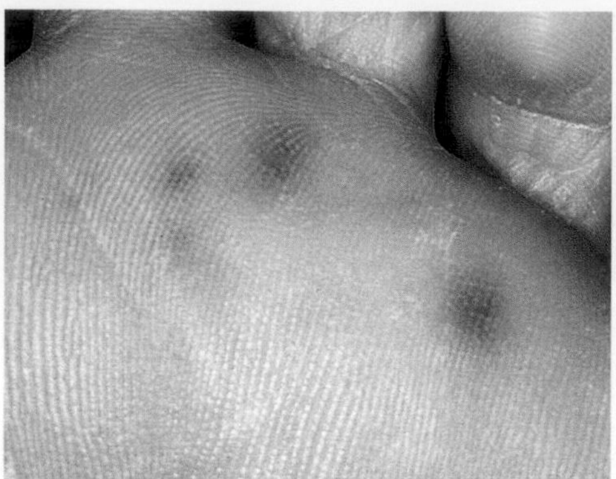

Fig. 10.10 Janeway lesions. Note the small (painless) nodules on the sole of a patient with bacterial endocarditis. (Source: *Zitelli and Davis' Atlas of Pediatric Physical Diagnosis*. 8th ed. 2023.)

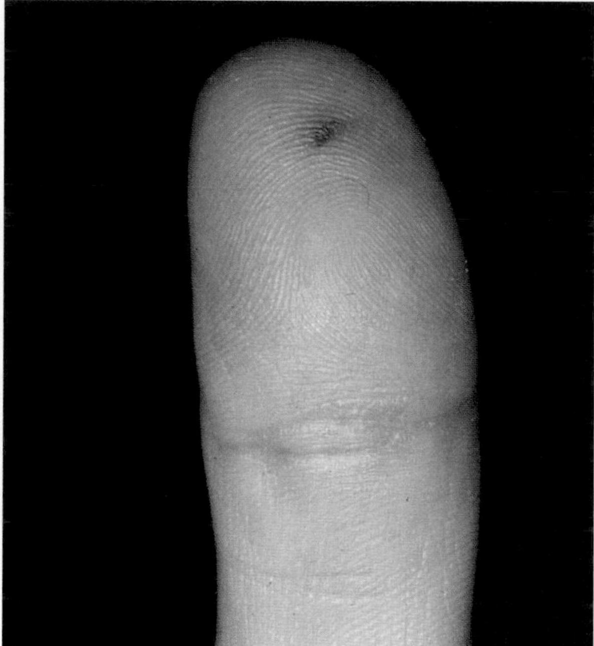

Fig. 10.11 Osler nodes. (Source: From Adams JG, et al. *Emergency Medicine, Clinical Essentials*. 2nd ed. Elsevier; 2013, 10.11.)

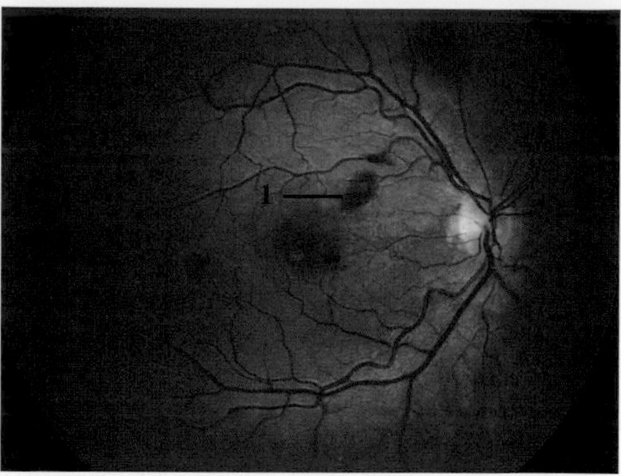

Fig. 10.12 Roth spots. A classic Roth spot, or white-centred hemorrhage is present within the superotemporal arcade (marked as 1). (Source: From Olsen TW. Retina. In: Palay D, Krachmer J, eds. *Primary Care Ophthalmology*. 2nd ed. Elsevier; 2005.)

or one major and three minor criteria. Minor criteria include a predisposing heart condition, fever above 38°C, Janeway lesions, Osler nodes or Roth spots or glomerulonephritis or a positive blood culture with an atypical organism.

Endocarditis is always a diagnosis to consider in a child with a prolonged fever without other obvious source. Repeated positive blood culture also prompts investigation of a cardiac source.

Rheumatic fever is now quite rarely seen and is diagnosed when Jones criteria are met. Symptoms and signs of rheumatic fever occur typically 1 to 3 weeks after streptococcal pharyngitis. Major Jones criteria include **P**ancarditis (with evidence of valvulitis), **A**rthritis (often migratory, involving large joints, quite painful but highly responsive to ibuprofen), **N**odules – subcutaneous, **E**rythema marginatum, **S**ydenham chorea – mnemonic **PANES**.[21] Two major criteria must be met to make the diagnosis. Those with carditis require long-term penicillin prophylaxis.

KEY LEARNING POINTS

Just under one percent of children have a congenital heart lesion, but many multiples of this are found to have a murmur when examined by their family doctor.

Infants who have a murmur picked up in the first 6 weeks of life should be reviewed in 2 weeks to ascertain whether the murmur is still present and to see if the infant has developed symptoms.

Ventricular septal defects usually become symptomatic at 4 to 6 weeks of age, and often a murmur is *not* evident on the newborn discharge examination.

Structural heart disease is more likely when murmurs have certain characteristics such as holosystolic, grade 3 or higher in intensity with a harsh-sounding quality, associated with a systolic click or present in diastole.

Ostium primum ASD is associated with a haemodynamically significant shunt and thus needs surgical closure.

Chest pain or syncope brought on by exercise should be taken seriously, especially if a family history of sudden cardiac death, cardiomyopathy or inherited arrhythmia.

Generally, hypertrophic cardiomyopathy (HCM) comes to light either as part of family screening or if a child or adolescent presents with symptoms such as breathlessness, angina or syncope that are related to exercise.

Long QT syndromes may present with sudden onset syncope or seizures but generally not palpitations or presyncope.

Supraventricular tachycardia (SVT) typically is sudden in onset, and the heart rate is described as too fast to count with a sensation of 'buzzing' under the fingertips.

In infancy, SVT is managed by vagal manoeuvres such as the use of crushed ice mixed with water in a sealed plastic bag held over the infant's forehead and nose for 10 to 15 seconds.

If the child has no symptoms, then a premature atrial contraction picked up on ECG is invariably benign. Premature ventricular contractions, in contrast, should be seen by a cardiologist.

Endocarditis is certainly a challenging diagnosis to make and is always a diagnosis to consider in a child with a prolonged fever.

Chief presenting symptoms of endocarditis are a persistent fever, malaise, arthralgias, splenomegaly and new or changing murmurs.

Symptoms and signs of rheumatic fever occur typically 1 to 3 weeks after streptococcal pharyngitis.

Delayed diagnosis of Kawasaki disease (KD) increases the risk of developing coronary artery aneurysms with each day of delay increasing the risk further.

REFERENCES

1. Van Oort A, Le Blanc-Botden M, De Boo T, Van Der Werf T, Rohmer J, Daniëls O. The vibratory innocent heart murmur in schoolchildren: difference in auscultatory findings between school medical officers and a pediatric cardiologist. *Pediatr Cardiol.* 1994;15(6):282–287. doi:10.1007/BF00798121.
2. Akrivopoulou G, Gkentzi D, Fouzas S, Vervenioti A, Dimitriou G, Karatza AA. Parental anxiety and misperceptions in children with innocent murmurs. *Pediatr Int.* 2021;63(10):1170–1174. doi:10.1111/ped.14664.
3. Ip FHL, Hay M, Menahem S. Impact of echocardiography on parental anxiety in children with innocent murmurs. *J Paediatr Child Health.* 2020;56(6):917–921. doi:10.1111/jpc.14775.
4. Ip HL, Menahem S. Does Echocardiography Have a Role in the Cardiologist's Diagnosis of Innocent Murmurs in Childhood? *Heart Lung Circ.* 2020;29(2):242–245. doi:10.1016/j.hlc.2019.02.003.
5. Writing Group for Echocardiography in Outpatient Pediatric Cardiology, Campbell RM, Douglas PS, et al. ACC/AAP/AHA/ASE/HRS/SCAI/SCCT/SCMR/SOPE 2014 appropriate use criteria for initial transthoracic echocardiography in outpatient pediatric cardiology: a report of the American College of Cardiology Appropriate Use Criteria Task Force, American Academy of Pediatrics, American Heart Association, American Society of Echocardiography, Heart Rhythm Society, Society for Cardiovascular Angiography and Interventions, Society of Cardiovascular Computed Tomography, Society for Cardiovascular Magnetic Resonance, and Society of Pediatric Echocardiography. *J Am Soc Echocardiogr.* 2014;27(12):1247–1266. doi:10.1016/j.echo.2014.10.002.
6. Arfanis K, Shillito J, Smith AF. Risking safety or safely risking? Healthcare professionals' understanding of risk-taking in everyday work. *Psychol Health Med.* 2011;16(1):66–73. doi:10.1080/13548506.2010.521566.
7. Øyen N, Poulsen G, Boyd HA, Wohlfahrt J, Jensen PK, Melbye M. Recurrence of congenital heart defects in families. *Circulation.* 2009;120(4):295–301. doi:10.1161/CIRCULATIONAHA.109.857987.
8. National Congenital Heart Disease Audit (NCHDA). 2021 Summary Report. The National Institute for Cardiovascular Outcomes Research (NICOR). Accessed at- https://www.nicor.org.uk/wp-content/uploads/2021/10/NCHDA-Domain-Report_2021_FINAL.pdf.
9. Ewer AK, Middleton LJ, Furmston AT, et al. Pulse oximetry screening for congenital heart defects in newborn infants (PulseOx): a test accuracy study. *Lancet.* 2011;378(9793):785–794. doi:10.1016/S0140-6736(11)60753-8.
10. Ainsworth S, Wyllie JP, Wren C. Prevalence and clinical significance of cardiac murmurs in neonates. *Arch Dis Child Fetal Neonatal Ed.* 1999 Jan;80(1):F43–F45. doi:10.1136/fn.80.1.f43. PMID: 10325811; PMCID: PMC1720873.

11. Lardhi AA. Prevalence and clinical significance of heart murmurs detected in routine neonatal examination. *J Saudi Heart Assoc.* 2010;22(1):25–27. doi:10.1016/j.jsha.2010.03.005.
12. Burd L, Deal E, Rios R, Adickes E, Wynne J, Klug MG. Congenital heart defects and fetal alcohol spectrum disorders. *Congenit Heart Dis.* 2007;2(4):250–255. doi:10.1111/j.1747-0803.2007.00105.x.
13. Lisowski LA, Verheijen PM, Copel JA, et al. Congenital heart disease in pregnancies complicated by maternal diabetes mellitus. An international clinical collaboration, literature review, and meta-analysis. *Herz.* 2010;35(1):19–26. doi:10.1007/s00059-010-3244-3.
14. Patorno E, Huybrechts KF, Bateman BT, et al. Lithium Use in Pregnancy and the Risk of Cardiac Malformations. *N Engl J Med.* 2017;376(23):2245–2254. doi:10.1056/NEJMoa1612222.
15. Hanson CL, Hokanson JS. Etiology of chest pain in children and adolescents referred to cardiology clinic. *WMJ.* 2011;110(2):58–62.
16. Sumski CA, Goot BH. Evaluating Chest Pain and Heart Murmurs in Pediatric and Adolescent Patients. *Pediatr Clin North Am.* 2020;67(5):783–799. doi:10.1016/j.pcl.2020.05.003.
17. Friedman KG, Kane DA, Rathod RH, et al. Management of pediatric chest pain using a standardized assessment and management plan. *Pediatrics.* 2011;128(2):239–245. doi:10.1542/peds.2011-0141.
18. McLeod KA. Syncope in childhood. *Arch Dis Child.* 2003;88(4):350–353. doi:10.1136/adc.88.4.350.
19. Postema PG, De Jong JS, Van der Bilt IA, Wilde AA. Accurate electrocardiographic assessment of the QT interval: teach the tangent. *Heart Rhythm.* 2008;5(7):1015–1018. doi:10.1016/j.hrthm.2008.03.037.
20. Wilde AAM, Amin AS, Postema PG. Diagnosis, management and therapeutic strategies for congenital long QT syndrome. *Heart.* 2022;108(5):332–338. doi:10.1136/heartjnl-2020-318259.
21. Medical mnemonics. https://knowmedge.com/blog/medical-mnemonics-major-and-minor-criteria-for-rheumatic-fever/

ADDITIONAL READING

Geva T, Martins JD, Wald RM. Atrial septal defects. *Lancet.* 2014;383(9932):1921–1932. doi:10.1016/S0140-6736(13)62145-5.

Gray H, Cornish J. Kawasaki disease: a need for earlier diagnosis and treatment. *Arch Dis Child.* 2019;104(7):615–616. doi:10.1136/archdischild-2018-316379.

Kelly A, Sales K, Fenton-Jones M, Tulloh R. Fifteen-minute consultation: Kawasaki disease: how to distinguish from other febrile illnesses: tricks and tips. *Arch Dis Child Educ Pract Ed.* 2020;105(3):152–156. doi:10.1136/archdischild-2019-316834.

McCrindle BW, Rowley AH. Improving coronary artery outcomes for children with Kawasaki disease. *Lancet.* 2019;393(10176):1077–1078. doi:10.1016/S0140-6736(18)33133-7.

Ntovolou AA, Ramesh P, Mikrou P. Evaluation of heart murmurs for the general pediatrician. *Paediatrics and Child Health.* 2020;31(2):85–88. doi:10.1016/j.paed.2020.11.004.

Ommen SR, Semsarian C. Hypertrophic cardiomyopathy: a practical approach to guideline directed management. *Lancet.* 2021;398(10316):2102–2108. doi:10.1016/S0140-6736(21)01205-8.

Uzun O, Kennedy J, Davies C, Goodwin A, Thomas N, Rich D, Thomas A, Tucker D, Beattie B, Lewis MJ. Training: improving antenatal detection and outcomes of congenital heart disease. *BMJ Open Qual.* 2018 Nov 24;7(4):e000276. doi:10.1136/bmjoq-2017-000276. PMID: 30555930; PMCID: PMC6267317.

Veselka J, Anavekar NS, Charron P. Hypertrophic obstructive cardiomyopathy [published correction appears in Lancet. 2017 Mar 25;389(10075):1194]. *Lancet.* 2017;389(10075):1253–1267. doi:10.1016/S0140-6736(16)31321-6.

von Alvensleben JC. Syncope and Palpitations: A Review. *Pediatr Clin North Am.* 2020;67(5):801–810. doi:10.1016/j.pcl.2020.05.004.

Wik G, Jortveit J, Sitras V, Døhlen G, Rønnestad AE, Holmstrøm H. Severe congenital heart defects: incidence, causes and time trends of preoperative mortality in Norway. *Arch Dis Child.* 2020;105(8):738–743. doi:10.1136/archdischild-2019-317581.

11

Fits, Faints and Funny Turns

Amre Shahwan

CHAPTER OUTLINE

BACKGROUND

In this chapter we stress the importance of a focussed history and relevant examination in a child with a suspected seizure and raise awareness of the differential diagnoses of seizures and epilepsy in childhood. Seizures are the most common neurological emergency presentation in children and can be very frightening for observers of seizures, particularly parents and families.

> Whereas approximately 1 in 20 children will experience a seizure, only 1 in 200 have epilepsy.

As in most areas of paediatrics and child health, a thorough, detailed history is essential, as the differential diagnosis of seizure mimics is broad. It is important to stress that events with associated altered level of consciousness or abnormal movements may not represent an epileptic seizure. A number of key seizure mimics will be described in detail.

While it is important to diagnose epilepsy in childhood or adolescence, it is as important to know and diagnose when epilepsy is not the diagnosis. It is actually worse to apply the label of epilepsy incorrectly to a child who does not have epilepsy, as many negative consequences will unfortunately follow. These include committing to antiseizure medication (ASM) long-term, unjustified restriction of certain activities and a negative impact on future job opportunities in life.

Diagnostic Approach – It Is All About the History

A child presenting with an epileptic seizure may be declaring the onset of epilepsy or may merely have an isolated seizure. Ask about a family history of epilepsy as genetic factors are of great importance in childhood epilepsy. If one parent has epilepsy the overall risk of epilepsy in their children is about 4%, and this rises to 10% if both parents are affected.

History is probably the most important tool in diagnosing epilepsy or seizure disorders.

Ask whether the child had prior episodes and the frequency of these episodes.

Find out where the episode occurred and what the child was doing at the time. Ask who witnessed the episode and ask what action, if any, was taken by those in attendance. Make efforts to contact witnesses to get a clear history.

Enquire about seizure onset seeking a history of possible subtle features seen before a larger seizure. These might include a history of witnessed minor features such as head or eyes turning to one side or unilateral limb stiffening or jerking before the more obvious seizure. Visual, auditory, sensory and autonomic, even gastric subjective symptoms expressed by an older child are very important, as they may point to a focal onset of seizures and help classify the seizure clearer. It is important to be aware that not all seizures (for instance, absence seizures) present with jerking movements.

Ask how long the episode lasted and how it ended. The duration and frequency of seizures will undoubtedly influence current and future treatment strategies. Ask about associated incontinence, tongue biting or injury, as the presence of these features supports the diagnosis of a likely epileptic seizure.

Ask about the condition of the child in the post-ictal phase. During the post-ictal phase (the period following an epileptic seizure), confusion, aphasia, a period of sleep or transient unilateral weakness which may last for hours with some of the more prolonged seizures.

When the history is not very clear, families, friends and school (with consent) should be encouraged to capture as many episodes onto smartphone videos as possible to help clarify or pin down the diagnosis.

Video recordings on smart devices taken by a witness (often a family member) are extremely helpful and are often the best diagnostic tool available to confirm or refute the diagnosis of an epileptic seizure.

As much as history is undoubtedly the most important tool when trying to diagnose or classify a seizure disorder or epilepsy type, clinical examination is also important. Uncovering focal neurological abnormalities is extremely important in directing your further approach to performing more specific investigations.

CLINICAL TIPS TO REMEMBER IN COMMON SEIZURE PRESENTATIONS IN CHILDREN

Febrile Seizures

Febrile seizures are the most frequent seizures seen in family practice. They often present as generalised tonic-clonic seizures but can present with more subtle features with minimal jerking and colour change. Febrile seizures are very common (1 in 20), may recur (at least 30% do recur), are usually short-lived under 5 minutes (but can be prolonged up to 15 minutes) and are most often generalised. However, some may exhibit focal features.

It is important to note that children with a diagnosis of epilepsy may have seizures with any intercurrent illness associated with fever.

Blood glucose, urinalysis and urine culture are the only mandatory investigations.

EEG or neuroimaging are *not* indicated unless other neurological concerns arise such as focal neurological signs on examination or other comorbidities raising concern for higher risk for epilepsy such as significant developmental delay, past history or known history of underlying neurological conditions associated with epilepsy.

Febrile seizures as an entity are a *diagnosis of exclusion*. Therefore, you must rule out other causes of seizures with fever, in particular CNS infection such as meningitis or encephalitis (Box 11.1).

SELF-LIMITED EPILEPSY WITH CENTRO-TEMPORAL SPIKES[2,3]

The peak age is 8 to 9 years with 75% of cases occurring between 7 and 10 years of age. Self-limited epilepsy with centro-temporal spikes (SeLECTS) accounts for 15% of all children presenting with seizures. Most are nocturnal or 'coming out of sleep' seizures. Symptoms include a feeling of tingling on one side of the face and mouth involving the tongue and lips with unilateral jerking/twitching of the face, drooling, numbness of the face and mouth with guttural sounds or speech arrest. SeLECTS can sometimes progress to a bilateral convulsive (tonic-clonic) seizure.

BOX 11.1 CLINICAL HISTORY

A Short-Lived Febrile Seizure Causing Widespread Panic in Family Doctor's Surgery

An 18-month-old male presents with an intercurrent viral illness associated with fever. He has no relevant past history, and all his developmental milestones have been met. There is a positive family history of febrile seizures.

He is about to be seen by you as his family doctor when, while in the waiting room, he has jerking involving all four limbs. Pandemonium ensues and he is rushed into your clinic room, and you rightly place him on his side on the examination couch. The episode stops spontaneously after 1 minute. You measure his temperature which is 39°C.

Clinical Pearls

Febrile seizures while benign by nature, are terrifying to watch by parents and carers. Thus, significant reassurance from a confident and calm doctor is required.

Correct positioning to protect the airway is important as is not attempting to place anything into the child's mouth.

With information and guidance, parents are helped to remain calm during what can be a very frightening experience. Supporting them with first aid management advice is very important.

Bringing the temperature down is important for the child's comfort but will not prevent a recurrence. Tepid sponging is no longer recommended.

Pitfalls to Avoid

If very prolonged (e.g. beyond 15 minutes or requiring intervention with rescue drugs to stop) or frequently recurrent with minimal temperatures (below 38°C and with minimal febrile illnesses), Dravet syndrome should be considered where seizures are provoked by warm ambient temperatures, hot baths, fever (often low grade) or vaccinations.[1]

It is important to empower the parents with advice on what to do should this recur at home.

You must request a *sleep-deprived* EEG for the diagnosis of SeLECTS in order to capture a period of sleep where the epileptic activity is activated.

The main differential diagnosis for SeLECTS is nocturnal frontal lobe epilepsy. Frontal lobe seizures are usually more explosive with hypermotor movements (rolling, yelling and fumbling, shuffling around), are usually very brief in duration (few seconds usually) and importantly children are mostly unaware of the seizures and have very little ability to explain or describe any symptoms.

In contrast, with SeLECTS, seizures usually last for a minute or two and awareness is often preserved, and the child is sometimes able to describe the symptoms they experience.

CHILDHOOD ABSENCE EPILEPSY (CAE)

Childhood absence epilepsy (CAE) is common with onset usually between 4 and 10 years of age and peak incidence around 8 years.[1] Seizures are characterised by sudden onset with loss of contact with surroundings, where the child stares blankly and is usually unresponsive. The *seizures are brief*, lasting 5 to 20 seconds.

Typically, seizures occur very frequently with multiple seizures daily before treatment. Oral and manual automatisms may occur including lip smacking, swallowing movements, lip pursing, hand plucking at clothes or clapping. There is no recollection of the event and no post-ictal phase. School performance is adversely affected if CAE is not recognised and treated because of the frequent interruptions caused by the brief seizures.

EEG shows characteristic regular 3 Hz generalised spike-wave activity (Fig. 11.1).

Absence epilepsy is not seen in infants, for example, an infant of 9 months having 'staring episodes' does NOT have absence epilepsy.

Absence seizures are SHORT (seconds) and FREQUENT (multiple daily). Therefore, a child having staring episodes for a minute or two a few times a week does NOT have absence epilepsy.

While in some types of epilepsy, ASM can be withdrawn without a repeat EEG, in CAE, it is important to repeat an EEG *with hyperventilation* before considering withdrawing ASM, as sometimes absence seizures are very subtle and may still be taking place without being obvious to observers at home or in the community.

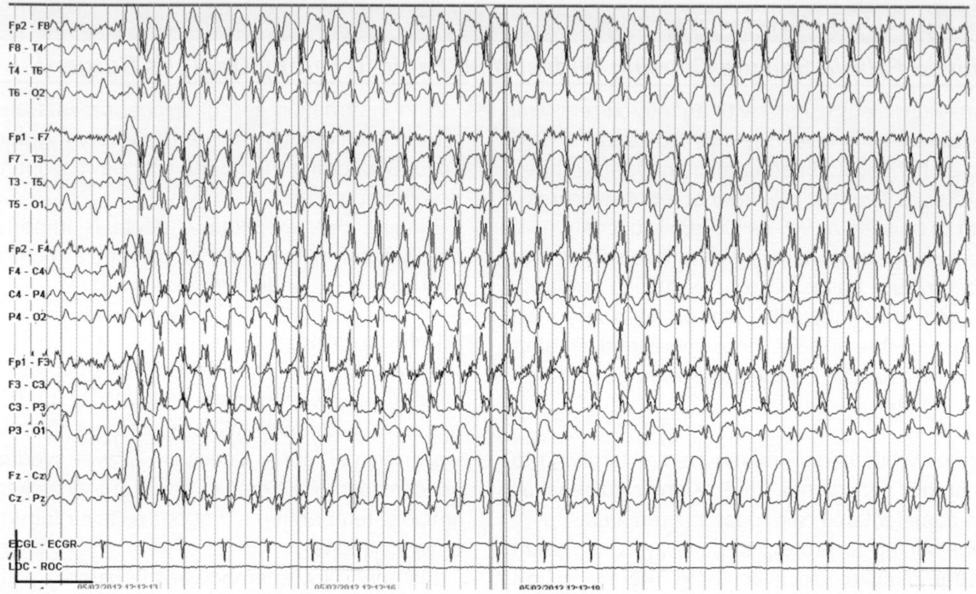

Fig. 11.1 Childhood absence epilepsy – EEG shows characteristic regular 3 Hz generalised spike and wave slow activity.

JUVENILE MYOCLONIC EPILEPSY (JME)

While it is a common feature of juvenile myoclonic epilepsy (JME) to have early morning myoclonus, patients with JME can experience in addition myoclonic seizures, generalised tonic-clonic seizures (GTCS) and occasionally very brief absence seizures.

Most often, the first presentation of JME is a generalised tonic-clonic seizure.

It is important to deliberately ask about morning myoclonus, as it may not be recognised by the parents as such. When asked, parents often comment that the young person (usually 12–18 years of age) has shakiness or clumsiness in the first 2 hours in the morning, perhaps spilling their cereal (the 'flying cornflakes') or dropping their toothbrush.

While in general photosensitive epilepsy is not that common, JME is one of the epilepsy syndromes often associated with photosensitivity (30% of patients). This can be confirmed during EEG testing by flashlight stimulation.

Sodium valproate is the preferred anticonvulsant in JME, but one should avoid using valproate in adolescent females in view of the risk of teratogenicity. Levetiracetam and zonisamide are suitable alternatives.

Seizures are well controlled in the vast majority, but *lifelong treatment* is often required. Carbamazepine and oxcarbazepine are contraindicated (as in CAE) as they can worsen myoclonic jerks.

INFANTILE SPASMS OR INFANTILE EPILEPTIC SPASMS SYNDROME (IESS)

Infantile spasms usually have onset between 4 and 12 months of age. They are characterised by typical movements that tend to be brief, 1 to 2 seconds, but occur in clusters. The infant may appear startled, drop their head and raise their arms as a typical example. Although brief, these movements are repetitive. West syndrome consists of a triad of infantile epileptic spasms, developmental delay or regression and hypsarrhythmia on EEG (Fig. 11.2).

Some parents may feel that infantile spasms may be related to feeding because spasm clusters often take place upon falling asleep or upon wakening times when there is often feeding taking place.

Symptoms such as presumed brief hiccoughs or startle seizures particularly on awakening or falling asleep with an associated developmental regression should prompt a neurology review and EEG (within 3 to 5 days) (Box 11.2).

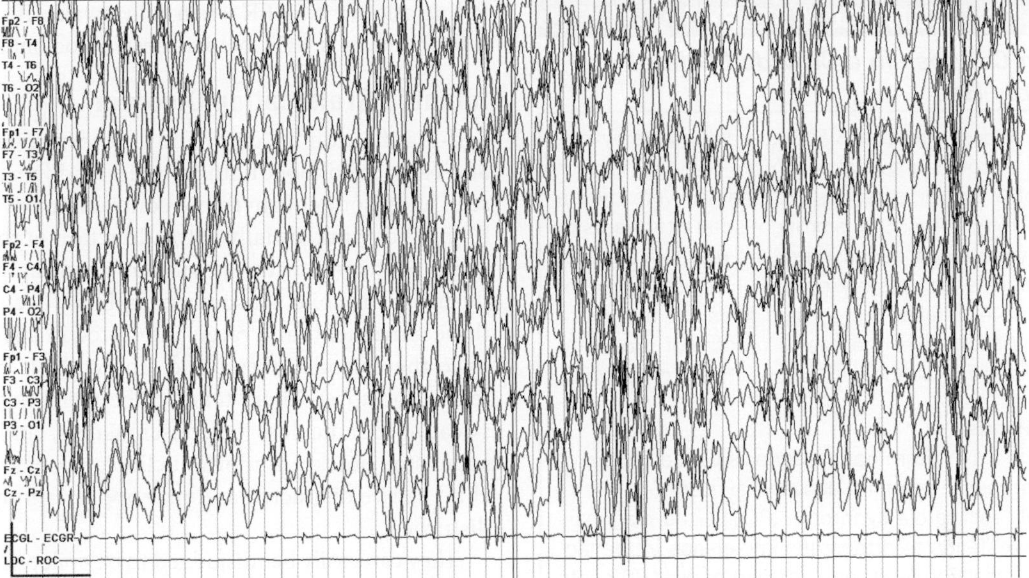

Fig. 11.2 EEG showing a disorganised EEG background overwhelmed with chaotic high amplitude epileptiform discharges.

BOX 11.2 CLINICAL HISTORY

6 Month Old With Clusters of Jerking

A 6-month-old male infant presents with episodes of clusters of repetitive arm and body jerks described as spasms or jolts by the parents. His arms extend and then flex repetitively. His legs sometimes come up to his trunk in the more noticeable spasms. They mainly occur on awakening. He is developmentally delayed and has poor muscle tone.

Clinical Pearls

The key feature that should draw attention to the possibility of the diagnosis of infantile spasms is *clustering*. In a cluster, an infant can have spasms one after the other over a short period of time (usually within 5–20 minutes). Clusters may recur several times a day but may occur only once a day. Spasms are usually seen on falling asleep or upon awakening from sleep.

Pitfalls to Avoid

Diagnostic confusion may occur as the infant may be thought to have infant distress or reflux.

Early referral for EEG and neurology review is important.

NONEPILEPTIC EVENTS WHICH MAY MIMIC EPILEPTIC SEIZURES

Syncope and Faints

The most frequently seen events that may be confused with seizures are simple faints or syncope. Syncope is a transient loss of consciousness usually leading to a fall. Vasovagal syncope is common with up to one in six children and adolescents under 18 years of age experiencing at least one episode. Vasovagal episodes (simple faints) may occur after a long period of standing or when seeing blood or sensing a strong chemical smell in a hospital.

Typical presyncopal symptoms include feeling faint, nausea, dizziness or feeling hot or being cold or sweaty. Mild syncope is associated with rapid recovery in under a minute.

In classical vasovagal syncope, there is a drop in blood pressure and bradycardia. Episodes occur when tired, hungry, stressed, unwell or feeling crowded (Box 11.3).

In terms of managing frequent episodes of vasovagal syncope, increasing fluid and dietary salt intake are relatively simple steps that may help reduce the frequency of episodes. Occasionally fludrocortisone is helpful if the above measures are unsuccessful.

BOX 11.3 CLINICAL HISTORY

Sudden Collapse in a Crowded School Assembly Hall

A 14-year-old girl appears very pale and suddenly collapses in a crowded school assembly. She has no prior history of a similar episode, and she recovers over a period of 15 minutes. She is brought soon afterwards to her family doctor for assessment and reassurance. Her examination is completely normal. Her astute doctor takes a more detailed history and finds out that there is a prior history over the past 3 months of moderate chronic disabling fatigue with frequent days off school.

Clinical Pearls

Syncope is a symptom not a diagnosis per se but by far the commonest reason is vasovagal syncope.

Postural tachycardia syndrome (POTS), the diagnosis in this case, leads to orthostatic intolerance in teenagers and typically a heart rate increase of over 30 beats per minute on standing.

Pitfalls to Avoid

Severe syncope may be associated with extensor spasms of the limbs, urinary incontinence and postepisode confusion. This is as a result of an anoxic seizure relating to the episode of syncope.

Syncope that takes place during exercise, while swimming, during sleep or upon awakening may be due to long Q-T syndromes. An ECG is thus required with assessment of the Q-T interval.

Benign Sleep Myoclonus in Early Infancy

This is relatively common and benign, often with an onset in the first few weeks of life. Myoclonic jerking of the limbs occurs in clusters exclusively while the infant is asleep. Rhythmical brief jerks of the limbs, generalised or focal, occur in brief or prolonged clusters, which could last minutes. The trunk and the face are usually not involved. The jerks cease on wakening and can be induced by rocking the crib while a baby is asleep. Sleep myoclonus resolves by 3 to 4 months of age. No investigations are required.

Obtain a smartphone video of the jerks and share with a neurologist who should be able to confirm the diagnosis.

An EEG should *not* be requested unless there is clinical uncertainty.

The MOST important feature of sleep myoclonus is its occurrence exclusively in sleep (including drowsiness/falling asleep). NEVER when fully awake. If seen when fully awake, it is NOT benign sleep myoclonus.

Infantile Gratification Disorder

Self-gratification is commonly observed in infancy and early childhood, both in males and females and is seen as episodes of rhythmic contractions of the lower limbs and trunk, usually with adduction of thighs with some posturing, with or without grunting and facial flushing. The child is usually completely occupied with these movements and rarely interested in anything else once the episode takes place. The child is never distressed or upset. There tends to be facial flushing and sweating but no loss of consciousness, and the episodes stop quickly. Important clinical clues are that the child can be distracted and may appear annoyed when disturbed.

They can easily be misjudged to be epileptic in nature to the inexperienced eye. Home smartphone videos are very helpful, and no investigation or treatment is required.

These episodes are purely behavioural and do not have any long-term implications.

Breath-Holding Spells

Breath-holding spells are very common especially in preschool children. The classical story is of a preceding physical or emotional provocation with first a cry followed by a brief pause resulting in a blue or pale colour change.

Breath-holding episodes are ALWAYS provoked.

Blue breath-holding spells are preceded by the child vigorously crying due to frustration, anger or pain, followed by holding their breath in expiration. The child stops breathing, becomes cyanotic, loses consciousness and becomes limp, and may experience a brief convulsion towards the end in the more extreme cases. There is quick recovery. Diagnosis is based on the history. Correction of associated iron deficiency anaemia helps reduce the frequency of recurrences.

Reflex Anoxic Seizures

These occur most often in the second year of life and may be precipitated by an unexpected bump to the head or a fall. Typically, the child will suddenly fall to the ground following a painful stimulus or shock, and they are often deadly white in colour. They may have body stiffening, limb jerking and eye deviation. The episode generally resolves within a minute.

Night Terrors

Night terrors are often familial, most commonly seen between 3 and 8 years of age.[4] They tend to happen during non-REM sleep early in the night. In a typical episode the child wakes up, suddenly screams while sitting in bed terrified, often crying and wide-eyed and often described as out of contact with surroundings. They appear quite frightened and often have profuse sweating.[5] Any attempts to wake the child up or bring them out of the episode are ineffective. They can last for minutes, then they go back to sleep. These episodes do not cause the child any harm despite the dramatic and 'scary' situation experienced by those witnessing the child and probably the fearful sensation the child may very well have during the episode. The child has no recollection of the event, and this distinguishes night terror from nightmares. This is considered to be a sleep disorder seen in toddlers and preschool children.

If you can pin down the specific time when night terrors take place, trying to wake the child some minutes before (maybe 20 minutes before the expected time) may help abort the occurrence of these episodes.

No investigations are generally required. Video EEG or telemetry may very rarely be required to differentiate night terrors from frontal lobe seizures.

Attempting to wake the child during a night terror is not advised, as this may aggravate the child further and add to their agitation.

Tics

Tics affect about one in five children with typical age of onset being 4 to 8 years of age. Eye blinking, facial grimacing and shoulder shrugging are the most frequently seen motor tics. Frequent vocal tics may include repeated throat clearing, coughing or sniffing. Tics are made worse by anxiety or stress and tend to disappear during sleep. Many have comorbidity including attention hyperactivity disorder or learning disability.

In more established tic disorders (such as Tourette's syndrome), vocal tics such as throat clearing and coprolalia may be very pronounced, making the diagnosis much easier.

Daydreaming

Daydreaming is very common but confusion with absence seizures may prompt referral. During a daydreaming episode, a clue to the diagnosis is that it is possible to interrupt them by touch or tickle, and episodes tend not to occur during interesting activities.[4]

Daydreaming must be distinguished from absence epilepsy.

With daydreaming, only a few episodes occur per day, and each episode may last many seconds to minutes. They are, of course, not induced by hyperventilation.

Migraine

Migraine variants may present with transient ophthalmoplegia or hemiplegia and therefore can be confused with seizures.

The aura in migraine is quite typical with linear or zigzag patterns in colour or black and white. The main overlap or confusion is seen with migraine versus occipital lobe epilepsy with visual phenomena.

When visual loss or visual phenomena occur transiently in occipital epilepsy, it tends to be very brief and unilateral, respecting the anatomical boundaries of the visual field corresponding to where seizures arise. Visual loss is also very brief.

Nonepileptic Attacks or Dissociative Seizures

These were formerly termed pseudoseizures, but this term is regarded as pejorative and is no longer used. They are seen mostly in adolescents but can occur (albeit rarer) in children as young as 5 years old. They are often misjudged as epileptic seizures. Attacks vary from very hypermotor or hyperkinetic erratic movements (trashing around!), nonrhythmic jerking to quieter episodes of more prolonged unresponsiveness or loss of contact with surroundings (Box 11.4).

BOX 11.4 CLINICAL HISTORY

A Girl With Frequent 'Seizures' and Admissions to Hospital

A 16-year-old girl presents with apparent seizure episodes while at school where she collapses and either lies motionless and unresponsive for over 15 minutes or has thrashing movements with side-to-side movements of her head. Invariably an ambulance is called, and she has now been admitted on six occasions over the past year to her local paediatric inpatient service. On two occasions she required further transfer to a tertiary hospital for paediatric intensive care (PICU).

She is commenced on a number of anticonvulsants but, despite apparent excellent compliance, the episodes continue to recur.

After her second admission to PICU, she undergoes video electroencephalographic monitoring, and after that a diagnosis of nonepileptic seizures is made. She is weaned off anticonvulsants over time. The diagnosis was explained to her and her parents, and cognitive behaviour therapy lead to a cessation of episodes some 6 months later.

Clinical Pearls

It is estimated that up to 20% of children and young people attending specialist services for apparent intractable epilepsy do not have epilepsy.

Helpful clinical clues indicating nonepileptic seizures include long duration of either complete stillness or nonrhythmic erratic thrashing movements, side-to-side head movements and tight eye closure during the episode.

Pitfalls to Avoid

Clues on examination include response to verbal requests, preserved corneal reflexes, responsive pupils and resistance to opening of the eyes if they are closed.[6]

These can be tricky to diagnose and video EEG recording may be required. A home smartphone video, nonetheless, is often sufficient for an experienced paediatric neurologist to diagnose with a high level of confidence.

KEY LEARNING POINTS

History is all important. Find out where the episode occurred and what the child was doing at the time. Ask who witnessed the episode and ask what action, if any, was taken by those in attendance.

Febrile seizures are very common (1 in 20), may recur (at least 30% do recur), are usually short-lived under 5 minutes (but can be prolonged up to 15 minutes) and are most often generalised.

Febrile seizures as an entity are a diagnosis of exclusion.

You must request a sleep-deprived EEG for the diagnosis of SeLECTS in order to capture a period of sleep where the epileptic activity is activated.

Typically, absence seizures occur with multiple very brief seizures daily, sometimes tens of seizures daily before treatment. Oral and manual automatisms may occur including lip smacking, swallowing movements, lip pursing, hand plucking at clothes or clapping.

Most often, the first presentation of juvenile myoclonic epilepsy (JME) is a generalised tonic-clonic seizure. It is important to deliberately ask about morning myoclonus, as it is not habitually recognised by the parents as such.

Infantile spasms usually have onset between 4 and 12 months of age. They are characterised by typical movements that tend to be brief, 1 to 2 seconds, but occur in clusters.

The most frequently seen events that may be confused with seizures are simple faints or syncope.

In benign sleep myoclonus, jerking of the limbs occurs in clusters exclusively while the infant is asleep. Rhythmical brief jerks of the limbs, generalised or focal, occur in brief or prolonged clusters, which could last minutes.

In infantile gratification disorder, the child is usually completely occupied with these movements and rarely interested in anything else once the episode takes place.

Breath-holding episodes are always provoked.

Night terrors are often familial, most commonly seen between 3 and 8 years of age. They occur during non-REM sleep.

Tics affect about one in five children with typical age of onset being 4 to 8 years of age.

With daydreaming, only a few episodes occur per day, and each episode may last many seconds to minutes.

Dissociative or nonepileptic seizures vary from very hypermotor or hyperkinetic erratic movements (thrashing around!), nonrhythmic jerking to quieter episodes of more prolonged unresponsiveness or loss of contact with surroundings. Clues on examination include response to verbal requests, preserved corneal reflexes, resistance to the opening of the eyes if closed and normally reactive pupils.

REFERENCES

1. Monrad P. Paroxysmal Disorders. In: Kleigman RM, Lye PS, Bordini B, Toth H, Basel D, eds. *Nelson Pediatric Symptom-Based Diagnosis*. Philadelphia: Elsevier; 2018:508–542.
2. Scheffer IE, Berkovic S, Capovilla G, et al. ILAE classification of the epilepsies: Position paper of the ILAE Commission for Classification and Terminology. *Epilepsia*. 2017;58(4):512–521. doi:10.1111/epi.13709.
3. Specchio N, Wirrell EC, Scheffer IE, et al. International League Against Epilepsy classification and definition of epilepsy syndromes with onset in childhood: Position paper by the ILAE Task Force on Nosology and Definitions. *Epilepsia*. 2022;63(6):1398–1442. doi:10.1111/epi.17241.
4. Bruni O, DelRosso LM, Melegari MG, Ferri R. The Parasomnias. *Child Adolesc Psychiatr Clin N Am*. 2021;30(1):131–142. doi:10.1016/j.chc.2020.08.007.
5. Prasad M, Babiker MO. Fifteen-minute consultation: when is a seizure not a seizure? Part 1, the younger child. *Arch Dis Child Educ Pract Ed*. 2016;101(1):15–20. doi:10.1136/archdischild-2015-308342.
6. Babiker MO, Prasad M. Fifteen-minute consultation: when is a seizure not a seizure? Part 2, the older child. *Arch Dis Child Educ Pract Ed*. 2015;100(6):295–300. doi:10.1136/archdischild-2015-308343.

ADDITIONAL READING

Agarwal M, Fox SM. Pediatric seizures. *Emerg Med Clin North Am*. 2013;31(3):733–754. doi:10.1016/j.emc.2013.04.001.

Berkovic SF. Epileptic encephalopathies of infancy: welcome advances. *Lancet*. 2019;394(10216):2203–2204. doi:10.1016/S0140-6736(19)31239-5.

Howell KB, Eggers S, Dalziel K, et al. A population-based cost-effectiveness study of early genetic testing in severe epilepsies of infancy. *Epilepsia*. 2018;59(6):1177–1187. doi:10.1111/epi.14087.

International League Against Epilepsy (ILAE) Classification of Epilepsies 2017. Available at: www.ilae.org or www.epilepsy.com.

Sullo F, Venti V, Catania R, et al. Non-Epileptic Paroxysmal Events: Clinical features and diagnostic differences with epileptic seizures. A Single Tertiary Centre Study. *Clin Neurol Neurosurg*. 2021;207:106739. doi:10.1016/j.clineuro.2021.106739.

12

Presentations of Endocrine Disease

Niamh McGrath

CHAPTER OUTLINE

In this chapter, we are going to focus on important endocrine conditions seen in childhood. Making the diagnosis of diabetes mellitus especially in children under the age of 5 can be particularly challenging and such children may present late with diabetic ketoacidosis.

Acquired hypothyroidism is relatively common in childhood and may present with a falloff in growth velocity. Another challenging diagnosis and a cause of short stature in girls is Turner's syndrome.

We know that, in the modern world, simple obesity is very common, but one should always be aware of children with obesity and short stature, where Cushing's syndrome needs to be considered.

Finally, we focus on adrenal insufficiency, whether it be a newborn with congenital adrenal hyperplasia (CAH) or an older child with adrenal insufficiency.

> Adrenal insufficiency is potentially life-threatening and so diagnosis and appropriate treatment are essential.

DIABETIC KETOACIDOSIS

The incidence of type 1 diabetes mellitus is increasing especially in younger children where the diagnosis can be more challenging.[1]

> Always consider and out rule diabetes in unwell toddlers and young children.

Secondary nocturnal enuresis is a common presenting symptom. Differential diagnoses also include urinary tract infection, appendicitis (diabetic ketoacidosis (DKA) may present with abdominal pain) and pneumonia (with rapid respirations) whereas, in DKA, Kussmaul's respiration is evident.

Diabetes mellitus is defined as either a random blood glucose over 11.1 mmol/L or a fasting blood glucose over 7.0 mmol/L. HbA1c levels are used to evaluate glycaemic control over the preceding 2 or 3 months and the aim is to keep HbA1c levels below 7.0% (53 mmols).

> Twenty-five percent of newly diagnosed children or adolescents with diabetes present in DKA, with a higher percentage of toddlers and younger children presenting with severe DKA at first presentation.

Most have a short history of classical symptoms (fatigue, weight loss, polydipsia and polyuria) but if the osmotic symptoms are unrecognised the first presentation may be with DKA. Symptoms in young children are often nonspecific due to their inability to articulate thirst and the fact that they are not toilet trained (Box 12.1).

BOX 12.1 **CLINICAL HISTORY**

Diabetic Ketoacidosis

A 2-year-old boy is referred by his family doctor to the paediatric emergency department with abdominal pain and vomiting for one day and a presumed diagnosis of appendicitis. The paediatric nurse who triaged the child notes a baseline tachycardia of 140 bpm and a raised respiratory rate of 40 bpm with deep sighing breaths. After consultation, a finger prick glucose and ketones are immediately performed which confirm a high glucose level of 23 mmol/L (normal 3.5–5.5) and an elevated ketone level of 5.2 mmol/L.

On direct questioning, the family confirm a throat infection three weeks previously and a one-week history of tiredness, excessive thirst, and urination with a 1 kg weight loss. His family history is negative for diabetes mellitus but there is a positive family history of coeliac disease.

Clinical Pearls

Firstly, consider the diagnosis of diabetes in any unwell child and perform point-of-care blood glucose and ketone testing with urinalysis. Delayed diagnosis means the child becomes more ill with progression to DKA.

There can be considerable diagnostic confusion in younger children with DKA who may present like an acute abdomen (as in this case) or pneumonia where the raised respiratory rate of acidosis can be misinterpreted as infection.

Pitfalls to Avoid

Cerebral oedema is **A LIFE-THREATENING EMERGENCY.** Its occurrence is more likely in younger children, during the first presentation, if severe dehydration or acidosis is present and with a longer duration of symptoms. Warning signs of idiopathic cerebral oedema include a slowing of the heart rate, a headache or change in neurological status (irritability, restlessness or increasing drowsiness), and if the child's blood pressure (BP) is starting to rise, mannitol or hypertonic saline should be available for immediate treatment.

About 0.3% to 1.0% of DKA episodes are complicated by cerebral oedema and the mortality from cerebral oedema is 20% to 25%.[1–5]

Delay in diagnosis is the leading cause of DKA for young children whereas omission of insulin is the leading cause amongst adolescents.

Point-of-care blood glucose or urinalysis allows the diagnosis to be made in most instances without delay. Refer all children with an elevated blood glucose for hospital treatment on *the same day* they present to primary care.

ACQUIRED HYPOTHYROIDISM

Acquired hypothyroidism is usually due to autoimmune thyroiditis with an increased prevalence in children with Down syndrome, diabetes mellitus, coeliac disease and Turner's syndrome.[6] Acquired hypothyroidism tends to present in older children and adolescents. The most common presentation is with a falloff in growth velocity. Other features include a goitre, coarse features and relative obesity (Fig. 12.1).

Suspect acquired hypothyroidism in any short child with a significant fall off in growth velocity and request basic investigations including Free T4, thyroid stimulating hormone (TSH) and thyroid autoantibodies and a left wrist X-ray for bone age.

The bone age is often significantly delayed. Blood tests in acquired hypothyroidism show an elevated TSH and a low or normal thyroxine (Free T4) level. Positive peroxidase and thyroglobulin antibodies are seen in autoimmune thyroiditis (Box 12.2).

SHORT STATURE AND A DELAYED PUBERTY IN A GIRL

Turner's syndrome is relatively common (1 in 2500) and is due to either an abnormality or absence of an X chromosome. In addition to short stature and ovarian failure, other features include neck webbing, a low posterior hairline, lymphoedema in newborns, wide carrying angles of the arms, renal and cardiac abnormalities (most especially coarctation of the aorta) (Figs. 12.2 and 12.3).

The mechanism of short stature in Turner's syndrome (45X0) is multifactorial but absence of one copy of the short stature homeobox gene (SHOX) is believed to play a major role.

Turner's syndrome in girls may be very difficult to diagnose until a falloff in growth velocity occurs or puberty is delayed.

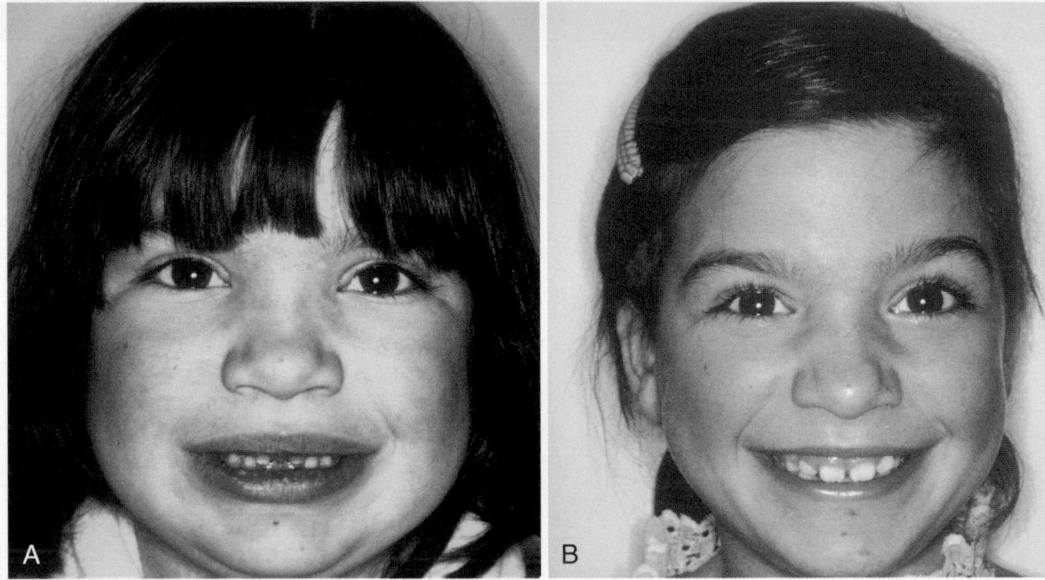

Fig. 12.1 Hypothyroidism. (A) The facial appearance of this 9-year-old child is due to the accumulation of tissue oedema secondary to severe hypothyroidism. (B) Same patient after 1 year of thyroid hormone replacement therapy. Note the eruption of the maxillary permanent teeth. (Source: *Oral and Maxillofacial Pathology*. 4th ed. 2016.)

BOX 12.2 **CLINICAL HISTORY**

A 10 Year Old With Vague Symptoms and a Falloff in Height

A 10-year-old girl presents with vague symptoms of loss of energy, fatigue, cold intolerance and dry skin over a three-month period. She has had a noted fall off in growth velocity over the past six months and her mother stated that her height had hardly changed at all during that period. You have no accurate measurements of prior heights, but she is on the 10th percentile for height once measured.

There is a family history of hypothyroidism. Her blood investigations show a low free T4 and high thyroid stimulating hormone (TSH) of 200 mU/L. Her thyroid peroxidase and antithyroglobulin antibodies are both positive confirming autoimmune thyroiditis as the diagnosis.

Clinical Pearls

Hypothyroidism is associated with often vague symptoms in childhood. Most cases are autoimmune in nature and may be linked to other autoimmune disorders.

Treatment is with daily L-thyroxine (on an empty stomach) and the goal of treatment is to maintain the TSH and free T4 levels in the normal range.

Pitfalls to Avoid

Always consider acquired hypothyroidism when there is a falloff in growth velocity.

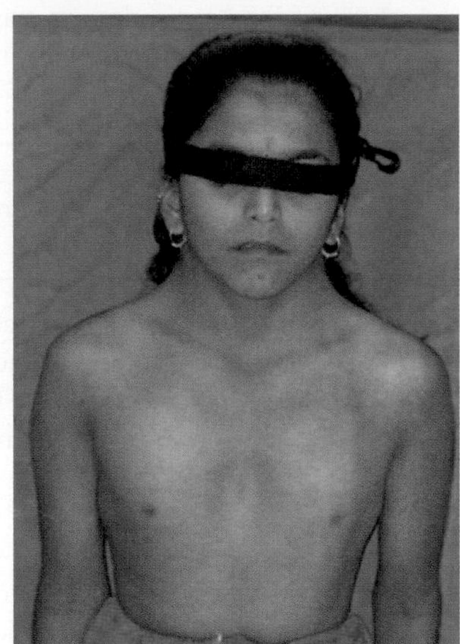

Fig. 12.2 Turner's syndrome case showing short stature and webbed neck. (From Gangane SD. *Human Genetics*. 6th ed. Elsevier; 2023.)

A karyotype should be performed in all girls with short stature and suboptimal growth velocity, in particular, if they are short for their mid-parental height (Box 12.3).

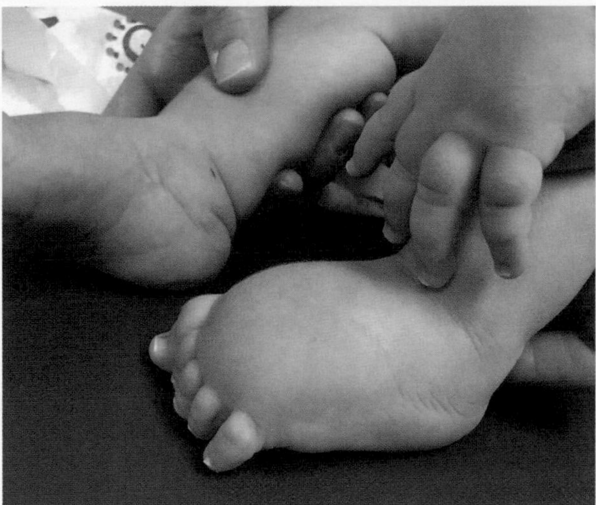

Fig. 12.3 Lymphedema associated with Turner's syndrome. (Source: Micheletti RG, et al. *Andrews' Diseases of the Skin Clinical Atlas*. 2nd ed. Elsevier; 2023.)

BOX 12.3 **CLINICAL HISTORY**

A Very Short Girl Who Has Pubertal Delay

A 14-year-old girl presented with pubertal delay. She was a full-term normal delivery with no pregnancy or perinatal complications. A cardiac murmur was noted at 15 months of age prompting paediatric referral from the community.

The cardiac murmur noted was assessed by a paediatric cardiologist who did perform a detailed examination and an echocardiogram which showed evidence of very mild aortic stenosis and a further cardiac review 2 years later was arranged.

Thereafter, she was reviewed at OPD on a six-monthly basis and, in accordance with best practice, height and weight measurements were performed on each occasion. Throughout her childhood years, her height was between the 9th and 25th centiles.

Subsequent annual outpatient appointments at the general paediatric OPD showed a slowing of growth velocity and delayed puberty.

In view of delayed puberty and primary amenorrhoea referral to a paediatric endocrinologist took place. Delayed pubertal development and almond-shaped eyes with a wide carrying angle were noted. FSH, LH and oestradiol and a karyotype were requested, and the LH and FSH were markedly elevated with a low oestradiol indicating primary ovarian failure. A pelvic ultrasound was requested, and the karyotype showed 45/46XX (SRY gene positive) and a diagnosis of Turner's syndrome was made. She was commenced on growth hormone therapy and ethinyloestradiol and, in view of the risk of gonadoblastoma, a bilateral oophorectomy was performed as a preventive measure.

Clinical Pearls

Short stature may be the sole finding in some girls with Turner's syndrome especially those who have chromosomal mosaicism.

Pitfalls to Avoid

In a child who is short and has symptoms of headaches, vomiting or visual disturbance consider craniopharyngioma as a possible diagnosis.

Crohn's disease and coeliac disease can also present with short stature and pubertal delay.

Hypochondroplasia is an allelic variant of achondroplasia that may manifest as short stature with less striking dysmorphic features. Again, a diagnosis that can be missed.

OBESITY AND SHORT STATURE

The rising incidence of obesity in children is starting to plateau in high-income countries (especially in northern Europe) but it is accelerating in Asia and Africa in line with marketing of unhealthy food, reduced physical activity and increased urbanisation.[7]

Growth hormone deficiency, Cushing's syndrome and hypothyroidism are all associated with obesity, but the distinguishing feature is a slowing of linear growth and consequent short stature.[7]

Cushing's syndrome can be a challenging diagnosis to make (Box 12.4). Always consider an endocrine cause of obesity if there is additional short stature (Fig. 12.4).

ADRENAL INSUFFICIENCY

Addison's disease is characterised by autoimmune destruction of the adrenal cortex. Addison's disease may occur in combination with other autoimmune conditions such as type 1 diabetes mellitus, hypothyroidism and premature ovarian insufficiency. The familial risk of Addison's disease is similar to the increased familial risk if one member of the family has coeliac disease.

Fatigue and lethargy are prominent features. A history of salt craving and a finding of orthostatic hypotension are often seen.

BOX 12.4 **CLINICAL HISTORY**

A 12 Year Old Who Is Both Short and Obese

A 12-year-old girl presents with obesity affecting the trunk, plethoric facies, purple striae and easy bruisability. She had difficulty climbing stairs and had apparent weakness of her muscles with a reduced muscle bulk. Her mother noted that she had some degree of hirsutism and she also developed acne. She is noted to be short and to be hypertensive on examination. She was admitted to hospital for investigation and a diagnosis of Cushing syndrome was made following an overnight dexamethasone suppression test.

Clinical Pearls

Cushing's syndrome needs to be distinguished from simple obesity.

Diagnosis is based on a high free cortisol on a 24-hour urine sample (never an easy task) or an overnight dexamethasone suppression test.

Pitfalls to Avoid

Clinical features not to miss include short stature, acne, virilisation, plethoric facies, hypertension, a buffalo hump and large purple striae.

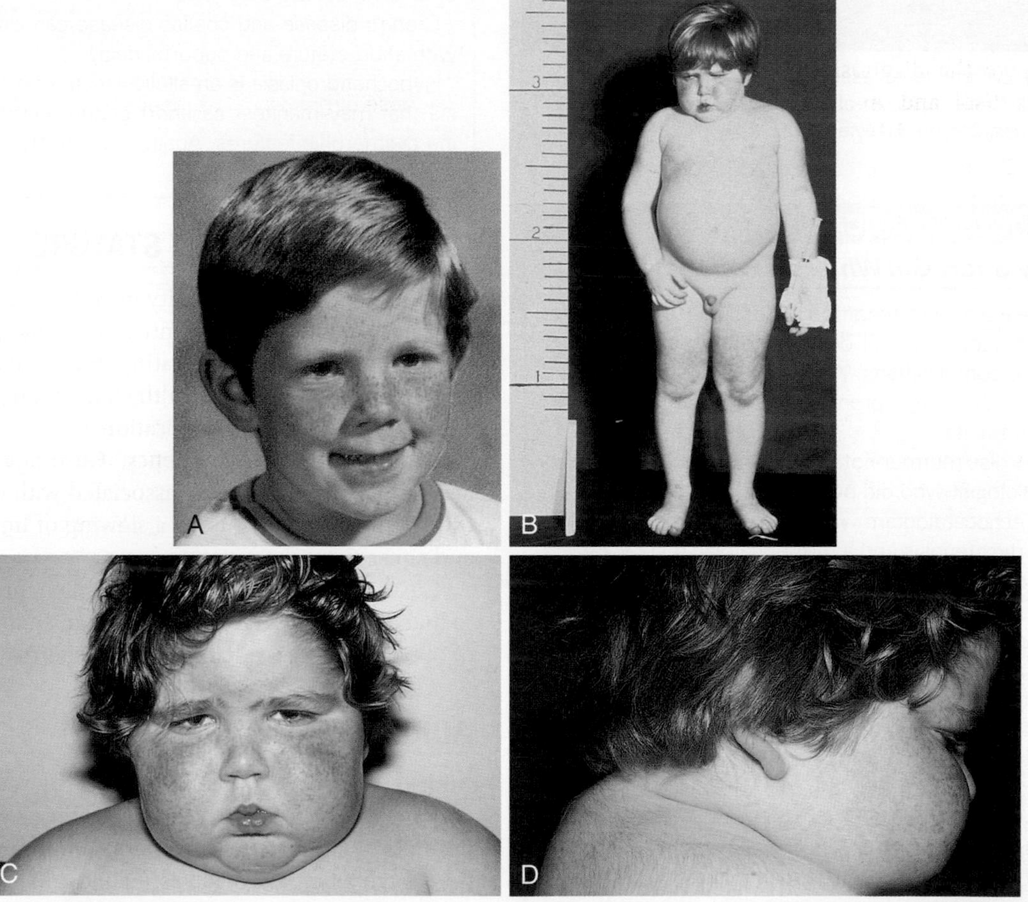

Fig. 12.4 Cushing's syndrome. These photographs show how dramatic the changes associated with Cushing's syndrome are and how rapidly they occur. (A) Patient before the onset of Cushing's syndrome. (B) Patient 4 months after photograph in (A) was taken. Note the centripetal obesity of the trunk compared with the extremities after the onset of Cushing's syndrome. (C) Moon facies, clearly demonstrated, should raise the diagnostic index of Cushing's syndrome. (D) Buffalo hump. Excessive adipose tissue over the lower cervical and upper thoracic spine is characteristic of Cushing's syndrome. (Source: Zitelli BJ, McIntire SC, Nowalk AJ, Garrison J, eds. *Zitelli and Davis' Atlas of Pediatric Physical Diagnosis*. Elsevier; 2018.)

Addison's disease typically has an insidious onset and vague symptoms such as weight loss, nausea, abdominal pain, joint pains and myalgia are seen.

Increased pigmentation of the skin and mucous membranes is a key feature.[8] This pigmentation is particularly evident in skin areas exposed to sunlight and areas of skin exposed to friction such as the elbows, knuckles and palmar creases (Fig. 12.5).

Another clue is the presence of associated conditions. Half of those with primary adrenal insufficiency have either Hashimoto's thyroiditis or Graves' disease and, in Scandinavia, 10% to 15% have coincident type 1 diabetes mellitus.[9] Low bone mineral density in Addison's may lead to osteoporosis and fractures.

To make the diagnosis request an early morning serum cortisol and ACTH. In adrenocortical insufficiency, the cortisol level will be low, and the ACTH level will be double the upper reference range. Positive adrenal autoantibodies will confirm the diagnosis of Addison's.

The key emergency to be aware of is acute adrenal crisis which is life threatening and requires immediate diagnosis and treatment.[7]

The most common precipitants of acute adrenal crisis are either gastroenteritis or food poisoning, but an adrenal crisis may follow other infections, surgery, dental procedures or poor compliance with treatment.

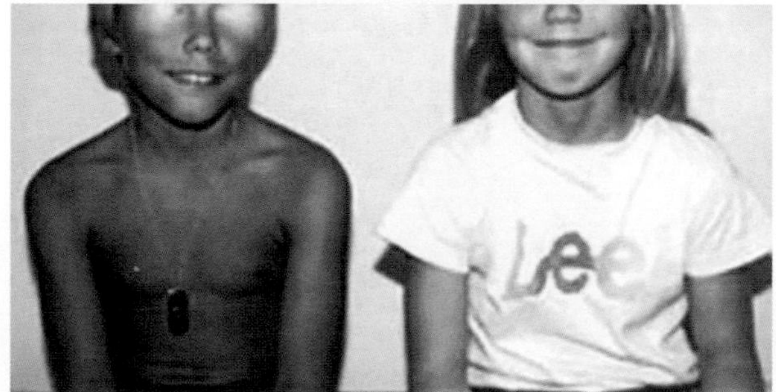

Fig. 12.5 A boy with Addison's disease, pictured with his sister, showing the diffuse hyperpigmentation typical of the disorder. (Source: *Pediatric Endocrinology: The Requisites in Pediatrics.* 1st ed. 2005.)

Acute adrenal crisis presents with nausea and vomiting, abdominal pain, marked malaise, headache, muscle cramps and evident dehydration.[10,11] Unrecognised, symptoms may progress to hypotension and shock, hypoglycaemia, confusion and later loss of consciousness (Box 12.5).

X-linked adrenoleukodystrophy (XLA) should be considered as a differential diagnosis for Addison's disease in young males even if neurological symptoms are not obvious at initial examination. Characteristically, in XLA there is an elevation of very long-chain fatty acids (VLCFA).

If in acute adrenal crisis, manage with intravenous saline, intravenous glucose and intravenous hydrocortisone. Long-term treatment is with both glucocorticoid and mineralocorticoid replacement.[12]

The dose of glucocorticoid needs to be trebled in times of acute illness and intravenous stress doses need to be given for general anaesthesia and surgery.

Patients and their families are taught how to inject intramuscular hydrocortisone in an emergency.

In treating adrenal insufficiency, hydrocortisone is the preferred medication, and a paediatric granulation formulation of hydrocortisone is now available in some countries.

Primary adrenal insufficiency is a very challenging diagnosis to make in family practice as the symptoms are relatively nonspecific and onset is often insidious. Be extra vigilant in situations where there is a family history of autoimmune primary adrenal insufficiency or in children who present with other autoimmune conditions.

Sick day rules state that during an intercurrent infection or gastroenteritis, triple the dose of hydrocortisone over a 24-hour period. Increases should also occur prior to procedures or surgery.

Once adrenal insufficiency is suspected (and that is the hard part), it is relatively easy to confirm or refute the diagnosis.

CONGENITAL ADRENAL HYPERPLASIA (CAH)

The vast majority of CAH cases are due to 21-hydroxylase (21-OH) deficiency.[13] Characteristic features include impaired cortisol and aldosterone production and androgen excess. Girls with classical CAH typically

BOX 12.5 CLINICAL HISTORY

A 10 Year Old With Unexplained Hypoglycaemia

A 10-year-old girl 'fainted' while out shopping with her parents. She was drowsy and difficult to rouse. An emergency ambulance was called, and she was taken to the local paediatric emergency department. On arrival her blood glucose was 0.8 mmol/L. She was given a bolus of 10% dextrose. She recovered quickly. She was observed in hospital overnight. Her 4-hourly blood glucose levels were all above 4 mmol/L. She was discharged later that day.

Three months later, in the early hours of the morning, she was found unconscious in bed by her parents. An emergency ambulance was called. The paramedical team found her blood glucose was 0.2 mmol/L and intravenous 10% dextrose was administered. She remained unconscious. Following arrival at the hospital she was still hypoglycaemic (glucose 2.0 mm/L) and had diagnostic endocrine tests for hypoglycaemia taken using the hypoglycaemia kit[14] (blood glucose, free fatty acids, insulin, C-peptide, beta OH butyrate, cortisol, lactate and blood gas).[15–17] Urine was sent for ketones and organic acids. She was given dextrose, intubated, ventilated and transferred to the PICU. Following an endocrinology workup, a diagnosis of Addison's disease was made.

Clinical Pearls

The key symptoms are unexplained weight loss, marked fatigue and lethargy and the key physical signs are postural hypotension and increased pigmentation.

The pigmentation of the skin is characteristically on the sun-exposed areas and areas exposed to friction, especially the palms and knuckles. If present, blue-black hyperpigmentation of the oral mucosa and tongue should raise the suspicion of Addison's disease.

Pitfalls to Avoid

Addison's disease in childhood is a very challenging diagnosis to make due to the nonspecific symptoms and its often-insidious onset.

Unexplained hyponatraemia or hypoglycaemia should always trigger the consideration of adrenal insufficiency.

In infants or children with unexplained hypoglycaemia, an essential diagnostic sample (includes serum cortisol measurement) should be taken at the time of presentation prior to glucose administration.

present with ambiguous genitalia at birth (Fig. 12.6), whereas boys have normal genitalia and may present with a salt-wasting crisis in early infancy.

Clinically, infants and children with 11βOH have hypertension rather than salt loss.

A 17-hydroxyprogesterone concentration above 30 nmol/L is diagnostic for 21-OH deficiency.

Children with CAH should receive hydrocortisone and, in salt-wasting forms of CAH, fludrocortisone daily. Encourage salt intake during hot weather conditions and consider seasonal adjustment of the fludrocortisone dose in countries with very hot summers.[13]

Give hydrocortisone by intramuscular, subcutaneous or intravenous routes if oral intake is not possible. Children with CAH should wear an emergency bracelet, receive education about sick day rules and have access to an emergency hydrocortisone kit (Box 12.6).

The classical biochemical features of acute adrenal crisis are hyponatraemia, hyperkalaemia and hypoglycaemia.

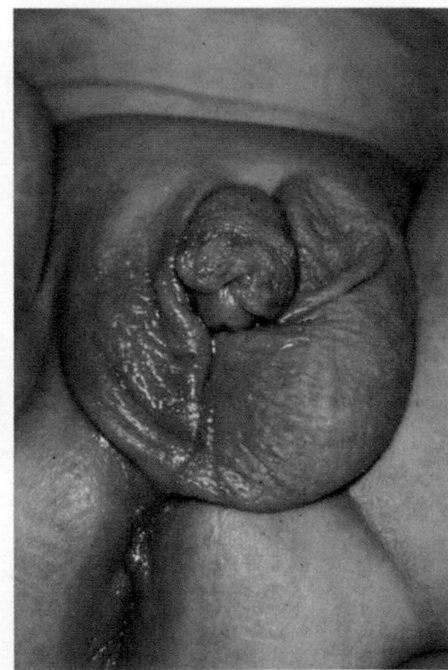

Fig. 12.6 Virilised external genitalia in a female infant with congenital adrenal hyperplasia caused by 21-hydroxylase deficiency. No gonads are present in the scrotum. (Crow, MK. *Goldman-Cecil Medicine*. 2nd ed. Elsevier; 2020.)

BOX 12.6 CLINICAL HISTORY

An Acutely Ill Child With a Background History of Congenital Adrenal Hyperplasia

A 2-year-old child was referred to the emergency department with an acute viral illness with low-grade fever and vomiting. She had vomited all her routine medications that morning. She had a background diagnosis of congenital adrenal hyperplasia diagnosed in the newborn period and was on maintenance therapy with regular outpatient follow-up. She looked very pale on arrival with an elevated heart rate of 160 per minute and delayed capillary refill over 3 seconds. Her blood glucose was 3.0 mmol/L and she was admitted for observation and further investigation.

Clinical Pearls

All children who are receiving glucocorticoid therapy are at risk of growth impairment and short stature and so always aim to treat children with the lowest possible effective dose.

Pitfalls to Avoid

There is an excess mortality in infants and children with congenital adrenal hyperplasia due to adrenal crises.

Advice is to triple the dose of hydrocortisone during an intercurrent illness or prior to surgery.

KEY LEARNING POINTS

Delay in diagnosis is the leading cause of DKA for young children whereas omission of insulin is the leading cause amongst adolescents.

Suspect acquired hypothyroidism in any child with a significant fall off in growth velocity and request basic investigations including Free T4, TSH and thyroid autoantibodies and a left wrist X-ray for bone age.

A karyotype is indicated in all girls with significant short stature.

Cushing's syndrome can be a challenging diagnosis to make. Always consider an endocrine cause of obesity if there is additional short stature.

Primary adrenal insufficiency is a very challenging diagnosis to make in family practice as the symptoms are relatively nonspecific and onset is often insidious.

Children with CAH should receive both hydrocortisone (divided into three doses) and fludrocortisone daily (if salt-losing). Give double or triple the dose of hydrocortisone during intercurrent illness or prior to surgery.

REFERENCES

1. Diabetes (type 1 and type 2) in children and young people: diagnosis and management NICE guideline [NG18] Published: 01 August 2015 Last updated: 29 June 2022. Accessed online at-https://www.nice.org.uk/guidance/ng18
2. Heddy N. Guideline for the management of children and young people under the age of 18 years with diabetic ketoacidosis (British Society for Paediatric Endocrinology and Diabetes). *Archives of Disease in Childhood - Education and Practice*. 2021;106:220–222. Published Online First: 24 Feb 2021. doi:10.1136/archdischild-2020-320076.
3. Peters MJ. Fluid resuscitation in diabetic ketoacidosis and the BPSED guidelines: what we still don't know. *Arch Dis Child Educ Pract Ed*. 2021;106(4):223–225. doi:10.1136/archdischild-2020-320078.
4. Tasker RC. Fluid management during diabetic ketoacidosis in children: guidelines, consensus, recommendations, and clinical judgement. *Arch Dis Child*. 2020;105(10):917–918. doi:10.1136/archdischild-2020-320164.
5. Wright N, Thomas R. BSPED guideline: what we know and why the guideline was changed. *Arch Dis Child Educ Pract Ed*. 2021;106(4):226–228. doi:10.1136/archdischild-2020-320077.
6. Chaker L, Bianco AC, Jonklaas J, Peeters RP. Hypothyroidism. *Lancet*. 2017;390(10101):1550–1562. doi:10.1016/S0140-6736(17)30703-1.
7. Murphy S. Understanding childhood and adolescent obesity. *Clinics in Integrated Care*. August 2022;13:100114. Doi:/10.1016/j.intcar.2022.100114.
8. Husebye ES, Pearce SH, Krone NP, Kämpe O. Adrenal insufficiency. *Lancet*. 2021;397(10274):613–629. doi:10.1016/S0140-6736(21)00136-7.
9. Dalin F, Nordling Eriksson G, Dahlqvist P, et al. Clinical and Immunological Characteristics of Autoimmune Addison Disease: A Nationwide Swedish Multicenter Study. *J Clin Endocrinol Metab*. 2017;102(2):379–389. doi:10.1210/jc.2016-2522.
10. Freitas PFS, Oliveira JM, Kater CE. Crisis? What crisis? Abdominal pain and darkening skin in Addison's disease. *Lancet*. 2020;396(10249):498. doi:10.1016/S0140-6736(20)31680.
11. Eyal O, Levin Y, Oren A, et al. Adrenal crises in children with adrenal insufficiency: epidemiology and risk factors. *Eur J Pediatr*. 2019;178(5):731–738. doi:10.1007/s00431-019-03348-1.
12. Bornstein SR, Allolio B, Arlt W, et al. Diagnosis and Treatment of Primary Adrenal Insufficiency: An Endocrine Society Clinical Practice Guideline. *J Clin*

Endocrinol Metab. 2016;101(2):364–389. doi:10.1210/jc.2015-1710.
13. El-Maouche, Diala, et al. "Congenital adrenal hyperplasia." *Lancet (London, England)* vol. 390,10108 (2017): 2194–2210. doi:10.1016/S0140-6736(17)31431-9.
14. NHSGGC Paediatrics for Health Professionals. Hypoglycaemia management, Paediatric Emergency Department. Accessed online at https://www.clinicalguidelines.scot.nhs.uk/nhsggc-guidelines/nhsggc-guidelines/emergency-medicine/hypoglycaemia-management-paediatric-emergency-department/.
15. The Royal Childrens Hospital Melbourne. Hypoglycaemia. Accessed online at https://www.rch.org.au/clinicalguide/guideline_index/Hypoglycaemia/.
16. Casertano A, Rossi A, Fecarotta S, et al. An Overview of Hypoglycemia in Children Including a Comprehensive Practical Diagnostic Flowchart for Clinical Use. *Front Endocrinol (Lausanne)*. 2021;12:684011. Published 2021 Aug 2. doi:10.3389/fendo.2021.684011.
17. Gandhi K. Approach to hypoglycemia in infants and children. *Transl Pediatr*. 2017;6(4):408–420. doi:10.21037/tp.2017.10.05.

ADDITIONAL READING

Berglund A, Viuff MH, Skakkebæk A, Chang S, Stochholm K, Gravholt CH. Changes in the cohort composition of Turner syndrome and severe non-diagnosis of Klinefelter, 47,XXX and 47,XYY syndrome: a nationwide cohort study. *Orphanet J Rare Dis*. 2019;14(1):16. Published 2019 Jan 14. doi:10.1186/s13023-018-0976-2.

Husebye ES, Anderson MS, Kämpe O. Autoimmune Polyendocrine Syndromes. *N Engl J Med*. 2018;378(12):1132–1141. doi:10.1056/NEJMra1713301.

Melmed S. Pituitary-Tumor Endocrinopathies. *N Engl J Med*. 2020;382(10):937–950. doi:10.1056/NEJMra1810772.

Saevik AB, Åkerman AK, Grønning K, et al. Clues for early detection of autoimmune Addison's disease – myths and realities. *J Intern Med*. 2018;283:190–199.

13

The Child With Abdominal Pain

Alan Mortell, Billy Bourke

CHAPTER OUTLINE

In this chapter, we describe two quite different scenarios where a child presents with abdominal pain. They require wholly different approaches.

Acute abdominal pain has a wide variety of differentials, but the key aim is to outrule a surgical cause, in particular acute appendicitis. Acute appendicitis may be a challenging diagnosis to make in the younger age groups, but it should be entertained in all ages who present with an acute abdomen. Clinical assessment is still the mainstay of diagnosis in acute appendicitis.[1] Not all acute abdominal pain relates to acute appendicitis, and an important lesson is described below.

Recurrent abdominal pain (now termed functional abdominal pain or FAP) is typically periumbilical and is also quite common. Children with FAP classically have an internalising personality – thus one should seek features such as being sensitive, anxious, conscientious, empathic, caring and high-achieving. Although clinically challenging, FAP is a very rewarding condition to manage as a family doctor or paediatrician.

ACUTE ABDOMINAL PAIN

Acute appendicitis is a very common general surgical emergency with an estimated lifetime risk of 7 to 8% and a peak incidence in the second or third decade of life. A family history of appendicitis increases the risk threefold. Interestingly, acute appendicitis is less often seen in non-white and ethnic minority groups who also have an increased risk of perforation.[1]

> An accurate preoperative diagnosis of appendicitis is challenging.

While appendicitis is relatively common in childhood, there are still many situations of diagnostic uncertainty especially in younger preschool children. Families are naturally upset when they present in good faith to their family doctor or local emergency department with their sick child and, if discharged home with a presumptive diagnosis of gastroenteritis, subsequently have to re-attend and a perforated appendicitis is diagnosed.

So, what are the 'golden rules' that enable safe practice and how can we maximise the chances of making the diagnosis of acute appendicitis?

Key Points in the History

Abdominal pain is a very common symptom in children and may reflect a wide variety of differential diagnoses.[2]

> Persistent abdominal pain presenting for more than 4 to 6 hours with associated persistent vomiting or protracted diarrhoea should be taken seriously, and one should always attempt to exclude a surgical cause.

Acute appendicitis is the most common surgical cause of an acute abdomen in children, but diagnostic delay is not infrequent. Diarrhoea is often present and may lead the clinician to a presumptive diagnosis of gastroenteritis. Delayed diagnosis is associated with a prolonged hospital stay (Box 13.1).

The risk of perforation increases with time, and younger children have a higher risk.

Individual clinical signs of appendicitis have a poor predictive value but, all together, the predictive value is far stronger. The Alvarado clinical risk score is stratified into low, intermediate and high risk and is based on symptoms, signs and laboratory tests. This score has good sensitivity, but low specificity, and it should not be relied upon to guide management.[3]

Making the Diagnosis of Appendicitis in Primary Care

Prehospital diagnostic delay, especially if over 48 hours, increases the risk of complicated appendicitis by four- to seven-fold, whereas there appears to be little negative

BOX 13.1 CLINICAL HISTORY

A 12 Year Old With Acute Abdominal Pain

A 12-year-old boy presented to an emergency department with a history of vomiting, low-grade fever, dysuria and abdominal pains. He was seen by his family doctor and was promptly referred to the emergency department for a surgical opinion. At the time he was noted to have stable vital signs with a low-grade temperature of 37.7°C.

He was admitted for observation, as he had some abdominal tenderness in the right iliac fossa and some possible guarding. The surgical opinion in the emergency department was of possible gastroenteritis, and a plain abdominal X-ray was ordered (normal) and blood tests were requested with the finding of an elevated white cell count (predominantly neutrophils) with an elevated CRP. His urinalysis was negative and stool culture was requested.

He had one spike in temperature up to 38.9°C on day 2 in hospital and had no further spikes in temperature prior to discharge.

Four days post-discharge, he re-presented to hospital. His presenting symptoms and signs on this occasion were severe abdominal pain, abdominal distension and coffee ground vomiting.

His examination reflected an unwell child, and he had a distended abdomen with generalised tenderness and guarding. He was felt to have an acute abdomen requiring urgent surgical review.

The immediate impression was of peritonitis secondary to perforation, and an urgent laparotomy was coordinated post-resuscitation. Laparotomy confirmed appendiceal perforation and pus in the peritoneum which was washed out.

He had a protracted and complex postoperative course and received broad-spectrum intravenous antibiotics and was commenced on total parenteral nutrition (TPN), which he remained on for an extended period.

He subsequently developed a pelvic collection requiring insertion of a pigtail catheter to drain a pelvic abscess. The abscess was successfully fully drained over the following 48 hours. He was finally discharged home 3 weeks later.

Clinical Pearls

Appendicitis can be a difficult diagnosis to make, and a confident preoperative diagnosis is still a challenge with clinical assessment the mainstay of diagnosis.[1]

There are significant limitations to both imaging and blood biomarkers in making the diagnosis.

Pitfalls to Avoid

It appears that some cases of acute appendicitis may be self-limiting and potentially respond to antibiotics alone whereas others, in particular young preschool children, may have perforation prior to reaching hospital.[1]

Overall mortality is low but, postoperative complications are common in complex appendicitis.[1]

impact of an in-hospital delay of 24 to 36 hours. There appear to be two entities of appendicitis, one that progresses to perforation often within a few hours and another that tends to be relatively self-limiting.[4]

> If the diagnosis is uncertain, active observation is a time-proven and safe management option, which yields improved diagnostic accuracy.[5]

Perforation still occurs in approximately 30% of cases. Spontaneous resolution may rarely occur in patients with low-grade appendicitis. Therefore, the incidence of complicated appendicitis is linked to the overall elapsed time from symptom onset to operation.[6] Prompt surgery will reduce pain and discomfort, avoid additional morbidity, enable faster recovery and reduce the length of time in hospital.

> Delayed diagnosis is linked to features such as an unresolved fever, diarrhoea and high CRP levels.

Differential diagnoses of acute appendicitis that can catch you out commonly include acute gastroenteritis or urinary tract infection. Be aware that a right lower lobe pneumonia can present with abdominal pain, but tachypnoea and grunting are usually evident.[7] Diabetic ketoacidosis may also present with abdominal pain as may nephrotic syndrome with hypovolaemia a feature in both.

Always consider Henoch Schönlein purpura (HSP) where the abdominal cramps can be very severe and predate the typical purpuric rash. No one wants to miss testicular torsion or an incarcerated inguinal hernia, so inspection of the scrotum and groin is mandatory in boys with acute abdominal pain (Box 13.2). Ovarian torsion should be considered in girls, as should an ectopic pregnancy in females of child-bearing age. Sickle cell disease can present with significant pain and distress but also a life-threatening splenic sequestration. Renal colic typically presents with excruciating pain in the flank, and pelvi-ureteric junction obstruction (PUJO) may also be associated with severe abdominal pain. Ileocaecal Crohn's disease (CD) may present with episodes of right-sided abdominal pain but may also have other features not least chronic diarrhoea, weight loss and perianal disease. Meckel's diverticulitis is another differential to be considered.

The Role of Investigations

Biomarkers, including the white cell count (WCC) and C-reactive protein (CRP), may be helpful. No inflammatory marker alone (such as the WCC, CRP or procalcitonin) can identify appendicitis with a high degree of sensitivity or specificity. However, if both the WCC and CRP are elevated, the likelihood of appendicitis is increased.

> If appendicitis is suspected but clinical signs are not clear cut, then an abdominal ultrasound is the preferred initial imaging technique.

Plain X-rays are generally unhelpful. Ultrasound is helpful but is operator dependent (Fig. 13.1). Abdominal CT yields excellent diagnostic accuracy but involves a moderate radiation dose, and currently magnetic resonance imaging (MRI) is not well studied but holds promise for the future in terms of diagnosing appendicitis in children.

There is now an increased emphasis on serial examination, particularly early in the course of illness. The diagnosis of appendicitis is particularly challenging in childhood, especially under 5 years of age. The main features linked to a delayed diagnosis of appendicitis in childhood are a short history of symptoms at the initial visit, attendance late at night, nondescript or vague physical findings and few investigations being performed.

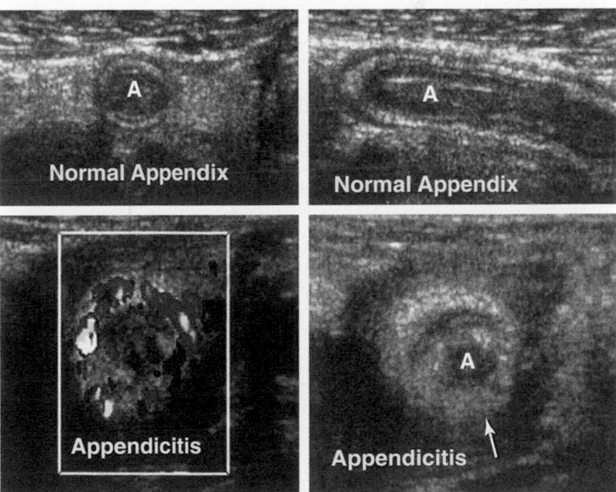

Fig. 13.1 Ultrasound image of a normal appendix (*top*) illustrating the thin wall in coronal (*left*) and longitudinal (*right*) planes. In appendicitis, there is distention and wall thickening (*bottom, right*), and blood flow is increased, leading to the so-called ring of fire appearance. *A*, Appendix. (Source: *Sabiston Textbook of Surgery: The Biological Basis of Modern Surgical Practice*. 21st ed. 2022.)

BOX 13.2 CLINICAL HISTORY

When You Hear Hoofbeats, Look for Horses, Not Zebras – But Occasionally You Will Be in for a Surprise

A 14-year-old male presented to hospital with a 6-hour history of significant left-sided lower abdominal pain with associated discomfort. He had no relevant past medical history. His examination revealed him to be apyrexial but in considerable distress, and thus he was admitted for surgical review and observation. His abdominal examination revealed no localising tenderness and no rebound tenderness, and thus he had both an abdominal ultrasound and plain X-ray performed, the latter showing mild constipation.

He was observed fasting overnight and was commenced on intravenous fluids. He remained apyrexial. Twelve hours later he was re-examined, and he had marked discolouration of the left hemiscrotum, and a diagnosis of testicular torsion was made. He went on to have a surgical exploration which showed a nonviable left testis, and thus an orchidectomy was performed, and the contralateral testis was stabilised (Fig. 13.2).

Clinical Pearls

Testicular torsion occurs most commonly at puberty but can occur at any age. Pain may be intermittent or be a dull ache of gradual onset, and the pain may be referred to the abdomen and be confused with acute appendicitis. Detorsion within 6 hours has a salvage rate of 90 to 100%.[21] Urgent scrotal exploration and bilateral testicular fixation should be performed in all cases of suspected testicular torsion.[21]

All clinically obvious cases of testicular torsion or those diagnosed by colour flow Doppler ultrasound should be treated as a surgical emergency. A colour flow Doppler study may be very helpful if testicular blood flow is absent, but findings may not be diagnostic in early or intermittent torsion.[21]

Scrotal exploration (ideally *within 4 hours* of the onset of symptoms) with detorsion of the affected side and bilateral testicular fixation should be performed. Emergency surgical exploration is necessary to avoid loss of the testis.[21]

Key differential diagnoses include acute epididymoorchitis and torsion of testicular appendages (more likely in prepubertal age group).

In torsion of the testicular appendages, the following features are distinctive, not least the child is afebrile and has normal vital signs, the scrotum may be erythematous and oedematous but usually appears normal, and the cremasteric reflex is usually present.

The testis should be nontender to palpation, and if present, tenderness is localised to the upper pole of the testis. The presence of a paratesticular nodule at the superior aspect of the testicle, with its characteristic blue-dot appearance, is pathognomonic for this condition (Fig. 13.3).

Pitfalls to Avoid

Always examine the groin in an adolescent presenting with acute abdominal pain.

Testicular torsion can occur at any age but is most commonly seen after puberty.

It is an acute surgical emergency, and if suspected, surgical exploration should be performed with great urgency and ideally within 4 hours of the onset of symptoms.

Key symptoms are testicular pain which may be referred to the abdomen, and the affected testis will be swollen and reddened.

Torsion of the testicular appendages (e.g. the Hydatid of Morgagni) is more likely in the prepubertal age group.

Colour flow Doppler is helpful if the diagnosis is not clear but should not delay surgical exploration.

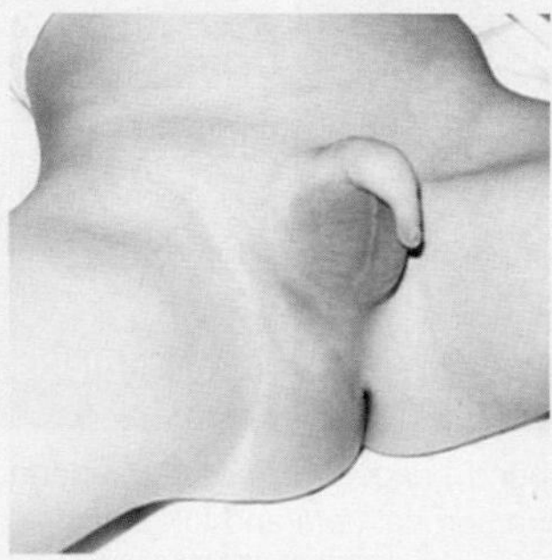

Fig. 13.2 Testicular torsion. (Abrahams PH, et al. *Abrahams' and McMinn's Clinical Atlas of Human Anatomy*. 8th edition, 2020, Elsevier Ltd.)

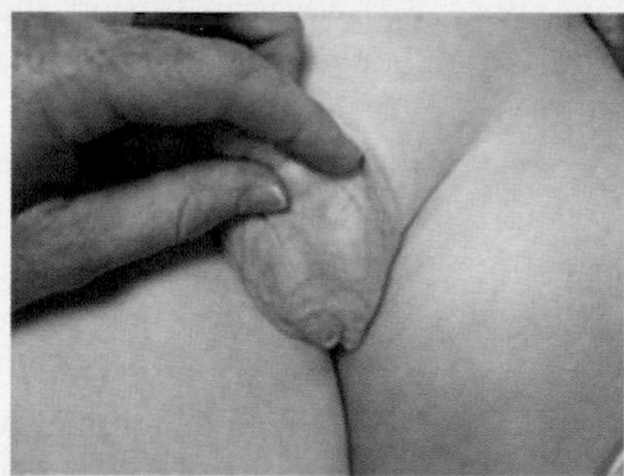

Fig. 13.3 Blue dot sign. Torsion of a testicular or epididymal appendage can mimic testicular torsion. Physical exam demonstrates localised tenderness at the superior pole of the testis or caput epididymis. In boys with thin scrotal skin, the classic 'blue dot' sign is seen, reflective of a necrotic appendix. (Partin AW, Dmochowski RR, Kavoussi LR, et al. *Campbell-Walsh-Wein Urology*, ed 12, Philadelphia, 2021, Elsevier. ISBN: 9780323546423.)

Operative Treatment

A recent meta-analysis found that short in-hospital delays of 12 to 24 hours in stable patients are not associated with an increased risk of perforation.[6] Repeated clinical assessment has been found to increase diagnostic accuracy without a concomitant increase in the risk of perforation.

> In general, nighttime appendicectomy operations should be avoided.

Laparoscopy is the preferred surgical approach with a shorter length of stay and reduced postoperative pain.

Laparoscopic appendicectomy is safe in children and adolescents with obesity and carries a relatively low-risk profile. Preoperative prophylactic antibiotics may be started once the child is diagnosed with appendicitis and is scheduled for surgery. Piperacillin or tazobactam are indicated if either perforation or complex appendicitis is suspected. Intravenous antibiotics are given for a minimum of between 3 and 5 days for either complicated or perforated appendicitis.

Normal appendectomy rates have fallen during the past 15 years but are variable between countries and are lower in Switzerland (where preoperative CT is routine) and the United States (with a high rate of preoperative CT) than in the UK where rates of about 20% are seen.[8]

Intraabdominal or pelvic abscess is seen in about 4% of those presenting with appendicitis, and the key physical sign can be a palpable mass with associated fever and elevated inflammatory markers. The management of an appendix mass (diagnosed clinically with or without ultrasound) is often nonoperative initially with broad-spectrum intravenous antibiotics and image-guided drainage of pus collections until the patient is clinically fit for discharge. Operative management of an appendix mass at initial presentation is generally a very challenging surgical procedure with a significant risk of complications occurring. Once an appendix mass has been managed conservatively then ideally, at least 6 weeks later, an interval laparoscopic appendicectomy can be performed with a short hospital stay postoperatively.[9]

RECURRENT ABDOMINAL PAIN

Recurrent (or functional) abdominal pain affects at least 10% of children – the vast majority of otherwise healthy children who present with abdominal pain in primary and secondary care will not have an underlying organic diagnosis.

Typically, FAP presents with central or peri-umbilical pain that is episodic and not consistently associated with any other significant gastrointestinal (GI) or systemic disturbance. However, other somatic symptoms such as nausea, headaches, dizziness and musculoskeletal pains do often accompany FAP. Pain may be very debilitating and in some even pervasive. In an otherwise well child, any pain that is described as present all the time is almost certainly functional. Persistent nausea or dyspepsia in the absence of other upper GI symptoms can be considered part of the spectrum of FAP.

> School absence is a marker of functional abdominal pain.

A careful history and full physical examination including plotting growth on a centile chart are essential, not just to evaluate the pain but as part of the establishment of the necessary therapeutic alliance that will facilitate acceptance of the diagnosis.

Abdominal examination will often elicit subjective tenderness that can be exquisite but from which the child is often distractable. Consistent tenderness in the right iliac fossa raises concern for Crohn disease (CD).

> It is important, then, to acknowledge that the pain is as real as organic pain and to provide a careful explanation to the child and parents of the biopsychosocial model of pain.

There are usually two overarching concerns for both the parents and the child when faced with any functional diagnosis, and these are that the doctors may be missing something serious and that, perhaps, a nonorganic diagnosis somehow invalidates the relevance of the problem.

While simple noninvasive tests addressing specific concerns may be justifiable, it is essential to avoid repeated unnecessary diagnostic tests which may promote a cycle of anxiety around symptoms, further health-seeking behaviour and inadvertent participation by the doctor as a cofactor in perpetuation of the problem.

In general, there is inadequate evidence to support either pharmacological or dietary interventions in FAP, and most practitioners advocate a psychological approach in the first instance.[10] Good data exists to support the efficacy of hypnotherapy, but this is not widely available. There are some studies that have shown benefit of other psychotherapeutic interventions such as cognitive behavioural therapy (CBT) or even mindfulness. These approaches also have the benefit of 'de-medicalising' the problem.[10,11] Antacids, antispasmodics, peppermint oil, 5HT inhibitors and even antidepressants have been used but may have adverse effects and efficacy generally has not been much better than placebo. A low FODMAP diet is not unreasonable if the child's symptoms fulfil the criteria for irritable bowel syndrome (IBS), but there remain inadequate studies to support its routine use in childhood.[12]

> Once there is acceptance of a biopsychosocial explanation for the abdominal pain, it may be useful to identify physical and psychological stress factors that may have an important role in the onset and persistence of the pain.[7]

Environmental factors may serve as reinforcers of the pain behaviour. Regular school attendance should be encouraged despite ongoing pain episodes. Parents and the school should work together to support the child. Attention should focus on the improvement of daily symptoms and quality of life emphasising the importance of the child returning to normal activities.[7]

DIFFERENTIAL DIAGNOSES TO CONSIDER

We are all aware that FAP is very commonly seen in family practice and that parents, and indeed children, are very aware of the possibility of an underlying organic illness. As FAP is so common, it may coexist with other diagnoses, and the issue of a 'second diagnosis' is always a challenge in primary care.

Several differentials need to be considered, but investigations should be kept to a minimum and should be reserved for red flag symptoms such as recent weight loss, effortless vomiting, dysphagia, nocturnal pain causing awakening or alteration of the bowel habit.

Inflammatory Bowel Disease

The key symptoms that may indicate inflammatory bowel disease (IBD) are anorexia with weight loss, nocturnal diarrhoea (with or without blood) and perianal disease (Box 13.3). The median time from symptom

BOX 13.3 CLINICAL HISTORY

Yet Another Functional Abdominal Pain

An 11-year-old boy presented with a 6-month history of recurrent episodes of central periumbilical pain. The episodes of pain were always periumbilical, and he had no alteration of bowel habit, nor did he have any nocturnal symptoms. His examination was normal, and his height and weight were both on the 75th centile for his age on the growth charts. His parents were recently separated, and his uncle had recently been diagnosed with bowel cancer, and it was recognised that he was an anxious, sensitive and conscientious boy. He was seen in outpatients, and a diagnosis of functional abdominal pain was made. His parents were unhappy that other diagnoses had not been formally excluded. He subsequently had an FBC, albumin, ESR and urinalysis which were normal and a coeliac screen which was found to be negative. He had one further visit to the outpatients 2 months later and was no better so was referred for psychological support. He continued to attend school despite the pain and remained a very high achiever in academic terms.

Nine months later, following the summer holidays, he had further episodes of severe abdominal pain. On this visit, his pain was both central and right sided, and his weight centile had slipped to below the 25th centile. He had nocturnal diarrhoea for 2 weeks. He looked a little pale and unwell. Investigations showed elevated inflammatory markers, a low albumin and a very high faecal calprotectin of over 1800. Subsequent endoscopy confirmed the diagnosis of Crohn's disease.

Clinical Pearls

FAP is a clinical diagnosis and can be made with confidence when the patients' symptoms and personality profile fit, and there are no 'red flag' features.

Pitfalls to Avoid

Early Crohn's can be subtle and organic diagnoses can coexist with nonorganic conditions.

In this case it is possible that the FAP symptoms were early manifestations of Crohn's, but it is more likely he had FAP at first presentation and then developed symptoms of Crohn's.

Re-evaluation of the child with FAP is recommended as it reassures the patient, family and the clinician. Being attentive to alterations in symptoms is important.

onset to diagnosis may be 7 months for CD (one in five wait up to 12 months for a diagnosis) with most delays being from the onset of symptoms to a referral to a specialist service.[13] In suspected IBD, the key initial investigations include a full blood count which may demonstrate iron deficiency anaemia, and a high platelet count suggestive of inflammation. Both the ESR and CRP may be elevated. Serum albumin and liver function tests should be requested, as hypoalbuminemia is typically seen in small intestinal CD. Diagnosis of IBD is confirmed at endoscopy (Fig. 13.4).

In general terms, ulcerative colitis (UC) presents with abdominal pain and bloody diarrhoea and tends to come to medical attention sooner. In CD, vague symptoms of nonbloody diarrhoea, fatigue, oral ulceration (Fig. 13.5), fever and weight loss are seen.[14] Extraintestinal symptoms such as erythema nodosum, uveitis, arthritis, pyoderma gangrenosum (Fig. 13.6) and primary sclerosing cholangitis may be seen.

Younger preschool children with CD may present with short stature and rectal bleeding.

The faecal calprotectin level is a good screening test for bowel inflammation.[15] However, calprotectin measures a protein found in neutrophils, so any inflammatory condition, including intestinal infection or any cause of blood in stools will result in elevation. In children a result less than 200 essentially excludes IBD. It is not a useful test in the first 2 years of life.

Eosinophilic Oesophagitis

Eosinophilic oesophagitis (EoE) should be considered if episodic abdominal pain is associated with dysphagia or a history of food impaction. The most common symptoms are food sticking in the oesophagus during swallowing and a sense of chest or abdominal discomfort when having a meal. In older children, abdominal pain and nausea with or without vomiting may become a prominent feature.[16] Children may adapt their eating behaviour to avoid solid foods and may consume excessive water or modify eating patterns by eating slowly. The diagnosis is confirmed by oesophagogastroduodenoscopy (OGD) and oesophageal biopsies.[16] Therapeutic options include swallowed topical steroids (e.g. fluticasone), proton pump inhibitors (PPIs) or elimination diets.

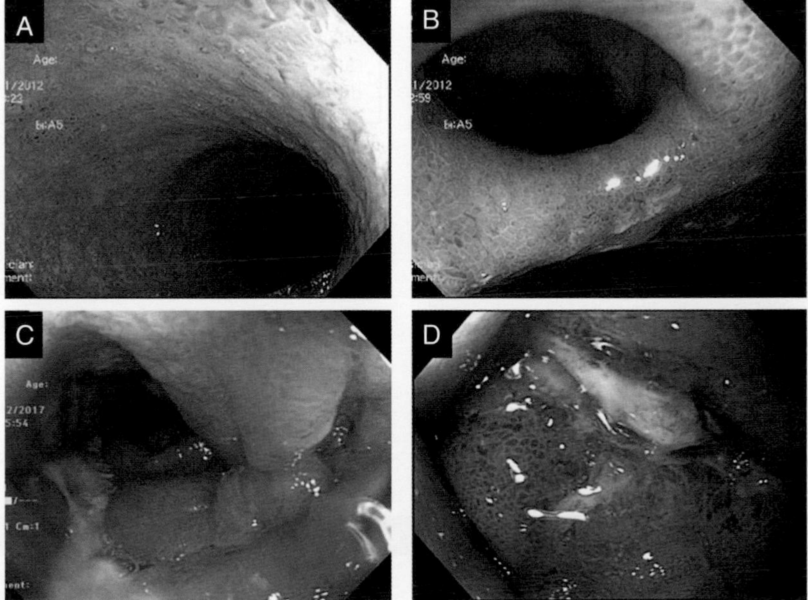

Fig. 13.4 Distribution of ileitis in ulcerative colitis and Crohn's disease. Diffuse colitis with granular, flat mucosa and loss of vascularity in the terminal ileum (i.e. backwash ileitis) (A) and widely patent or 'fish mouth' – shaped configuration of the ileocecal valve (B) in ulcerative colitis. Linear ulcers and mucosal oedema of the terminal ileum (C) and ulcerated, strictured and deformed ileocecal valve (D) in Crohn's disease. (Bo Shen. *Atlas of Endoscopy Imaging in Inflammatory Bowel Disease.* 1st ed. Academic Press, 2020, Elsevier Inc.)

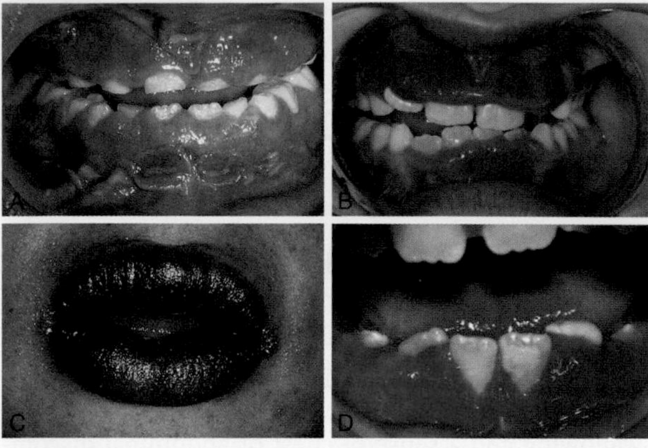

Fig. 13.5 Presentations of orofacial granulomatosis/Crohn disease. (A) The intraoral appearance is pathognomonic with swelling of the gingivae; the patient also had a cobblestone appearance of the buccal mucosa and ulceration of the labial and buccal sulci. (B) A different presentation with bright red swollen gingivae. (C) The patient initially presented with a painless swelling of the lips and had evidence of malabsorption, perianal fissuring and bowel problems and was diagnosed with Crohn disease. Management was with systemic corticosteroids. (D) Crohn disease. This child has recurrent flare-ups of his disease that is characterized by concurrent deterioration of his oral disease. (Source: Widmer RP, Cameron AC, Georgiou A. *Handbook of Pediatric Dentistry*, 5th ed. Elsevier Ltd; 2022.)

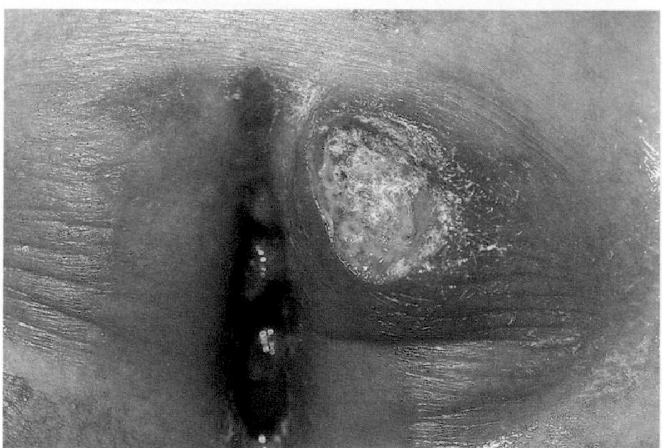

Fig. 13.6 Pyoderma gangrenosum. Painful ulcer on the vulva of a girl with Crohn's disease. (Source: Paller AS, Mancini AJ. *Hurwitz Clinical Pediatric Dermatology: A Textbook of Skin Disorders of Childhood and Adolescence*. 6th ed. Elsevier; 2022.)

Coeliac Disease

Coeliac disease is common, affecting up to 1% of certain populations, and may present at any age.[17,18] The prevalence of coeliac disease is increasing rapidly in developed countries. Typical features include symptoms and signs of malabsorption, including diarrhoea, steatorrhoea, constipation, vomiting, weight loss or growth failure, abdominal pain or bloating. However, the most consistent symptoms are fatigue and irritability, as abdominal pain on its own is rarely caused by coeliac disease.

Coeliac disease is seen more frequently in children with type 1 diabetes mellitus or Down syndrome. Young children with a first-degree relative with coeliac disease, have a **7%** risk of coeliac disease and, for this reason, serological testing should be considered even without symptoms in children with a positive family history. Immunoglobulin A-tissue transglutaminase (IgA-tTG) titre is the serological test of choice. A normal IgA-tTG and total IgA (to exclude IgA deficiency, which will give a false negative result) result excludes coeliac disease if there is a low clinical index of suspicion for coeliac disease.

The presence of typical coeliac changes on duodenal histology with clinical improvement on a gluten-free diet confirms the diagnosis.

> Children with symptoms consistent with coeliac disease and a high IgA-tTG titre (above 10 times the normal range) and a positive antiendomysial antibody may be diagnosed without a small intestinal biopsy.[19]

Helicobacter pylori/Peptic Ulcer Disease

H. pylori is acquired in very early childhood and colonisation in the absence of a peptic ulcer does NOT cause FAP.[20] Ulcers cause pain but are rare in childhood and extremely unusual before adolescence.

> Checking for *H. pylori* (stool or breath tests) is NOT recommended for the investigation of FAP.

KEY LEARNING POINTS

Acute Abdominal Pain

Acute appendicitis is the most frequently seen surgical emergency in children.

The sequence typically is periumbilical pain **followed by** anorexia **followed by** nausea or sometimes vomiting **followed by** the shifting of the pain to the RIF over the subsequent 2 to 8 hours.

Gastroenteritis is a key differential and typically nausea or vomiting and diarrhoea are **followed by** abdominal pain.

Reluctance to jump or tenderness or wincing with pain on jumping can also indicate some peritoneal irritation and is worth exploring.

If abdominal pain lasts for more than 4 to 6 hours or is associated with persistent vomiting or protracted diarrhoea, a surgical cause needs to be excluded.

Equipping the parents with the knowledge of what an evolving appendicitis presentation may look like, empowers them to return early if concerning symptoms arise, or if the symptoms are not resolving as anticipated.

The missed appendicitis rate is 5% and, when appendicitis is missed at the initial consultation, the risk of perforation is 50% by the time of the second visit.

Toddlers pose unique diagnostic challenges, and a toddler with diarrhoea and abdominal pain is a red flag for appendicitis.

In terms of ultrasound and acute appendicitis, a positive report helps confirm the diagnosis, but a negative report does not exclude appendicitis. When the appendix is visible on ultrasound, it is usually inflamed with a characteristic appearance of a thickened noncompressible wall and a dilated lumen. When there is continued clinical uncertainty, the next steps are CT or possibly MRI scan.

The main features associated with a late diagnosis of appendicitis in childhood were found to be late night attendance, nondescript or vague physical findings and few investigations being performed.

If a child with abdominal pain does not settle quickly, appendicitis should be excluded by early and, if necessary, repeated surgical consultations.

Always examine the groin in cases of acute abdominal pain and look for testicular torsion. If suspected, urgent surgical opinion and exploration is required.

Recurrent (or Functional) Abdominal Pain

FAP is very common (10–15%) whereas inflammatory bowel disease is very rare, and both may coexist. Signs to watch out for in suspected Crohn's disease include perianal disease, severe mouth ulcers, arthropathy, uveitis or evident erythema nodosum.

Coeliac disease is common, affecting up to 1% in certain populations, and may present at any age. When coeliac disease causes FAP there are usually other symptoms as well, especially fatigue and feeling miserable.

Safety netting and empowering parents to return early if ongoing concerns is an essential aspect of an abdominal pain consultation.

REFERENCES

1. Bhangu A, Søreide K, Di Saverio S, Assarsson JH, Drake FT. Acute appendicitis: modern understanding of pathogenesis, diagnosis, and management [published correction appears in Lancet. 2017 Oct 14;390(10104):1736]. *Lancet*. 2015;386(10000):1278–1287. doi:10.1016/S0140-6736(15)00275-5.
2. Cappendijk VC, Hazebroek FW. The impact of diagnostic delay on the course of acute appendicitis. *Arch Dis Child*. 2000;83(1):64–66. doi:10.1136/adc.83.1.64.
3. Ohle R, O'Reilly F, O'Brien KK, Fahey T, Dimitrov BD. The Alvarado score for predicting acute appendicitis: a systematic review. *BMC Med*. 2011;9:139. doi:10.1186/1741-7015-9-139. Published 2011 Dec 28.
4. Andersson RE. Does Delay of Diagnosis and Treatment in Appendicitis Cause Perforation? *World J Surg*. 2016;40(6):1315–1317. doi:10.1007/s00268-016-3489-y.
5. Alvarado A. Clinical approach in the diagnosis of acute appendicitis. In Garbuzenko DV (Ed.), *Current Issues in the Diagnostics and Treatment of Acute Appendicitis*. IntechOpen; 2018. doi:10.5772/intechopen.75530.
6. Li J, Xu R, Hu DM, Zhang Y, Gong TP, Wu XL. Effect of delay to operation on outcomes in patients with acute appendicitis: a systematic review and meta-analysis. *J Gastrointest Surg*. 2019;23(1):210–223. doi:10.1007/s11605-018-3866-y.
7. Miranda A. Abdominal pain. In: Kleigman RM, Lye PS, Bordini B, Toth H, Basel D, eds. *Nelson Pediatric Symptom-Based Diagnosis*. Philadelphia: Elsevier; 2018:161–181.
8. Kim SH, Choi YH, Kim WS, Cheon JE, Kim IO. Acute appendicitis in children: ultrasound and CT findings in negative appendectomy cases. *Pediatr Radiol*. 2014;44(10):1243–1251. doi:10.1007/s00247-014-3009-x.
9. Forsyth J, Lasithiotakis K, Peter M. The evolving management of the appendix mass in the era of laparoscopy and interventional radiology. *Surgeon*. 2017;15(2):109–115. doi:10.1016/j.surge.2016.08.002.
10. Andrews ET, Beattie RM, Tighe MP. Functional abdominal pain: what clinicians need to know. *Arch Dis Child*. 2020;105(10):938–944. doi:10.1136/archdischild-2020-318825.

11. Thapar N, Benninga MA, Crowell MD, et al. Paediatric functional abdominal pain disorders. *Nat Rev Dis Primers*. 2020;6(1):89. doi:10.1038/s41572-020-00222-5. Published 2020 Nov 5.
12. Altobelli E, Del Negro V, Angeletti PM, Latella G. Low-FODMAP Diet Improves Irritable Bowel Syndrome Symptoms: A Meta-Analysis. *Nutrients*. 2017;9(9):940. doi:10.3390/nu9090940. Published 2017 Aug 26.
13. Ashton JJ, Harden A, Beattie RM. Paediatric inflammatory bowel disease: improving early diagnosis [published correction appears in Arch Dis Child. 2019 Sep;104(9):925]. *Arch Dis Child*. 2018;103(4):307–308. doi:10.1136/archdischild-2017-313955.
14. Oliveira SB, Monteiro IM. Diagnosis and management of inflammatory bowel disease in children. *BMJ*. 2017;357: j2083. doi:10.1136/bmj.j2083. Published 2017 May 31.
15. Ricciuto A, Griffiths AM. Clinical value of fecal calprotectin. *Crit Rev Clin Lab Sci*. 2019;56(5):307–320. doi:10.1080/10408363.2019.1619159.
16. Ahmed M, Mansoor N, Mansoor T. Review of eosinophilic oesophagitis in children and young people. *Eur J Pediatr*. 2021;180(12):3471–3475. doi:10.1007/s00431-021-04174-0.
17. Lebwohl B, Sanders DS, Green PHR. Coeliac disease. *Lancet*. 2018;391(10115):70–81. doi:10.1016/S0140-6736(17)31796-8.
18. ESGHAN. New guidelines for the diagnosis of paediatric coeliac disease. 2020. Accessed online at https://www.espghan.org/knowledge-center/publications/Clinical-Advice-Guides/2020_New_Guidelines_for_the_Diagnosis_of_Paediatric_Coeliac_Disease
19. BMJ Best practice. *Coeliac Disease*. Accessed online at https://dev.bp-frontend.tf.aws.bmjgroup.com/topics/en-gb/636/diagnosis-approach
20. Seo JH, Bortolin K, Jones NL. Review: Helicobacter pylori infection in children. *Helicobacter*. 2020;25(Suppl 1):e12742. doi:10.1111/hel.12742.
21. Somani BK, Watson G, Townell N. Testicular torsion. *BMJ*. 2010;341:c3213. doi:10.1136/bmj.c3213. Published 2010 Jul 27.

ADDITIONAL READING

Almaramhy HH. Acute appendicitis in young children less than 5 years: review article. *Ital J Pediatr*. 2017;43(1):15. doi:10.1186/s13052-017-0335-2. Published 2017 Jan 26.

Al-Toma A, Volta U, Auricchio R, et al. European Society for the Study of Coeliac Disease (ESsCD) guideline for coeliac disease and other gluten-related disorders. *United European Gastroenterol J*. 2019;7(5):583–613. doi:10.1177/2050640619844125.

Choi JY, Ryoo E, Jo JH, Hann T, Kim SM. Risk factors of delayed diagnosis of acute appendicitis in children: for early detection of acute appendicitis. *Korean J Pediatr*. 2016;59(9):368–373. doi:10.3345/kjp.2016.59.9.368.

Hall NJ, Eaton S, Stanton MP, Pierro A, Burge DM. CHINA study collaborators and the Paediatric Surgery Trainees Research Network. Active observation versus interval appendicectomy after successful non-operative treatment of an appendix mass in children (CHINA study): an open-label, randomised controlled trial. *Lancet Gastroenterol Hepatol*. 2017;2(4):253–260. doi:10.1016/S2468-1253(16)30243-6.

Lawton B, Goldstein H, Davis T, Tagg A. Diagnosis of appendicitis in the paediatric emergency department: an update. *Curr Opin Pediatr*. 2019;31(3):312–316. doi:10.1097/MOP.0000000000000749.

14

Pneumonia in Children

Desmond Cox

CHAPTER OUTLINE

BACKGROUND

Viruses are the most common cause of community acquired pneumonia (CAP) in preschool children, so in general, antibiotics are not required for the majority of cases.

Children under 12 years of age have up to 10 respiratory tract infections (RTIs) per year, and RTIs are the single most frequent reason why parents consult their family doctor.[1] It is quite commonplace for family doctors to have to distinguish between upper and lower RTIs. For an upper respiratory tract infection (URTI), about half will still have nasal discharge or cough 7 days after the initial consultation so patience on the part of the parents is required. Some parents may choose to reconsult their family doctor because their infant or child is not better despite an improvement in their overall condition. Parents do require accurate information about the expected time to full recovery (often up to 14 days) and what to look out for.

> A lower respiratory tract infection (LRTI) or community-acquired pneumonia (CAP) is typically characterised by fever, cough and tachypnoea.

There is no uniform definition for CAP, and many guidelines base the definition on the clinical presentation. Most cases of CAP can be managed in the community and do not require hospitalisation.

AVOIDING UNNECESSARY ANTIBIOTICS

Doctors tend to be sensitive to perceived parental pressure, and this may lead on to unnecessary prescribing of antibiotics.

The key aim of the initial and subsequent assessments is to determine whether the child has a mild or severe CAP. Most family doctors are very well able to recognise both mild and severe CAP with an initial rapid pattern recognition and subsequent deductive reasoning. Thus, a family doctor will use an initial fast, intuitive assessment based on prior experience of dealing with children with CAP and may 'double check' with a more analytical approach if the child fails to get better.[1] How long you wait before the latter and the ability to cope with uncertainty and change direction if there is no improvement are key factors. For most family doctors, the presence of an ongoing fever, an ill-appearing child who is not improving, should and generally do lead to either commencement of antibiotics or hospital referral.

A high fever (>38.5°C), toxicity, tachypnoea, grunting and moderate to severe subcostal recession all point to a severe CAP requiring either or both of the above options.

Equally challenging is the ability to distinguish a viral (the great majority) from a bacterial CAP.[2] This difficulty leads to a wide variation in antibiotic prescribing, referral to hospital and referral for radiological testing. Antibiotics are still frequently prescribed (a rate of 40% in the UK and even higher in the United States) and may contribute to medicalisation of illness and antibiotic resistance. Management decisions are made based on the severity of illness and the potential for complications.[3] A recent trial of children aged from 6 months to 12 years showed that those with uncomplicated CAP did not benefit from treatment with antibiotics. This multicentre trial concluded that, in treating CAP in children, an expectant approach avoiding investigation and treatment with antibiotics is the correct one.[4]

> Antibiotics are *not* routinely indicated for most cases of uncomplicated CAP.

Therefore, family doctors should offer safety netting advice and not routinely offer antibiotics for children presenting with a chest infection.[5]

Contrary to popular myth, most parents are primarily seeking a medical opinion of their child and defer treatment decisions to their family doctor. Clinical uncertainty has far greater influence than parental pressure in relation to antibiotic prescribing.

LENGTH OF ANTIBIOTIC TREATMENT

A recent study looked at the ideal dose and duration of antibiotic treatment in childhood pneumonia.[5] The World Health Organization recommends a 3-day course. Guidelines across Europe recommend 5 to 10 days, and the National Institute for Health and Care Excellence recommends 5 days. This randomised trial showed that the 3-day course of amoxycillin was as effective as the 7-day course.[5]

> Several national and international guidelines do not recommend chest radiography (CXR) in children with pneumonia who are well enough to be treated as outpatients.

INDICATIONS FOR INVESTIGATIONS

A chest X-ray (CXR) should be reserved for children who have been admitted to hospital with severe symptoms, whose saturations are below 92% and if a complicated pneumonia is suspected.[6] Chest radiography has many limitations, not least poor inter-observer reliability, and thus point-of-care ultrasound and rapid sequence magnetic resonance imaging (MRI) have both emerged as potential alternatives. Point-of-care ultrasound is promising as an alternative to CXR in the emergency department and it does have potential as a screening test. Rapid sequence MRI is less well studied and may be reserved for children with severe pneumonia or if associated complications.

Current British Thoracic Society (BTS) guidelines[7] recommend microbiological testing only in children with severe pneumonia, but others recommend testing for influenza and other common respiratory viruses for children in the emergency department or those admitted to hospital. Nasopharyngeal samples are taken for common respiratory viruses and for pertussis. The viruses most often detected are respiratory syncytial virus (RSV), influenza, parainfluenza and human metapneumovirus. Blood cultures are indicated for children with pneumonia who are in hospital or who have complicated pneumonia.

A recent meta-analysis evaluated the ability of biomarkers to identify bacterial pneumonia.[8] The authors conclude that, although C-reactive protein (CRP) and procalcitonin performed better than the white blood cell count, they still had a sensitivity and specificity of just 60% to 70%. Therefore, current BTS guidelines do not recommend ordering acute phase reactants (such as CRP and procalcitonin) to distinguish viral from bacterial pneumonia.

MAKING THE DIAGNOSIS IN PRIMARY CARE

Diagnosis of CAP can be challenging in primary care, as many infants and young children develop upper respiratory tract symptoms of coughing, coryza and fever. Consider the assessment of clinical severity as well as the age of the child to determine your management strategy.

Infancy

If under 12 months of age, acute bronchiolitis is the most likely cause of a lower respiratory infection, and referral to hospital may be indicated based on the degree of

BOX 14.1 CLINICAL HISTORY

Acute Bronchiolitis in an Ex-Preterm Infant

A 5-month-old infant was admitted to hospital with increasing respiratory distress, a cough and episodes of apnoea requiring stimulation. His feeding had significantly decreased over the previous 24 hours.

He was born at 29 weeks gestation and spent the first 7 weeks of his life in the neonatal nursery in a tertiary neonatal unit far from his home. He required nasal CPAP for the first 7 days of life and had a patent ductus arteriosus treated with ibuprofen.

He was quite distressed with rapid respirations (over 70 per minute), subcostal and intercostal recession and his oxygen saturations were 87% on arrival to a regional paediatric department.

His parents were extremely concerned about his condition.

He was commenced on humidified oxygen via nasal prongs, intravenous fluids and a chest X-ray was ordered. His nasopharyngeal aspirate yielded respiratory syncytial virus (RSV) and thus he was isolated. His chest X-ray showed significant atelectasis and possible consolidation and therefore intravenous antibiotics were commenced. As he was quite unwell, he received intravenous hydrocortisone and nebulised salbutamol with no obvious benefit. Twelve hours post-admission he was transferred to a tertiary care paediatric centre for ongoing care.

Clinical Pearls

Evidence-based guidelines for managing acute bronchiolitis recommend primarily supportive care with oxygen and nasogastric feeds if tolerated, but many unnecessary treatments (as above) are well documented.

Family education including the recognition of signs of respiratory distress and the avoidance of unproven treatments are critical.

SpO_2 measurement under 92%, tachypnoea over 60 breaths per minute, apnoea and severe respiratory distress with inadequate fluid intake are all indications for admission to hospital.

Pitfalls to Avoid

Overtreatment with antibiotics, bronchodilators and unnecessary ordering of chest X-rays are still problematic. Quality improvement initiatives have been shown to work to reduce unnecessary investigations and treatments.

Following inpatient care, one should consider discharge if the infant is tolerating feeds and has had SpO_2 over 92% for at least 4 hours including a period of sleep.

Chest X-rays (CXR) are *not* routinely performed and can often confuse the clinical picture leading to the inappropriate prescribing of antibiotics. Nasal suctioning is recommended in infants with coincident nasal blockage causing respiratory distress.

There is no evidence that hypertonic saline is of added benefit.

respiratory distress, the fluid intake and if any evidence of desaturations. Infants with chronic lung disease, preterm infants born before 32 weeks gestation, congenital heart disease, neuromuscular disease and immunodeficiency are more likely to have severe disease.

Acute bronchiolitis is commonly seen in infants in temperate climates during the winter months and most relate to infection with RSV (Box 14.1). Key signs are chest retractions with head bobbing, wheeze and fine crackles on chest auscultation. Antibiotics are not indicated either in primary care or in hospital.[9] Pertussis may occur, particularly in unimmunised infants (Box 14.2).

> Bronchiolitis is treated with supportive therapy such as supplemental oxygen via nasal prongs and nasogastric feeds if inadequate oral intake.

Preschool Age Group

> Viruses are the most common cause of CAP in preschool children, so in general, antibiotics are not required for the majority of cases.

In children with signs of severe CAP, bacterial infection should be suspected. If your clinical examination reveals bilateral wheeze on auscultation, then you can safely assume that the cause of this infection is viral in nature. Most young children who wheeze do not have a coexisting bacterial infection. In the absence of fever, the chance of a wheezing child having a bacterial infection is less than 2%. Therefore, in general, children who present with a wheezing episode do not need antibiotics.

BOX 14.2 **CLINICAL HISTORY**

Coughing Paroxysms With Apnoea in a Young Infant

A 2-month-old male infant presents to hospital with a one-week history of coughing, and both the nursing staff, and the parents have become very concerned over a period of 24 hours, as they have witnessed pauses in his breathing. The consultant on-call is asked to review the infant in view of his clinical deterioration. On further history, the cough was noted to be paroxysmal and very distressing, and the infant appeared to go blue with some of the episodes. A nasopharyngeal aspirate confirmed *Bordetella pertussis* infection. The infant remained in hospital for over 3 weeks and was empirically treated with oral azithromycin. After 1 week in hospital the infant was transferred to the paediatric intensive care for repeated apnoea with cyanosis requiring oxygen and bag and mask ventilation.

Clinical Pearls

Pertussis in early infancy can be prevented by a maternal vaccination programme during pregnancy in nonimmune mothers.

Symptoms may steadily worsen in hospital despite commencement of azithromycin, and coughing spasms may last up to 3 months.

Pitfalls to Avoid

Azithromycin is used to stop nasopharyngeal carriage but does not change the clinical course.

Infants under 3 months are especially vulnerable to severe pertussis.

Children of this age group can inhale foreign bodies, and this differential including asking about a history of choking must be remembered (Box 14.3; Fig. 14.1).[10]

School-Aged Children

In an older child, the most important symptom is tachypnoea with grunting, and the most important sign is the presence of a raised respiratory rate with evidence of respiratory distress. Dullness to percussion may or may not be evident, and defined features of either consolidation (reduced air entry with increased vocal fremitus and possibly bronchial breathing) or effusion (marked dullness, reduced air entry and reduced vocal fremitus) are always much easier to elicit once a CXR has been performed and shows significant changes.

BOX 14.3 **CLINICAL HISTORY**

Coughing Following a Choking Episode in a Toddler

A 3-year-old presents to his family doctor with a 6-week history of a dry and persistent cough. His mother recalled an acute episode where he had a violent episode of coughing while eating popcorn 6 weeks ago. His family doctor commences him on both inhalers and oral antibiotics, but he is largely unresponsive. He is referred to hospital for chest X-ray and specialist opinion.

Clinical Pearls

Foreign body inhalation is mostly seen in children aged 1 to 4 years. The most common objects inhaled include popcorn, peanuts, seeds, carrots, beans, small toy parts and baby teeth.

Children with suspected foreign body inhalation should be referred for a rigid bronchoscopy where the foreign body can be identified and removed.

Pitfalls to Avoid

An inhaled foreign body in a child can easily be missed, particularly if a history of choking or coughing is not forthcoming.

A CXR will only detect radio-opaque foreign bodies, so a normal chest X-ray does not rule out foreign body aspiration.

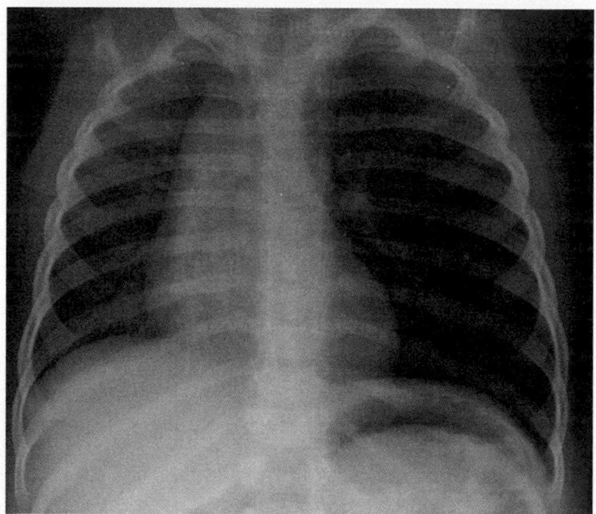

Fig. 14.1 Inhaled foreign body. An 18-month-old toddler who had dyspnoea after eating peanuts. Chest X-ray shows expansion and hyperlucency of the left lung with mediastinal shift to the right. A bit of peanut was found in the left main bronchus on bronchoscopy. (Courtesy Prof Stephanie Ryan.)

It is perfectly reasonable to treat with antibiotics when a CAP is suspected in an older child but equally important to review after 48 hours to ensure progress is being made and the child is improving on treatment.

If not improving after 48 to 72 hours, then referral to hospital for a CXR and clinical assessment is indicated.

COMPLICATED PNEUMONIA

Complicated pneumonia (CCAP) is characterised by a parapneumonic effusion or empyema, necrotising pneumonia or a lung abscess with the child also being highly pyrexial.[11] These children are quite unwell with often a pleural effusion detectable on clinical examination. They may develop progressive respiratory distress and rarely septic shock.

Risk factors for CCAP in previously healthy children include being under 24 months of age, having fever for several days prior to hospitalisation, unilateral pleuritic chest pain, high acute phase reactants and a low white cell count at presentation and a prior history of iron deficiency anaemia. Worldwide, CCAP is the greatest cause of death in infants over 1 month up until 5 years of age.[12]

If a complicated pneumonia is suspected, ask about a history of prolonged fever and whether pleuritic chest pain is present. The typical history is of a child who is unwell for several days despite starting antibiotics.

It is important to state that almost all children with CCAP are previously healthy without an underlying lung cystic malformation or immunodeficiency, and almost all make a full and complete recovery. The protracted nature of the illness and long duration of stay in hospital is very challenging for the family, and they may point to perhaps an earlier diagnosis in the community leading to a more rapid recovery. CCAP has reduced in prevalence but does still occur and the main focus is on reviewing the child with CAP after 48 hours to ensure that they are getting better. If not, then referral for radiological testing is indicated (Box 14.4).

One needs to suspect a complicated community-acquired pneumonia (CCAP) in any child with suspected bacterial pneumonia not responsive to appropriate antibiotics within 48 to 72 hours.[10]

BOX 14.4 CLINICAL HISTORY

A 4-Year-Old With Complicated Pneumonia

A 4-year-old presents to his family doctor with a 3-day history of fever and a cough. His examination reveals mild respiratory distress with tachypnoea and crackles heard on the right side of the chest. His family doctor commences him on co-amoxiclav orally and reassures his parents. Forty-eight hours later his parents are concerned that his temperature has not settled and bring him back for review. His examination is essentially unchanged, and the family are advised to continue oral antibiotics. After a further 48 hours, he is still pyrexial and ill and now looks pale with significant listlessness. The family re-present to the family practice and on this occasion, he is referred to the local emergency department. His chest X-ray (CXR) shows extensive consolidation on the right side, and an ultrasound performed the following morning shows a significant pleural effusion. He is now quite unwell and requires supplemental oxygen therapy. After a series of discussions and a further 24-hour observation, he has a follow-up chest ultrasound showing extension of the pleural effusion.

Transfer to a paediatric tertiary centre takes place and, later that evening, a chest drain is inserted, pleural fluid drained and urokinase instilled into the pleural cavity. All initial cultures are negative, but pleural fluid PCR is positive for *Streptococcus pneumoniae*. He is treated with intravenous cefotaxime for 10 days in total and a further 3 weeks of oral antibiotics, spending in all 11 days in hospital. At outpatient follow-up 4 months later he is perfectly well with no respiratory symptoms and a normal CXR.

Clinical Pearls

One of the 'golden rules' is that if a family keep re-presenting with their child and are concerned about the lack of improvement that, time and time again, their instincts are correct, and you need to change direction, revisit the diagnosis or consider referral to hospital.

Children with a complicated pneumonia will look very ill and have a high fever, a rapid respiratory rate and may have desaturations requiring oxygen therapy.

Pitfalls to Avoid

Children with complicated pneumonia should be referred to a paediatric tertiary centre. Initial imaging should include chest X-ray and ultrasound with chest CT being reserved for selected patients.[12]

Most require chest drain insertion with intrapleural fibrinolytic therapy. Complicated pneumonia is thus characterised by severe illness, prolonged hospitalisation with, thankfully, most children making a full recovery.

CCAP is usually caused by either *Streptococcus pneumoniae* or *Staphylococcus aureus* with *Haemophilus influenzae* and *Mycoplasma pneumoniae* occurring less often.

A parapneumonic effusion is the most frequently seen manifestation of CCAP. The presence of a parapneumonic effusion makes a bacterial cause six times more likely. Most cases of parapneumonic effusion resolve with antibiotics alone. However, effusions that are enlarging or causing respiratory compromise should never be managed with just antibiotics.[13] Occasionally a parapneumonic effusion can progress to a pleural empyema which is defined as pus in the pleural space. In necrotising pneumonia, consolidation with necrosis develops and leads to cavitation with the formation of pneumatocoeles in the affected lung (Fig. 14.2). Lung abscess formation is rarely seen and may occur with a preexisting cystic lung malformation or background immunodeficiency. Studies in Europe have shown a decline in the incidence of these complications following the introduction of the PCV 13 pneumococcal conjugate vaccine.[11]

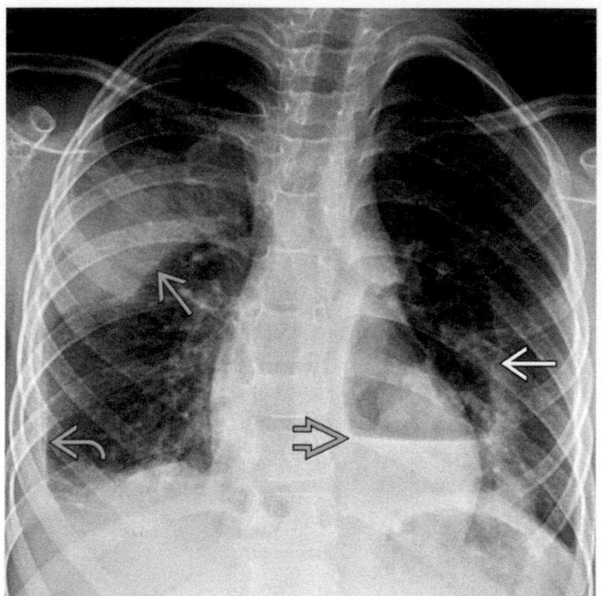

Fig. 14.2 Lung abscess/cavitary necrosis. PA radiograph in a 6-year-old with complicated pneumonia shows a cavitary mass in the left lower lung with an air-fluid level, suspicious for an abscess. Other signs of infection are present, including a right upper lung opacity and a right pleural effusion. (Source: ExpertDDX: *Pediatrics*. 2nd ed. 2020.)

The choice of antibiotics in CCAP should be based on local guidelines and sensitivity patterns. Intravenous antibiotics should be continued until the child is clinically improving, remains afebrile for at least 24 hours and/or the chest drain is removed.

Pleural drainage (ultrasound-guided) is recommended in children with an effusion that is evolving or who have respiratory distress. A minimally invasive drain is preferred, and the instillation of intrapleural fibrinolytics such as urokinase may shorten hospital stays. Video-assisted thoracoscopic surgery can also be considered as an alternative treatment modality depending on the level of surgical expertise.

Most children with CCAP make a complete recovery with often 7 to 14 days in hospital, but long-term complications can result in a small number of children.

The Role of Investigations in CCAP

In complicated pneumonia, the chest X-ray may show evidence of a parapneumonic effusion with blunting of the costophrenic angle and a rim of fluid ascending the lateral chest wall (the so-called meniscus sign) (Fig. 14.3) or, if a large effusion, a complete 'white out'.[12]

> Ultrasound is the investigation of choice for suspected pleural empyema.

Chest ultrasound can differentiate between consolidation and pleural fluid, estimate the size of the pleural effusion, detect the presence of fibrinous septations and provide guidance on the optimal chest drain insertion site (Fig. 14.4). A CT thorax is not routinely used in the management of pleural empyema unless in complicated cases or cases of necrotising pneumonia or lung abscess.

Detection of pneumococcal PCR in pleural fluid is very helpful in making treatment decisions with a pleural empyema. Serial measurements of the CRP are of help in monitoring the response to treatment.

RECURRENT PNEUMONIAS

In countries with neonatal cystic fibrosis screening, primary ciliary dyskinesia (PCD)[14] and common variable immunodeficiency (CVID)[15] are the two diagnoses to consider in children with recurrent bacterial pneumonia severe enough to require admission to hospital.

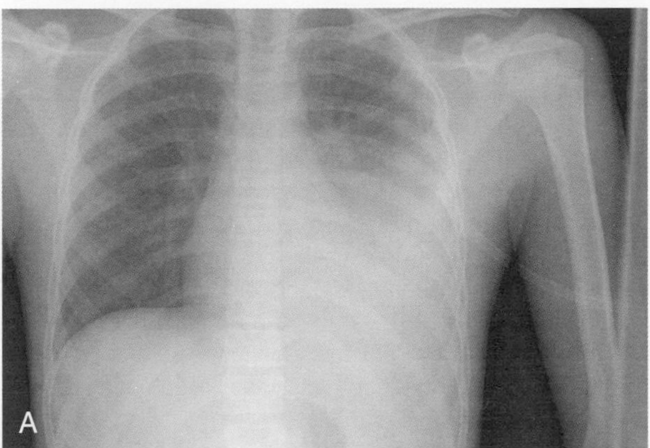

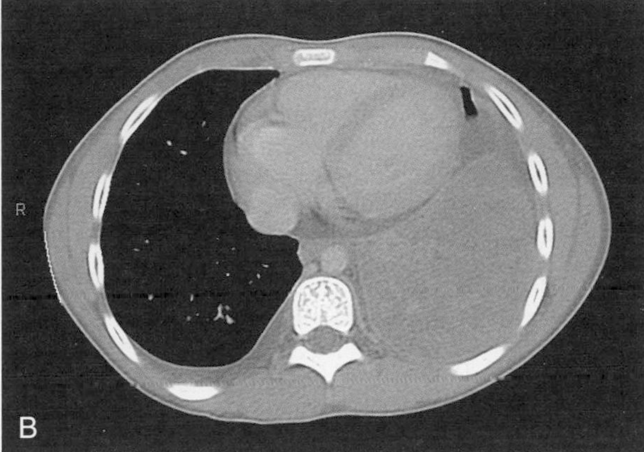

Fig. 14.3 (A) Radiograph and (B) computed tomography (CT) of the chest of a 13-year-old girl with *Mycoplasma pneumoniae* complicated by parapneumonic effusion. The radiograph demonstrates opacification of the left lung base with a moderate pleural effusion. Concurrent CT also demonstrates a small right-sided pleural effusion and a trivial pericardial effusion. (Kimberlin D, et al. *Principles and Practice of Pediatric Infectious Diseases.* 6th edition, 2023, Elsevier Inc.)

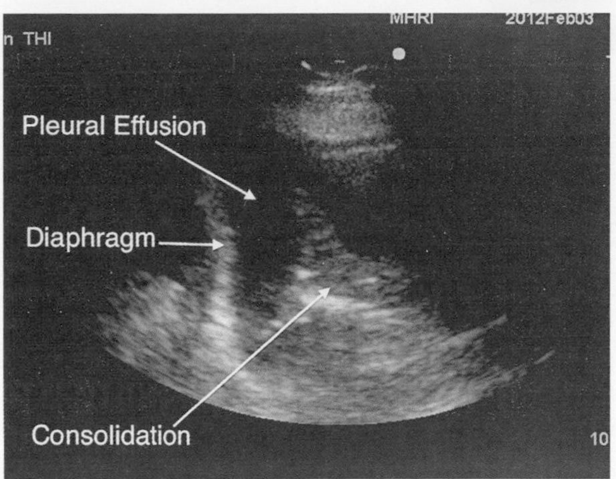

Fig. 14.4 Ultrasound image of the lung depicts the diaphragm, a pleural effusion and an infiltrate. (Edward J. Wing, Fred J. Schiffman. *Cecil Essentials of Medicine.* 10th edition, 2021, Elsevier Inc.)

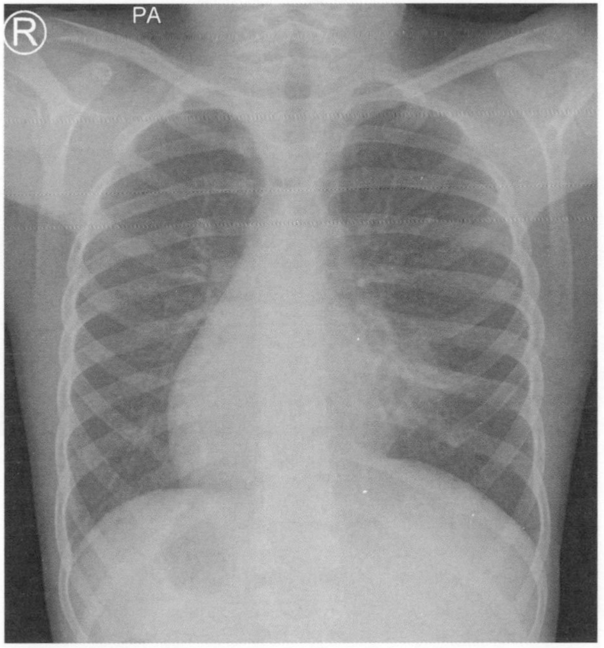

Fig. 14.5 Primary ciliary dyskinesia. A 7-year-old boy with recurrent respiratory tract infection. He has situs inversus (note the heart and the stomach bubble are on the right). Density in the left middle lobe blurring the left heart border is due to bronchiectasis. (Courtesy Prof Stephanie Ryan.)

Always investigate children with repeated confirmed bacterial pneumonias requiring intravenous antibiotics and consider CVID and other inborn errors of immunity.

In PCD, cilia in the airways, nasal lining and reproductive tract have impaired movement. This leads to poor airway clearance, recurrent infections, a chronic wet cough from an early age and thereafter bronchiectasis (Fig. 14.5; Box 14.5).

BOX 14.5 CLINICAL HISTORY

Recurrent Pneumonias Needing Hospitalisation

A 3-year-old boy had three hospital admissions over the previous 12 months with radiologically proven pneumonias all requiring intravenous antibiotics. He has a longstanding history of a persistent wet fruity cough from 6 months of age. He had a persistent watery nasal discharge from early infancy. He also had a history of conductive hearing loss requiring bilateral grommet insertion.

In his birth history he was born at term and was admitted to the neonatal intensive care unit (NICU) with progressive respiratory distress which required mechanical ventilation for 48 hours.

Investigations included a CT thorax which showed significant bronchiectasis. His sweat test was normal.

His serum IgA, IgM and IgG levels were normal, and he had satisfactory specific antibody responses to primary vaccinations (Hib, tetanus, pneumococcus). Nasal ciliary brushings were sent for electron microscopy, and a diagnosis of primary ciliary dyskinesia (PCD) was confirmed.

Clinical Pearls

Children with PCD often present with a typical clinical presentation as outlined above.

The presence of a *chronic wet cough is abnormal* and should prompt further investigation for causes of bronchiectasis.[16] Newborn cystic fibrosis screening is in place in most EU countries but consideration of CF as a diagnosis may depend on the child's age, as some presenting were born prior to national screening or in countries where national screening is not in place.

PCD typically presents (as in this case) early in life. The reported frequency of PCD is 1 in 10,000, and conductive hearing loss is seen in 80% of cases.

About 50% of children with PCD have situs inversus or heterotaxy syndromes which may be associated with congenital heart disease, asplenia or polysplenia.[11] Male and female infertility are common in PCD.

The key features of PCD are neonatal respiratory symptoms, daily nasal congestion, daily wet cough and laterality defects.

Pitfalls to Avoid

No single test will diagnose every child with PCD but examination of ciliary samples by electron microscopy has been regarded as the gold standard. Children with PCD are noted to have reduced nasal nitric oxide measurements, and this test is useful for screening tool in children over 5 years of age. Where the diagnosis is uncertain, ciliary samples can be sent for a more detailed high-speed video microscopy test which assesses cilia beat frequency and patterns. Genetic testing via whole exome sequencing has been used to identify candidate genes associated with PCD.[14]

Airway clearance techniques with chest physiotherapy and nebulised mucolytics as well as aggressive treatment of exacerbations with antibiotics are the mainstays of treatment.

KEY LEARNING POINTS

Respiratory tract infections are very common in children and viruses are the commonest cause.

Clinical assessment should focus on distinguishing a mild and severe CAP.

Neither chest radiography nor clinical examination findings distinguish a viral from a bacterial lower respiratory tract infection.

If your clinical examination reveals bilateral wheeze on auscultation, then it is likely that the cause of this infection is viral in nature.

One needs to suspect a complicated community-acquired pneumonia (CCAP) in any child with suspected bacterial pneumonia not responsive to appropriate antibiotics within 48 to 72 hours.[12]

All children with CCAP should be discussed with a respiratory paediatrician and ideally referred to a tertiary centre.

The long-term prognosis is excellent, and a complete recovery is expected, and families should be assured of a favourable prognosis.

REFERENCES

1. Jeremy H, Christie C, Alastair DH, Jenny I. Primary care clinician antibiotic prescribing decisions in consultations for children with RTIs: a qualitative interview study. *Br J Gen Pract*. 2016;66(644):e207–e213. doi:10.3399/bjgp16X683821.
2. Florin TA. Differentiating Bacterial From Viral Etiologies in Pediatric Community-Acquired Pneumonia: The Quest for the Holy Grail Continues. *J Pediatric Infect Dis Soc*. 2021;10(12):1047–1050. doi:10.1093/jpids/piab034.
3. Thornton HV, Blair PS, Lovering AM, Muir P, Hay AD. Clinical presentation and microbiological diagnosis in paediatric respiratory tract infection: a systematic review. *Br J Gen Pract*. 2015;65(631):e69–e81. doi:10.3399/bjgp15X683497.
4. Little P, Francis NA, Stuart B, et al. Antibiotics for lower respiratory tract infection in children presenting in primary care in England (ARTIC PC): a double-blind, randomised, placebo-controlled trial. *Lancet*. 2021;398(10309):1417–1426. doi:10.1016/S0140-6736(21)01431-8.
5. Saul H, Gursul D, Cassidy S, Bielicki J. A short course of antibiotics is effective for treating pneumonia in children. *BMJ*. 2022;378:cd17671.
6. Zar HJ, Andronikou S, Nicol MP. Advances in the diagnosis of pneumonia in children. *BMJ*. 26 Jul. 2017;358:j2739. doi:10.1136/bmj.j2739.
7. British Thoracic Society. Paediatric Community Acquired Pneumonia. Accessed online at https://www.brit-thoracic.org.uk/quality-improvement/clinical-resources/paediatric-community-acquired-pneumonia/
8. Gunaratnam LC, Robinson JL, Hawkes MT. Systematic Review and Meta-Analysis of Diagnostic Biomarkers for Pediatric Pneumonia. *J Pediatric Infect Dis Soc*. 2021;10(9):891–900. doi:10.1093/jpids/piab043.
9. Montejo M, Paniagua N, Saiz-Hernando C, Martinez-Indart L, Mintegi S, Benito J. Initiatives to reduce treatments in bronchiolitis in the emergency department and primary care. *Arch Dis Child*. 2021;106(3):294–300. doi:10.1136/archdischild-2019-318085.
10. Helen W. Inhaled foreign bodies. *Arch Dis Child*. 2005;90:ep31–ep33. doi:10.1136/adc.2005.080259.
11. de Benedictis FM, Kerem E, Chang AB, Colin AA, Zar HJ, Bush A. Complicated pneumonia in children. *Lancet*. 2020;396(10253):786–798. doi:10.1016/S0140-6736(20)31550-6.
12. GBD 2016 Lower Respiratory Infections Collaborators. Estimates of the global, regional, and national morbidity, mortality, and aetiologies of lower respiratory infections in 195 countries, 1990–2016: a systematic analysis for the Global Burden of Disease Study 2016'. *Lancet Infect Dis*. 2018;18(11):1191–1210. doi:10.1016/S1473-3099(18)30310-4.
13. Breuer O, Picard E, Benabu N, et al. Predictors of Prolonged Hospitalizations in Pediatric Complicated Pneumonia. *Chest*. 2018;153(1):172–180. doi:10.1016/j.chest.2017.09.021.
14. Horani A, Ferkol TW. Understanding Primary Ciliary Dyskinesia and Other Ciliopathies. *J Pediatr*. 2021;230:15–22.e1. doi:10.1016/j.jpeds.2020.11.040.
15. Yazdani R, Habibi S, Sharifi L, et al. Common Variable Immunodeficiency: Epidemiology, Pathogenesis, Clinical Manifestations, Diagnosis, Classification, and Management. *J Investig Allergol Clin Immunol*. 2020;30(1):14–34. doi:10.18176/jiaci.0388.
16. Brodlie M, Graham C, McKean MC. Childhood cough. *BMJ*. 6 Mar. 2012;344:e1177. doi:10.1136/bmj.e1177.

ADDITIONAL READING

Clark JE, et al. Children with pneumonia: how do they present and how are they managed? *Arch Dis Child*. 2007;92(5):394–398. doi:10.1136/adc.2006.097402.

Erlichman I, Breuer O, Shoseyov D, et al. Complicated community acquired pneumonia in childhood: Different types, clinical course, and outcome. *Pediatr Pulmonol*. 2017;52(2):247–254. doi:10.1002/ppul.23523.

Hay AD, Wilson AD. The natural history of acute cough in children aged 0 to 4 years in primary care: a systematic review. *Br J Gen Pract*. 2002;52(478):401–409.

Jankauskaite L, Oostenbrink R. Childhood lower respiratory tract infections: more evidence to do less. *Lancet*. 2021;398(10309):1383–1384. doi:10.1016/S0140-6736(21)01955-3.

Shapiro DJ, Hall M, Lipsett SC, et al. Short- Versus Prolonged-Duration Antibiotics for Outpatient Pneumonia in Children. *J Pediatr*. 2021;234:205–211.e1. doi:10.1016/j.jpeds.2021.03.017.

15

Mental Health Issues in Adolescence

Fiona McNicholas

CHAPTER OUTLINE

BACKGROUND

Adolescence is a time of great opportunity and change, an exciting and enjoyable time filled with new activities and responsibilities. Key developmental tasks include the establishment of autonomy and gaining independence from one's parents by spending more time with peers.

Adolescents are wired for impulsivity and action, rebellious and risky behaviours, extremes of emotions without the more mature benefits of restraint, impulse control, careful judgments, error correction and emotion regulation of later years. Happily, many adolescents navigate this period well and develop adaptive coping strategies and resilience for challenges in later life. For others, this transition can be associated with significant stress and pressure and contribute to mental health (MH) difficulties.

Furthermore, there is a growing awareness of increased pressure on adolescents associated with modern-day living. The current economic and occupational climate means that, for many adolescents, establishing autonomy from parents, socially, economically and physically is delayed as they stay longer in education, and experience difficulties accessing affordable housing. Not only is the period of adolescence extended by a delayed exit, but it may also commence earlier, as younger children are increasingly being exposed to adult content via social media.

Navigating these developmental challenges of autonomy, awaiting the development of the prefrontal cortex of the brain to allow for improved and more controlled executive functioning, can be difficult and present with varying degrees of behavioural, emotional, physical and psychological symptoms. For most adolescents these represent brief periods of feeling sad, anxious, stressed or self-conscious or risk-taking behaviours, and when well-managed, often with the support of peers and family, lead to resilience. However, there are a significant number in whom experiences are more severe, longer lasting and associated with significant impairment in personal, social or educational functioning, meeting criteria for mental illness.

> The World Health Organisation has estimated that mental illness accounts for almost half of the disease in adolescents and young adults, and at any one time 25% of those aged between 12 and 25 years will meet diagnostic criteria for a mental health disorder.

It is also recognised that for most adult mental illnesses, their origins begin in adolescence, 50% by the age of 18 years and 75% surfacing by the age of 25 years. Despite this high level of morbidity, most adolescents with mental illness do not attend specialist services. As such, it is important that paediatricians and family practitioners are familiar with signs and symptoms of mental illness, can distinguish these from transient adolescent distress and where necessary offer appropriate intervention or onward referral to specialist Child and Adolescent Mental Health Services (CAMHS).

KEY ISSUES

Apart from injuries and a small number of acute or chronic illnesses, the main reason a family doctor will see a young adolescent is with psychological difficulties.

> These presentations include self-harm, eating disorders of various types, anxiety and depression, ADHD and functional symptoms including chronic disabling fatigue.

This chapter offers a review of the main mental health difficulties that adolescents face and might come to the attention of a paediatrician or family doctor. It also outlines how best to approach these conditions as a first responder and presents a useful assessment framework including when to refer for specialist help.

ASSESSMENT OF PSYCHOLOGICAL DISTRESS AND MENTAL HEALTH ISSUES: THE IF-ME MODEL OF ASSESSMENT

This assessment follows a biopsychosocial model, with the recognition that many mental health difficulties are multifactorial in nature and influenced by individual and genetic risk factors, the context in which the child or adolescent lives, such as family, school, peers and biological factors including any medical illness or medication. Over the course of the assessment, a range of issues are explored with the young person's current and past difficulties, early developmental difficulties, including adverse childhood experiences, medical problems or medication use.

Family history is explored to incorporate any relevant presence of mental health difficulties. Academic progress and social support network are important to explore including the presence of any adverse social experiences or risky behaviours. Information is elicited from the young person, their parents and school records as appropriate. It is important to have clearly established the limits of confidentiality ahead of any individual discussion, such that the adolescent and parent are aware that the clinician is unable to keep private information obtained which suggests that the adolescent is at risk of self-harm, harm by others or intention to harm others. Failure to do so risks therapeutic disengagement. Both clinical observations, questionnaires and structured observations assist in the overall comprehensive assessment. A helpful model to consider when assessing youth's mental health is to consider the mnemonic, ***IF-ME,*** IF it were ME going for an assessment, how would I like to be assessed (Table 15.1) and treated (Table 15.2). Focusing on these four areas, ***Individual, Family, Medical and Environmental,*** allows the clinician to gather pertinent information in a timely and structured way, identifying risks and strengths in each area and considering targeted support. Supplementing a multiinformant clinical assessment with questionnaires is also very helpful. The strengths and difficulties questionnaire

TABLE 15.1 IF-ME Domains and Focus of Enquiry

Individual	Family
Establish presenting symptoms, history of same and conduct systems review to establish if other comorbid symptoms present. *Remember presentation will not always be self-initiated or wanted.*	Ask about family composition, relationships, parenting style and any family history of psychiatric illness.
Medical	**Environmental**
Take a developmental history, including medical illness or use of medication. Establishing presence of any feeding or eating difficulties, and measuring current and past weight, height, calories and exercise levels is key if suspicion of an eating disorder.	School is the main environmental influence for youth. Ask about getting corroboration from teachers, difficulties with behaviour, academic ability and social skills. Socioeconomic disadvantage or poor choice of peer groups should also be considered and asked about.

TABLE 15.2 **General Multimodal Therapeutic Approaches Using IFME Framework**

Disorder Type	Individual	Family	Medication*	Environmental
Anxiety	Cognitive behavioural therapy (CBT) Relaxation training	Psycho-educational Identify family history of anxiety and offer support as needed	SSRI (for example, Sertraline)	School supports Exposure treatments
Depression	CBT or Interpersonal therapy (IPT)	Psycho-educational Identify family history of depression or conflict and offer support if necessary	SSRI (for example, fluoxetine)	Identify and address life events such as bullying, academic difficulties, peer pressures
Attention-deficit/ hyperactivity disorder (ADHD)	Study and organisational skills	Psycho-educational Parenting Identify family history of ADHD and offer appropriate support as necessary	Psychostimulants such as methylphenidate or lisdexamphetamine	Classroom support and individual educational plan Examination accommodations
Eating Disorder (ED)	**CBT, IPT	Psycho-education and carer support Family-based treatment (FBT)	Weak evidence of effectiveness in core ED psychopathology, including high-dose fluoxetine in Bulimia Nervosa (BN); lisdexamphetamine in Binge Eating Disorder (BED)+ Low-dose antipsychotics in Anorexia Nervosa (AN) if high anxiety or obsessional behaviours	Consider limiting or monitoring activities such as exercise/school Supervision of meals Examination accommodations Attention to pressures from social media
Psychosis	Supportive psychotherapy, CBT	Psycho-education and carer support Encouraging low-expressed emotion	Second-generation antipsychotic medication with regular metabolic and cardiovascular review	Risk assessment, minimising stressors, examination and school accommodation and caution against substance abuse
Psycho-somatic disorders such as chronic fatigue syndrome (CFS)	Supportive psychotherapy, relaxation, CBT, hypnotherapy	Parental reassurance and support, advice on responding to adolescents' symptoms and seeking of further investigation	Advice on nutrition, sleep and activity scheduling Medications such as analgesics, antispasmodics or antidepressants as required	Identifying and managing school-related stressors, individualised educational plan

*Suggested as first line with doses adjusted based on weight, tolerability and effectiveness.
**Typically following weight restoration and trial of FBT.
+is for less evidence for eating disorder medication.

(SDQ), self, teacher and parent report, is a widely used, freely available and psychometrically sound mental health screen and has recently been advocated for the assessment of emotional and behavioural problems in adolescents.

ANXIETY ISSUES

The experience of stress in life is ubiquitous, linked to the exposure to stressors, internal or external, real or imagined and related to positive or more often negative events. This innate stress response may activate a healthy response of fight or flight. For those who feel unable to cope, either due to the magnitude of the stressor or the developmental age they are at, this may lead to ongoing stress and anxiety.

> Significant levels of anxiety are present in as many as 10 to 25% of young people, with a mean age of onset at age 11.

Physical symptoms include shortness of breath, palpitations, gastrointestinal symptoms such as nausea, vomiting or diarrhoea, tremulousness, pain or discomfort. Cognitive components can include fear of failure, abandonment, anticipated disasters and fear of serious illness or even death. When the cognitive component is absent or unconsciously suppressed, the focus on somatic symptoms alone might lead to prolonged, unnecessary and even harmful medical investigations and delayed intervention.

Many anxiety symptoms start in early life and follow a developmental progression, linked to their typical experiences. Separation anxiety commences at about 6 to 9 months of age and signals the positive and protective attachment of the infant to their parent, is short-lived but can occasionally re-emerge at times of other transitions or life events, such as starting school. It is not suggestive of any pathology. Only when being separated from a loved one persists over time and limits the young person's functioning does it become pathological. Young children also often develop specific fears with accompanying avoidance behaviour, such as fear of the dark, dogs or storms. These also generally fade with age with few remaining into the adolescent years.

A child may be shy, fearing scrutiny or undue focus, and hesitant to talk in the presence of strangers. Such behaviour typically improves with age but for a certain cohort of children is replaced by social anxiety becoming more prominent in adolescent years. Young people with social anxiety (previously referred to as social phobia) are uncomfortable meeting unfamiliar people, typically of the same age and experience physical and cognitive symptoms. They fear they will not know what to say, how to behave, how to dress and they worry they will be judged unfavourably and excluded or ridiculed. Depending on the intensity, such fears may lead to an adolescent developing physical symptoms at the start of the school week, school avoidance, refusing or unable to accept invitations to events and reducing social contact to carefully selected and often constricted groups. Some adolescents may continue to attempt social engagement, despite the anxiety, by relying on medication or alcohol. Untreated, significant social anxiety can lead to substance misuse and depression and loss of academic or occupational potential. Some adolescent fears are more pervasive, and they worry about 'everything', and this is referred to as general anxiety. They may present with incapacitating levels of cognitive and physical components of anxiety referred to above. Should they reach a crescendo and symptoms become intense, physical symptoms may escalate to the point that they feel unable to cope with the shortness of breath, rapid heart rate, and fears of imminent death or serious incapacitation. These symptoms constitute a panic attack. When the fear of recurring panic attacks becomes part of the general anxiety, this is referred to as a panic disorder and is rare before puberty.

OBSESSIVE-COMPULSIVE DISORDER

Obsessive-compulsive disorder (OCD) is another type of anxiety disorder, present in 1% of adolescents, characterised by the experiences of recurring thoughts or images which are associated with certain compulsive behaviours aimed to reduce the associated anxiety. The age of onset is typically in early adolescence and, unlike the female predominance for most anxiety disorders, this affects boys and girls equally.

The treatments of all adolescent anxiety disorders can easily be understood referring back to the IFME model outlined above (see Table 15.2). Individual work includes cognitive behavioural therapy (CBT), the mainstay of treatment especially with developmental cognitive maturity, relaxation training and mindfulness.

Directing parents to suitable reading materials, so that they do not unwittingly re-enforce or overly accommodate OCD or anxiety behaviours, is essential.

As many anxiety disorders in young people are often inherited, parental insight into their own anxiety state is helpful and leads to optimal modelling and parenting.

Medication is considered second line to CBT, although the evidence base is strong and medication, often off-label or off-licence, typically a selective serotonin reuptake inhibitor (SSRI), is recognised to be effective.

DEPRESSION

A recent study from the United States showed that a universal screening programme for depression identified that 2.5% of adolescents aged 12 to 17 years of age attending a large emergency department for a variety of symptoms were found to have moderate to severe depression. Most did not present with psychiatric symptoms. Thus, depression is very common among young people and may first present to a family doctor or paediatrician.

The experience of feeling sad is a normal emotional response often linked to loss, whether to a person, place or object. However, the experience of a pervasive sense of sadness, with physical and physiological components, experienced most days for a 2-week period, accompanied by negative thoughts about oneself ('I am not attractive/kind/clever'), the world about them ('no one cares for me, I don't have good friends') and their future ('I have nothing to look forward to, this will never change, I would be better off dead') signals the presence of a major depressive disorder.

> During a depressive episode the young person may feel tired, lacking in energy and concentration, with a decline in academic ability.

They may have poor sleep, often interrupted by negative ruminative thoughts. Their appetite may be lost with consequent weight loss, or some may overeat in an effort to experience some pleasure to compensate. They may retreat from social and family activities, finding little enjoyment in previously pleasurable activities. Such isolation and inactivity further remove them from peer and family support and is likely to reinforce the idea that they have nothing to live for and lead to suicidal thoughts or behaviours. They may engage in other acts of self-harm, such as cutting or substance use, to find relief, either temporarily or permanently, from the unpleasant and perceived intolerable state they are in.

Depression associated with psychotic features, especially command hallucinations ordering them to end their life, merits urgent specialist assessment, often in an inpatient setting. The presence of self-harming behaviours or thoughts raises the level of risk and urgency of careful assessment and treatment.

For mild depression, a family doctor may offer individual supportive therapy or group CBT for 2 to 3 months.

> Clinical guidelines for treatment of adolescent depression include CBT as first line as individual treatment and the addition of medication 6 weeks later if no response.

Fluoxetine, an SSRI, is the medication of choice, with the adage of starting low and going slow to reach an expected therapeutic dose. Side effects are typically benign, and mainly gastrointestinal given the predominance of serotonin receptors in the gut.

> The use to initiation of medication for the treatment of adolescent depression should remain within specialist Child and Adolescent Mental Health Services (CAMHS).

Family-focused treatment includes giving the parents information on depression, advice about safe management of self-harm risks, minimising any intrafamilial conflict or heightened expressed emotion and establishing presence of any ongoing family stressors or adverse life events, including parental mental illness that might benefit from treatment.

SELF-HARM

Rates of self-harm (SH) are high in adolescence and have been increasing. National biennial surveys of high school students 14 to 18 years of age attending schools across the United States consistently report high rates of having 'made a plan to self-harm' (15%), 'engaged in SH' (9%) and 'engaged in SH that required medical attention' (3%) in the prior year. Self-cutting is the most common method of self-harm in community settings and quite often goes unreported. Deliberate poisoning is the most common method in hospital presentations. There is an increased risk of self-harm in poor families, if there is domestic violence or excess alcohol use by parents and if there are prior childhood adverse events.

> For adolescents with depression and either active suicidal thoughts or episodes of self-harm, referral to Child and Adolescent Mental Health Services (CAMHS) is warranted.

Similar statistics are reported in many other countries, with rate of self-harm among females consistently higher than males. Prevalence rates of SH across large EU studies are 5% of males and 15% of females.

> Community studies highlight the reality that hospital attendances for self-harm are only a small subset of all SH cases and more likely to be following an overdose.

It is important to distinguish acts of SH with or without suicidal intent. In themselves self-harming behaviours, such as cutting or substance abuse do not confirm the presence or absence of a psychiatric disorder. However, careful assessment is needed to help establish the co-occurrence of a treatable mental illness or psychiatric disorder, such as depression, anxiety or an eating disorder and to assess the level of immediate risk, including a need to refer on to CAMHS for further assessment and treatment.

While SH is more frequently seen in females, completed suicide is more common in males.

A family history of SH or suicide, past or current adverse childhood experiences (including abuse, bullying, loss), comorbid psychiatric illness and risky peer behaviours should all be enquired about. Identifying positive aspects of personal and family functioning is equally important and offers important treatment opportunities.

Any presentation of SH needs to be considered carefully, irrespective of stated intent. A therapeutic assessment may indicate a need for subsequent specialist support. Risk scales for suicide in those presenting with self-harm are not sufficiently accurate (Box 15.1).

Sensible daily living advice, such as attention to nutrition, exercise and sleeping habits are vitally important. In the presence of significant self-harming behaviour with suicidal intent and/or psychotic features, a period on inpatient admission might be necessary.

ATTENTION DEFICIT HYPERACTIVITY DISORDER

Attention deficit hyperactivity disorder (ADHD) is considered to reflect neurodiversity rather than disability and, as such, individuals with ADHD have both strengths

BOX 15.1 CLINICAL HISTORY

Self-Harm

A 13-year-old girl presents with peri-umbilical abdominal pain that has been ongoing for the past 3 years. It has no known triggers but occurs up to twice per week, with increasing severity over the past 3 months causing her to be unable to attend school. Her menses are regular, last 5 days and are associated with cramps.

She lives at home with her mother and younger sister. Her father passed away unexpectedly 3 years ago, and she is not sure of the cause of his death. She has no close friends and does not like any of her teachers. She used to play the piano and go swimming but has stopped in the past year. She has not started dating and is not sure if she is interested in boys or girls. She has never engaged in any sexual activity. She has never tried alcohol, cigarettes or any drugs. She describes her mood as quite low and informs you that she has deliberately cut herself on her inner thighs and forearms with a razor blade on two occasions in the past 3 months following arguments with her mother about her not wanting to go to school.

On examination she has well-healed horizontal linear scars on her inner thighs and forearms. Otherwise, her physical examination is unremarkable.

Clinical Pearls

The loss of her father, the lack of engagement with school, her disengagement from activities she previously enjoyed are all potential contributors to her low mood and self-harm.

Common forms of self-harm (SH) include cutting the arms or legs with a sharp object, taking an overdose of medication (often paracetamol) or alcohol or illicit drug intoxication.

Although depression is a common comorbidity, treatment with antidepressants has not been shown to lessen the risk of a repeat episode in young people treated in hospital for SH. Conduct disorder and attention deficit hyperactivity are common comorbidities in SH.

Deliberate self-poisoning (over 80%), followed by self-cutting (10%) are the most common presentations of SH to hospital.

Specialist SH multidisciplinary teams enhance both the service to the young person and their family and enable the professional development of the clinical team.

For adolescents, self-motivation to change, positive parenting and healthy sleeping habits all exert a positive effect. Family involvement is critical.

Pitfalls to Avoid

The most seen SH treated in hospital is deliberate self-poisoning, and this may be associated with suicidal ideation. Up to 15% of those presenting with SH have a repeat episode within 12 months.

Self-injury (in particular, cutting or biting) is the main cause of SH seen in the community and is often repeated but has a very low risk of suicide. If the young person is deemed to be low risk, this should not result in delayed assessment or reduced access to aftercare in the community.

and weaknesses. International prevalence studies suggest a rate of 5.5% in childhood and adolescence reducing to 3% in adulthood. Recognising and treating ADHD in childhood is important from a public health perspective as adults with ADHD have a shortened life expectancy.

Core symptoms of ADHD include pervasive hyperactivity (always on the go, inability to sit still, fidgetiness), impulsivity (unable to wait their turn, engaging in dangerous activities without due regard to consequences, blurting things out) and inattention (difficulty with staying focused on task, concentrating for long periods, following through on instructions, remembering) that are *present and impairing in a number of domains*, such as school, after school activities, with peers and at home.

The typical age of diagnosis corresponds to timing and nature of academic challenges, such as entering formal education or at the time of transition to secondary school as the academic load intensifies. Equally 'transparency' of symptoms is dependent on IQ and gender, with girls often presenting with the less obvious inattentive type more often, and those with a high IQ managing to retain adequate academic functioning until the academic load increases. Untreated ADHD is a risk factor for subsequent conduct disorder, substance misuse, criminal activity, early school dropout, poorer academic attainment and comorbid depression and self-harm.

Treatment of adolescent ADHD using the IF-ME guiding principles includes cognitive strategies to help with personal and study organisation; adolescent-specific parenting programs to encourage nonpunitive but firm authoritative parenting, emphasising structure and consistency (see Table 15.2).

First-line medication is with methylphenidate or long-acting amphetamine-based products with regular monitoring of weight, height, blood pressure and heart rate with educational supports based on individual assessments and learning needs. The flexibility of ADHD medication management allows more autonomy to be gradually shifted toward the adolescent with age as they become skilled in their own management of dosing depending on daily activities.

EATING DISORDERS

With the advent of social media, ideal body images are viewed and presented on an almost continuous basis, sharpening any personal dissatisfaction and intensifying any insecurities that a person may have. Given the importance of physical attractiveness in adolescents and the commencement of romantic relationships, adolescents may be especially vulnerable to these messages.

> It is thus no surprise that the peak age of onset of an eating disorder is in adolescence.

Large-scale community studies in the United States and Europe have cited prevalence rates of anorexia nervosa (AN) and bulimia nervosa (BN) of between 1–1.5% of females and 0–0.3% to 0.1–0.5% of males. Binge eating disorder (BED) presents less often in adolescence and is typically diagnosed in adults and equally common in men and women. The prevalence of concerning eating behaviours falling short of any of these criteria is as high as 5%.

Disordered eating patterns differ by group. In BN and BED excessive amounts of food are consumed in a short period of time with a sense of lack of control and accompanied by extreme guilt, disgust and distress, occurring on a weekly basis. In those with BN, they are accompanied by compensatory behaviours of vomiting, laxative or diuretic use, bouts of fasting or excessive exercise. Young people with BN are often of normal or slightly higher weight, and those with BED are most often of higher weight.

> Those with anorexia nervosa have an intense fear of weight gain and restrict their food intake in an effort to lose weight, which is often accompanied by excessive exercise regimes.

Although some young people with AN may engage in episodic binging, they remain underweight. Prior diagnostic criteria for AN include a BMI under 18.5, or more than 15% body weight loss (or body mass index of 85%) and amenorrhea have now been removed due to the need for developmentally sensitive weight parameters to be referenced and the growing awareness of AN presenting in males. DSM-5 also introduced a new eating disorder classification called Avoidant Restrictive Food Intake Disorder or ARFID. Although this may present in adulthood, it is more often a childhood diagnosis often presenting first to paediatricians. Such children may present with restrictive or avoidant eating behaviours accompanied by serious weight loss or nutritional deficiency but in the absence of body image disturbance.

> The assessment and management of eating disorders require a paediatrician to first and foremost conduct a full history and careful examination.

It is essential to establish the child's premorbid weight (not always available) and whether the child was either overweight, of normal weight or underweight relative to peers. This enables clinicians to establish the target restorative weight. Careful plotting on appropriate weight, height and BMI charts is essential. Always check the lying and standing blood pressures and the heart rate. Be aware that young people with low weight are typically bradycardic. Therefore, a young person with a normal or fast heart rate may be more unwell.

The MARSIPAN guidelines (now superceded by Medical Emergencies in Eating Disorders or MEED) and checklist are a very useful framework for clinicians to use.

Early and aggressive treatment is essential to ensure both medical and psychological wellbeing. A twin-track approach of nutritional restoration and psychological work is essential for those with AN and weight loss commencing with medical stabilisation. The treatment of choice for both AN and BN is outpatient-based family treatment or FBT, which takes a very practical and behavioural approach in assisting parents refeed their child and in the case of BN, limiting binges and compensatory behaviours. A clinician and parent's manual are available. Co-occurring mental illness is often expected to resolve with weight restoration. Addressing interpersonal and family issues is delayed until adequate restoration of weight. In the presence of significant family dysfunction or extreme carer fatigue, interpersonal therapy or CBT might be more appropriate as first line treatment for the older adolescent. FBT is also recommended as the treatment of choice for those with ARFID. Reverting to the IFME model (Table 15.2), there is little evidence to support medication in the treatment of eating disorders, other than in the presence of comorbid psychiatric illness. Most eating disorders have varying degrees of comorbid anxiety and depression, occasionally OCD and carry a very high morbidity and indeed mortality. Environmental considerations might include cessations of sporting activities, reduced school attendances and social media use monitoring. Parents and young people may benefit from the eating disorder support associations (Box 15.2).

PSYCHOSIS

The experience of isolated auditory or visual hallucinations can be relatively common in childhood, but they are generally transient and self-limiting and dissipate over time. Many children describe an imaginary friend with whom they find comfort. The child often finds it hard to give accurate or convincing descriptions of these experiences, being often poorly defined and vague.

However, for a small group they might signal subsequent psychotic disorders. Such a young person might describe the voices in detail, identifying them as male or female, singular or multiple, coming from outside of their head, conversing with each other and describing their actions (suggestive of third-person auditory hallucinations). They may occur in the presence of delusions, fixed beliefs, held with conviction and out of keeping with the person's cultural background. Delusions may be grandiose (often in mania), such as believing one can fly, paranoid (often in schizophrenia), such as a belief someone is trying to poison them, nihilistic (in depression), such as they are empty or rotting from inside. The mistaken belief that radio advertisements are giving them a special message is often suggestive of schizophrenia. Abnormalities of thought may also be evidenced such that it may be difficult to understand what the person is saying, to follow their train of thought or to engage them in conversation.

> The presence of psychotic symptoms, especially when paired with anxiety, distress or persistence suggests an urgent need to refer to CAMHS for assessment and management.

There is often a period of gradual deterioration, with negative symptoms, such as increasing social isolation, lack of attention to self-care preceding frank psychotic symptoms. Whilst all first-onset psychosis should have a medical workup, this is most urgent in those with a sudden onset to outrule any organic cause.

CHRONIC DISABLING FATIGUE OR CHRONIC FATIGUE SYNDROME

Key symptoms of chronic disabling fatigue or chronic fatigue syndrome (CFS) include postexertional malaise, cognitive dysfunction, sleep disturbance, muscle pain, joint pain, general malaise, headaches, sore throat, dizziness, painful lymph nodes, nausea and palpitations.

Younger children have a different set of symptoms with less cognitive or sleep problems. Tender lymphadenopathy and dizziness are more likely in preadolescents. Those with 'mild' symptoms are generally able to carry on everyday activities, such as school, but to do so they may have to give up hobbies to allow extra time for rest. Those with 'moderate' symptoms can usually no longer attend

BOX 15.2 CLINICAL HISTORY

An Adolescent With an Eating Disorder

A 16-year-old female presents to the paediatrician with secondary amenorrhea of 6 months and physical complaints of fatigue, and syncope. The history offered by her is of stress related to pursuit of academic excellence, juggling her busy sports commitments (school hockey and club soccer). When asked about body image, she is quite vague and reports being 'somewhat chubby' previously and currently. She became vegetarian a year ago and vegan in the last 3 months and reports rarely feeling hungry with some unquantified weight loss. She emphasises her desire to maintain a high fitness level assisted by her careful meal planning and veganism. Developmental history from parents suggests normal premorbid development, with excellent physical health, academically able with a good peer group. Parents noticed irritability around food preparation and intake in the last few months and are unaware of exact weight loss as she generally wears baggy clothes. There is no history of binging, purging or laxative use. She achieved menarche at age 12, was perceived as of normal stature, wearing size 10 to 12 clothes over the last year. Current weight was unknown. On review of systems, she is cold all the time, feels tired and becomes dizzy on standing.

On examination her height is 167 cm, on the 75th percentile and her weight is 43 kg, on 3rd percentile for age. Her BMI is 15.4 (0.5th percentile). Her vital signs show a postural diastolic drop in BP of 15 mmHg and an orthostatic increase in heart rate from 52 to 78 per minute and a temperature of 36°C. She is emaciated with sunken eyes and pale skin, and she had thinning of her hair. She has delayed peripheral capillary refill of 3 seconds and cool mottled extremities. Examination of her oral cavity showed extensive erosion of the dental enamel. Bloods and ECG requested by her family doctor are normal.

Clinical Pearls

The most likely diagnosis is anorexia nervosa (AN). The history of energy intake and weight loss is vague and needs to be validated with reference to prior family doctor or school records and a more detailed account of foods eaten to establish both the extent and rapidity of weight loss. This is essential to evaluate whether outpatient refeeding is safe and the speed of calorie replacement. The Junior MARSIPAN or MEED guideline has a helpful checklist and traffic-light system to quantify risk.

Specific eating psychopathology is often denied or minimised at initial presentation and requires a high index of suspicion in the presence of significant weight loss and change in eating habits, including eating alone. The vagueness of history here, lack of concern about weight loss and amenorrhea and attribution to other causes is not infrequently seen. Given this girl's secondary amenorrhea of 6 months, it is likely that weight loss has been present for 9 to 12 months. The physical symptoms and cardiovascular compromise also suggest significant weight loss. This highlights the importance of establishing accurate premorbid weights and requesting parents obtain these from the family doctor or any prior school, club or hospital records, even if 2 to 3 years prior. Awareness of typical calorie requirements based on age, gender and activity levels is also necessary to establish specific requirements to allow a weekly weight gain of 0.5 to 1.0 kg.

Treatment is initially focused on weight restoration and medical stability, with the gold standard being family-based treatment (FBT), where the responsibility to refeed is placed firmly with the parents. Frequent clinic reviews are needed to monitor daily intake, weight gain and vital signs. Serial electrolytes may be needed if refeeding syndrome is a risk or as in this case purging is considered. Following progress with weight restoration targeted therapeutic work with both the adolescent and the family can proceed. Medication has little role in the treatment of eating disorders unless significant comorbid anxiety or depression.

Pitfalls to Avoid

Anorexia nervosa is a potentially life-threatening condition as the standardised mortality ratio is six times that of the general population. To minimise behaviour as typical adolescent dieting or delay treatment carries significant risks, including risk of chronicity.

Anorexia nervosa is a diagnosis of exclusion and other diagnoses do need to be actively considered including malignancy, inflammatory bowel disease or endocrine disorders including hyperthyroidism and Addison's disease.

Suggested target outpatient weight gain ranges from 0.5 to 1.0 kg per week and to be cautious regarding the risk of refeeding syndrome. Key biochemical monitoring for refeeding syndrome includes the measurement of serum potassium, phosphate, magnesium and calcium. Clinical features include a depressed level of consciousness, fluid overload, muscle weakness, diarrhoea and electrolyte derangement.

Anthropometric measurements need to be carefully taken with documentation of weight and height centiles and age and gender normed charts referenced.

school and sleep a lot during the day. Finally, those with 'severe' symptoms may be house- or bed-bound, and it takes them a long time to recover from an activity involving extra effort. Long-term follow-up has confirmed the importance of the child or adolescent remaining engaged in education in addition to social contacts as being central to their ability to cope with this illness.

CFS is the leading cause of prolonged school absence in adolescence with 1% of secondary school children missing a day a week yet only 1 in 10 have been given a diagnosis.

About 1 in 1000 adolescents are so severely affected they do not attend school at all. All symptoms experienced (the key one being profound fatigue) should be assessed in terms of severity, onset and course. A sleep diary should be taken. A family history, looking for a history of chronic illness or similar symptoms in either parent is important. Twin studies show a moderate genetic risk.

Examination should focus on weight and height centiles, lying and standing blood pressure and heart rate (looking for evidence of postural orthostatic tachycardia syndrome), a detailed neurological examination and palpation for lymphadenopathy or hepatosplenomegaly.

Referral from family practice to a paediatric or adolescent service is warranted if symptoms are severe. A paediatrician should be able to make a diagnosis, exclude other causes, treat symptoms, provide advice about sleep and activity and consider if severe, referral to a specialist paediatric or psychiatric service.

Advise against over-sleeping and to anchor wake-up time to avail of the cortisol surge in the morning. Prolonged bed rest or complete inactivity should also be avoided as the associated physical deconditioning is likely to exacerbate the fatigue.

There is strong evidence for the effectiveness of cognitive behaviour therapy (CBT) especially in younger children and adolescents, in those with significant depression and anxiety, in athletes and in those with high levels of pain (see Table 15.2). Pain is often a dominant symptom and, where simple analgesics and CBT are ineffective, referral to a specialist pain management clinic is warranted. Antidepressant drugs should only be used in those that have a severe mood disorder and fluoxetine should be considered as first choice. It is important to allow adequate time to assess for a response. In terms of long-term prognosis, most recover by 6 months with specialist treatment whereas less than 10% recover without specialist treatment.

KEY LEARNING POINTS

At any one time 25% of those aged between 12 and 25 years will meet diagnostic criteria for a mental health disorder. The IF-ME framework provides a helpful and comprehensive approach to both the assessment and treatment of young people with mental health issues.

Significant levels of anxiety are present in as many as 10 to 25% of young people, with a mean age of onset at age 11.

During a depressive episode the young person may feel tired, lacking in energy and concentration, with a decline in academic ability. Always ask about a history of self-harm and if any suicidal ideation.

Clinical guidelines for treatment of adolescent depression include CBT as first line as individual treatment and the addition of medication 6 weeks later if no response.

The use of medication (such as fluoxetine) for the treatment of adolescent depression should remain within specialist Child and Adolescent Mental Health Services (CAMHS).

Community studies highlight the reality that hospital attendances for self-harm (SH) are only a small subset of all SH cases and more likely to be following an overdose.

Whilst SH is more frequently seen in females, completed suicide is more common in males.

The presence of past SH is the greatest predictor of future behaviour and, if linked to active wishes to end one's life, carries the greatest risk of suicidal behaviour.

Core symptoms of ADHD include pervasive hyperactivity (always on the go, inability to sit still, fidgetiness), impulsivity (unable to wait their turn, engaging in dangerous activities without due regard to consequences, blurting things out) and inattention (difficulty with staying focused on task, concentrating for long periods, following through on instructions, remembering) that are *present and impairing in a number of domains*, such as school, after school activities, with peers and at home.

Those with anorexia nervosa (AN) have an intense fear of weight gain and restrict their food intake in an effort to lose weight, which is often accompanied by excessive exercise regimes.

When the presentation is suggestive of eating psychopathology, it is essential to establish the degree of weight loss, establish the target restorative weight and to reference the weight centiles and an ideal body weight.

In assessing an eating disorder, a thorough physical examination is required, and it is essential to establish the

Continued

KEY LEARNING POINTS—CONT'D

premorbid weight, and this enables the doctor to establish the target restorative weight. Check both standing and lying blood pressures and heart rate looking for any cardiac compromise with the MARSIPAN or MEED guidelines providing a useful framework for clinicians to use.

The presence of psychotic symptoms, especially when paired with anxiety, distress or persistence suggests an urgent need to refer to CAMHS for assessment and management.

Chronic fatigue syndrome (CFS) is the leading cause of prolonged school absence in adolescence with 1% of secondary school children missing a day a week yet only 1 in 10 have been given a diagnosis.

In CFS, there is strong evidence for the effectiveness of cognitive behaviour therapy (CBT) especially in younger children and adolescents, in those with significant depression and anxiety, in athletes and in those with high levels of pain.

FURTHER READING

American Psychiatric Association. *Diagnostic and statistical manual of mental disorders*. 5th edition Arlington, VA: American Psychiatric Association; 2013.

Black CJ, Drossman DA, Talley NJ, Ruddy J, Ford AC. Functional gastrointestinal disorders: advances in understanding and management. *Lancet*. 2020;396(10263):1664–1674. doi:10.1016/S0140-6736(20)32115-2.

Carter G, Page A, Large M, et al. Royal Australian and New Zealand College of Psychiatrists clinical practice guideline for the management of deliberate self-harm [published correction appears in Aust N Z J Psychiatry. 2018 Jan;52(1):98-99]. *Aust N Z J Psychiatry*. 2016;50(10):939–1000. doi:10.1177/0004867416661039.

Crandal BR, Aguinaldo LD, Carter C, Billman GF, Sanderson K, Kuelbs C. Opportunities for Early Identification: Implementing Universal Depression Screening with a Pathway to Suicide Risk Screening in a Pediatric Health Care System. *J Pediatr*. 2022;241:29–35.e1. doi:10.1016/j.jpeds.2021.10.031 .

Faltinsen E, Zwi M, Castells X, Gluud C, Simonsen E, Storebø OJ. Updated 2018 NICE guideline on pharmacological treatments for people with ADHD: a critical look. *BMJ Evid Based Med*. 2019;24(3):99–102. doi:10.1136/bmjebm-2018-111110.

Hawton K, Saunders KE, O'Connor RC. Self-harm and suicide in adolescents. *Lancet*. 2012;379(9834):2373–2382. doi:10.1016/S0140-6736(12)60322-5.

Hayden JC, Kelly L, McNicholas F. A clinician's guide to self-poisoning with paracetamol in youth: The what, when and why? *Acta Paediatr*. 2020;109(11):2237–2242. doi:10.1111/apa.15414.

Hill C, Waite P, Creswell C. Anxiety disorders in children and adolescents. *Paediatrics and Child Health*. 2016;26(12):548–553. ISSN 1751-7222. https://doi.org/10.1016/j.paed.2016.08.007 Available at https://centaur.reading.ac.uk/66854/.

Ivey-Stephenson AZ, Demissie Z, Crosby AE, et al. Suicidal Ideation and Behaviors Among High School Students – Youth Risk Behavior Survey, United States, 2019. *MMWR Suppl*. 2020;69(1):47–55. doi:10.15585/mmwr.su6901a6. Published 2020 Aug 21.

Katzman DK. *Neinstein's adolescent and young adult health care: a practical guide*. Lippincott Williams & Wilkins; 2016.

Knipe D, Padmanathan P, Newton-Howes G, Chan LF, Kapur N. Suicide and self-harm. *Lancet*. 2022;399(10338):1903–1916. doi:10.1016/S0140-6736(22)00173-8.

Lock J, Le Grange D. Family-based treatment: Where are we and where should we be going to improve recovery in child and adolescent eating disorders. *Int J Eat Disord*. 2019;52(4):481–487. doi:10.1002/eat.22980.

Marikar D, Reynolds S, Moghraby OS. Junior MARSIPAN (Management of Really Sick Patients with Anorexia Nervosa). *Arch Dis Child Educ Pract Ed*. 2016;101(3):140–143. doi:10.1136/archdischild-2015-308679.

McMahon EM, Keeley H, Cannon M, et al. The iceberg of suicide and self-harm in Irish adolescents: a population-based study. *Soc Psychiatry Psychiatr Epidemiol*. 2014;49(12):1929–1935. doi:10.1007/s00127-014-0907-z.

Mitchell JE, Peterson CB. Anorexia Nervosa. *N Engl J Med*. 2020;382(14):1343–1351. doi:10.1056/NEJMcp1803175.

National Confidential Enquiry into Patient Outcome and Death. Better mental health services for young people (2019). Accessed online at- https://www.ncepod.org.uk/2019ypmh.html

Nuffield trust. International comparisons of health and wellbeing in adolescence and early adulthood report. 2019. Accessed online at- https://www.nuffieldtrust.org.uk/research/international-comparisons-of-health-and-well-being-in-adolescence-and-early-adulthood

Patton GC, Sawyer SM, Santelli JS, Ross DA, Afifi R, Allen NB, Arora M, Azzopardi P, Baldwin W, Bonell C, Kakuma R, Kennedy E, Mahon J, McGovern T, Mokdad AH, Patel V, Petroni S, Reavley N, Taiwo K, Waldfogel J, Wickremarathne D, Barroso C, Bhutta Z, Fatusi AO, Mattoo A, Diers

J, Fang J, Ferguson J, Ssewamala F, Viner RM. Our future: a Lancet commission on adolescent health and wellbeing. *Lancet.* 2016 Jun 11;387(10036):2423–2478. doi:10.1016/S0140-6736(16)00579-1 Epub 2016 May 9. PMID: 27174304; PMCID: PMC5832967.

Royal College of Psychiatrists. Medical emergencies in eating disorders (MEED) Guidance on recognition and management CR233, May 2022. Accessed online at https://www.rcpsych.ac.uk/improving-care/campaigning-for-better-mental-health-policy/college-reports/2022-college-reports/cr233

Spielmans GI, Spence-Sing T, Parry P. Duty to Warn: Antidepressant Black Box Suicidality Warning Is Empirically Justified. Front Psychiatry. 2020;11:18. Published 2020 Feb 13. doi:10.3389/fpsyt.2020.00018

The Lancet. Health and wellbeing in adolescence and early adulthood. *Lancet.* 2019;393(10174):847. doi:10.1016/S0140-6736(19)30401-5.

The Lancet. Making the most out of crisis: child and adolescent mental health in the emergency department. *Lancet.* 2016;388(10048):935. doi:10.1016/S0140-6736(16)31520-3.

Theunissen MHC, de Wolff MS, Reijneveld SA. The Strengths and Difficulties Questionnaire Self-Report: A Valid Instrument for the Identification of Emotional and Behavioural Problems. *Acad Pediatr.* 2019 May-Jun;19(4):471–476. doi:10.1016/j.acap.2018.12.008. Epub 2019 Jan 10. PMID: 30639760.

Turecki G, Brent DA. Suicide and suicidal behaviour. *Lancet.* 2016;387(10024):1227–1239. doi:10.1016/S0140-6736(15)00234-2.

Walsh O, Nicholson AJ. Adolescent health. *Clinics in Integrated Care.* 2022;14(100123). ISSN 2666–8696, https://doi.org/10.1016/j.intcar.2022.100123.

ADDITIONAL READING FOR PARENTS AND/OR PROFESSIONALS

Clark L. *SOS help for emotions: Managing anxiety, anger, and depression.* SOS Programs & Parents Pres; 2001.

Creswell C, Parkinson M, Thirlwall K, Willetts L. *Parent-led CBT for child anxiety: helping parents help their kids.* Guilford Publications; 2019 Apr 23.

Lock J, Le Grange D. *Help your teenager beat an eating disorder.* Guilford Publications; 2015 Jan 20.

McDougall T, Armstrong M, Trainor G. *Helping children and young people who self-harm: An introduction to self-harming and suicidal behaviours for health professionals.* Routledge; 2010 Jul 12.

Rief SF. *The ADHD book of lists: A practical guide for helping children and teens with attention deficit disorders.* John Wiley & Sons; 2015 Jun 15.

Steinberg L, Silk JS. Parenting adolescents. In: Bornstein MH, ed. *Handbook of. Parenting.* Lawrence Erlbaum Associates Publishers; 2002:103–133.

16

Neonatal Intensive Care – A Challenging Arena

John Murphy

CHAPTER OUTLINE

THE IMPORTANCE OF NEONATOLOGY

Neonatology is the speciality that cares for infants from birth until 28 days. In essence there are four categories of newborn infants. First is the healthy term infant who remains with their mother throughout their stay in hospital. Second is the term infant who is admitted briefly to the neonatal unit with a minor problem such as transient tachypnoea. Third is the sick term infant or the infant with a major malformation requiring immediate attention and treatment. Finally, we have the preterm infant requiring various levels of treatment and intensive care depending on their degree of prematurity.

Neonatology is described as the general medicine of the newborn. Unlike other paediatric subspecialties, it is not organ specific. The doctor must be capable of taking care of the whole infant. This makes the specialty both interesting and challenging.

KEY POTENTIAL PITFALLS

The biggest risk factor is **time**. Things move quickly and change rapidly in neonatology. You as a health professional must be able to readily identify the altered clinical condition of the infant and speedily respond. It is not sufficient to do things in the correct order, they must be done within the time frame that maximises their effectiveness. A slow response to a critical situation can result in an adverse result.

The second is **anticipation.** Knowledge and experience teach one to be able to predict what will happen next to the ill infant. If this principle of predictive practice is applied case-by-case, many of the common neonatal complications can either be modified or prevented. The neonatal motto is 'always be one step ahead of the infant'.

The third is the **accurate recording** and documentation of clinical measures. Fluid intake and urine output, weighing the infant, heart rate, respiratory rate, blood pressure, temperature and level of alertness are the pillars on which the specialty has been built. These recordings are critically important in the early and timely identification of the deteriorating infant.

The fourth is the ability to **interpret a basic suite of blood tests** and **plain films** such as a chest X-ray and an abdominal film. The common blood tests include a blood sugar, urea and electrolytes, blood gas, full blood count, blood culture, urine culture and LP results. 'Know them and act on them'.

THE UNIQUE FEATURES OF NEWBORNS

Newborn infants have limited respiratory reserves. The tidal volume of a term infant is 18 mL and as little as 4 mL in very preterm infants. They tolerate respiratory distress poorly, become tired and lapse into respiratory failure in a matter of hours. It is important to recognise when intervention such as assisted ventilation is necessary.

Newborns have limited ability to maintain their blood pressure and circulation in the face of sepsis. They tend to respond disproportionately by increasing their heart rate as they cannot mount a high vascular resistance. A persistent tachycardia is a red flag in relation to an infant's clinical status.

The neonatal brain is prone to injury which can result in long-term neurodisability. It has a high energy requirement and is vulnerable to both hypoxia and hypoglycaemia. It is adversely affected by the collection of toxic substances such as bilirubin and the accumulation of metabolites associated with inborn errors of metabolism.

Newborn infants are more prone to central nervous system (CNS) infections than any other paediatric age group. Bacterial meningitis takes a high toll. Within hours of the meninges becoming infected, a vasculitis of the cerebral blood vessels takes place. The vasculitis leads to multiple areas of cerebral ischaemia. There must be a low threshold for screening for meningitis.

SAFE PRACTICE IN NEONATAL INTENSIVE CARE UNIT (NICU)

A culture of safety should pervade the unit and indeed the maternity hospital. Everyone in the team should play their part. As in healthcare in general, errors in the neonatal intensive care unit (NICU) are often system errors. The key mantra in NICU should be to learn all the time from the mistakes of others.

> Maintaining competency is another key strategy, as there are a multitude of technical procedures in NICU that require high levels of skill.

Volume is a key factor and simulation of procedures such as line insertion (both umbilical and PICC), successful intubation and resuscitation ensures that trainees, advanced nurse practitioners and consultants develop and maintain their skills over time.

Neonatal transport adds a further layer of complexity and requires regional and national transport teams, close collaboration and support of smaller units, so-called retro transfers to enable growing infants to be repatriated closer to home and national resuscitation guidelines and courses.

> Appropriate documentation is important, and in many NICUs, it is via an electronic health record.

Careful, accurate and factual notes should be entered regularly into the casefile with avoidance of the temptation to 'cut and paste' prior entries by others. Timing of interventions is essential, and all significant changes should be clearly documented.

GOOD COMMUNICATION

The care provided by teams in modern NICU is highly complex, and communication and good teamwork are vital. Good communication is key to provide safe care, enables efficient handover between healthcare professionals and keeps the parents and family up to speed with the infant's progress in NICU. Communication starts before the infant is born with an exchange between the obstetrical team in the referring or tertiary hospital and the neonatal team and enables a timely transfer or delivery that ensures appropriately trained staff are available to offer prompt and expert resuscitation. Handover in the morning and in the evening is important and should be both formal and efficient to ensure staff coming on duty have a very clear understanding of the infant's current condition. Rushed or incomplete handovers can lead to vitally important information not being shared or passed on. Family members, especially parents, should be made to feel that they are a vital element of the team caring for their infant.[1] They often feel overwhelmed at first by the technology and the incredibly small size of their infant. They may be a long way from their home following a neonatal transfer and thus require accommodation near the hospital. Better rapport with parents tends to promote improved compliance with handwashing and infection control measures in NICU, a greater likelihood of providing breast milk to nourish the infant, improved compliance with policies of the unit (such as a quiet hour where infants can rest, and the lights are dimmed) and possibly a greater willingness to inform nursing and medical teams of subtle changes in their infant. Generally, families are eternally grateful for the work and professionalism of staff within NICU, and the lines of communication should always be kept open to take them on the journey. This work should continue following discharge from NICU with a detailed discharge plan, advice regarding immunisations and appropriate developmental and general follow-up.

Not infrequently, there may be misunderstanding or disagreement between the family and healthcare professionals in terms of management, especially in infants with a poor prognosis or life-limiting conditions.

> In end-of-life care situations, excellent communication with the family and relatives is of paramount importance.

In order to improve communication and minimise conflict with parents and families, general advice would support the early use of palliative care teams and the recognition that parents are under extreme stress and should be offered appropriate pastoral support. Be cognisant also that staff are under significant stress. It is best to have a designated lead clinician to provide continuity of clear information to the family and seek second opinions or external advice (both ethical and legal) as required. Also consider the earlier involvement of mediation services if conflict is anticipated or becoming evident.

In general terms, try to resolve disputes by discussion, consultation and consensus. It is important to remember that these discussions about limiting care are taking place when the family are under enormous stress.

MANAGEMENT IN THE DELIVERY SUITE

It is essential that all staff (both medical and nursing) successfully complete a Neonatal Resuscitation Programme every 2 years to ensure they have the requisite up-to-date skills to resuscitate an ill newborn. The team awaiting the delivery of an infant with potential issues at birth should reflect the likely needs of the infant and clearly if the infant is markedly preterm then a more experienced team is required.

> If intubation is deemed to be likely in the delivery suite, the resuscitation team should include senior personnel who are particularly skilled at intubation.[1]

Call senior personnel in advance if a markedly preterm infant or multiple preterm births are being delivered or if events such as a prolapsed cord or a non-reassuring CTG trace are noted. The establishment of adequate ventilation is the most important aspect of resuscitation of the newborn. This is achieved by means of properly performed mask and T-piece ventilation or intubation. Successful intubation is evidenced by a rapid rise in the heart rate or evidence of the delivery of an adequate tidal volume to the infant (Fig. 16.1). The evidence for the latter is usually an adequate chest rise, the auscultation of breath sounds bilaterally or the exhalation of carbon dioxide as shown by a CO_2 detector[1] (Fig. 16.2) with a colour change if the tube is in the airway.

> Simulation training plays a critical role in upskilling residents and advanced nurse practitioners in intubation.

A tiny number of flat newborns (perhaps 1 in 1000) require chest compressions or medications such as adrenaline (via ET or intravenously) in the delivery suite.

Care of the Preterm Infant

In the delivery room management of a preterm infant under 28 weeks gestation, delayed cord clamping for 1 minute and placement in a polyurethane bag to maintain temperature are the first steps.

> Gentle resuscitation with a neopuff and blended oxygen are given. Start nasal CPAP early with later administration of surfactant if the infant has increasing respiratory difficulties.

0.3% of all births are extremely preterm (23–26 weeks gestation) and advances in NICU for infants born at the margins of viability have led to greatly improved

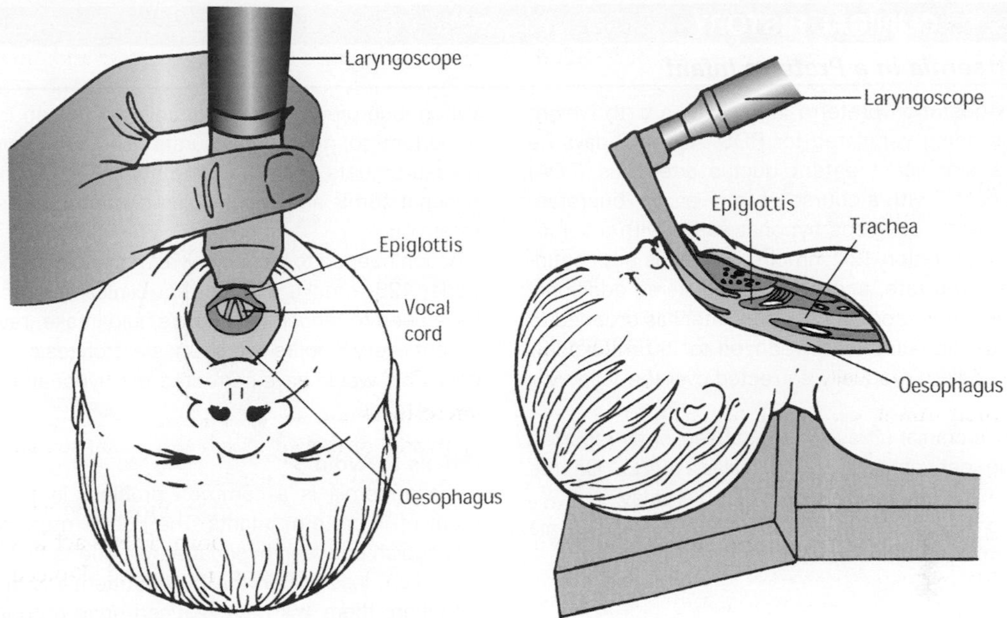

Fig. 16.1 Neonatal intubation. (Source: Reproduced with permission from Henderson C, Macdonald S. *Mayes' Midwifery – A Textbook for Midwives.* 13th ed. Bailliere Tindall; 2004.)

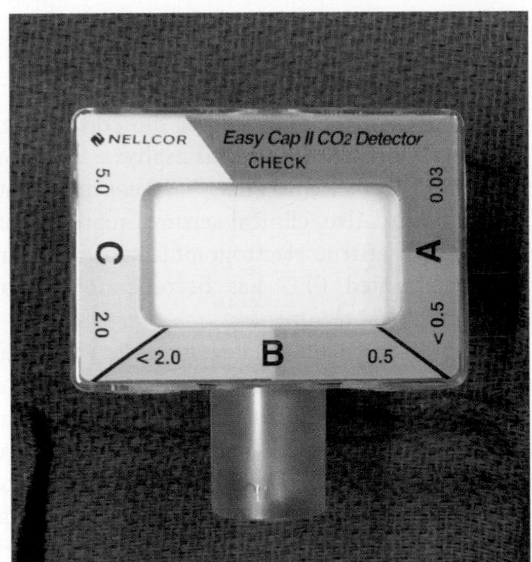

Fig. 16.2 Colorimetric CO_2 detector with yellow colouring indicating an end-tidal CO_2 concentration greater than 2%, or 15 mmHg. (Source: *Hagberg and Benumof's Airway Management.* 5th ed. 2023.)

survival, but these infants are more likely to have long-term morbidity and do use healthcare extensively, especially in the first 2 years of life.[2]

Events in the first few hours after birth affect both neonatal mortality and morbidity. Skilled resuscitation, maintaining normothermia, controlling acid-base status and rapidly obtaining intravenous access to prevent hypoglycaemia and electrolyte imbalance (Box 16.1) are all important. Ventilation strategies have changed with the increased use of continuous positive airway pressure. High oxygen saturation is avoided in an effort to reduce lung inflammation from oxygen toxicity.[2]

The most important variable affecting mortality in extremely preterm infants (under 26 weeks gestation) is gender (yet again girls do better!). Therefore, for infants born at or under 26 weeks gestation, postnatal survival increases steeply in the first few postnatal days and varies by gestational age in days, even within a category of completed gestational age in weeks[3] (so each day in utero counts!).

Neonatal Encephalopathy and Therapeutic Hypothermia

Neonatal encephalopathy (NE) is a condition seen in term infants with an altered level of consciousness and is often accompanied by seizures and a failure of spontaneous breathing. The causes are diverse, but the majority of cases are due to decreased delivery of blood or oxygen

BOX 16.1 CLINICAL HISTORY

Hyponatraemia in a Preterm Infant

A 28-week-gestation preterm infant with a birth weight of 1.0 kg is being ventilated for RDS. At age 5 days he develops a significant patent ductus arteriosus (PDA) which is treated with a course of intravenous ibuprofen. He subsequently develops hyponatraemia with a serum sodium concentration 124 mmol/L. His fluids are continued at the same rate, and he is administered additional sodium. The serum sodium 24 hours later has dropped to 115 mmol/L. His fluids were reduced to 100 mL/kg/day. His serum sodium gradually corrected over the following 24 hours.

The infant's cranial ultrasound is subsequently reported as showing periventricular leukomalacia (PVL). On follow-up the baby develops diplegic cerebral palsy.

There is a known association between hyponatraemia and periventricular leukomalacia.

Clinical Pearls

The management of the fluid and electrolyte balance is the central issue in this case. Renal impairment is a well-recognised complication of ibuprofen administration. The impairment can lead to fluid retention and hyponatraemia. When ibuprofen is being administered to an infant, it is important to maintain accurate fluid input and output measurements and weigh the infant. The combination of hyponatraemia and weight gain confirms excessive fluid retention.

Action needed to be taken when the serum sodium was under 128 mmol/L. The correct clinical response would have been to reduce the infant's fluid intake, review urine output every 8 hours and check electrolytes at least twice daily. This would have corrected the hyponatraemia at an earlier stage.

Pitfalls to Avoid

Hyponatraemia is a common problem in the management of ill preterm infants. The doctor must be able to distinguish between hyponatraemia due to fluid retention or sodium loss. When the hyponatraemia is due to fluid retention, there will be a reduced urine output, and the infant's weight will have increased.

The key next step is to reduce the infant's fluid intake by 20 to 25%.

to the foetal brain during labour, termed hypoxic-ischaemic encephalopathy.

The mainstay of treatment is **effective resuscitation** and **supportive measures** which aim to ensure adequate delivery of blood, glucose and oxygen to the brain and thereby prevent further injury. It is vital to maintain normal blood gases, in particular normal CO_2 levels (Box 16.2), normal glucose and electrolytes.

A Cochrane meta-analysis has demonstrated that therapeutic hypothermia (TH) (Fig. 16.3) given in the first 6 hours after birth will help to mitigate the effects of hypoxic-ischaemic encephalopathy.[4] Other studies have shown TH reduces death rates and improves outcome.[5] There remains controversy about suitable screening tests.[6]

There is very good evidence that therapeutic hypothermia (TH) prevents adverse motor outcomes at 18 months in moderate to severe NE.

TH offered after 6 hours has limited or no value, so **time** is vitally important. There are several issues with this strict six-hour window in that the cord pH may not reflect the degree of perinatal asphyxia, and some infants do not show features of neonatal encephalopathy for several hours. Also, clinical seizures represent only a small fraction of true electrographic seizures. Hence amplitude-integrated EEG has become popular and picks up subclinical seizures.

Infants born in smaller maternity units will require transfer to a tertiary unit for TH, and such infants are passively cooled (turning off the radiant heater and removing blankets) prior to the arrival of the neonatal transport team. Active cooling can be initiated as soon as the transport team arrives. Active cooling can take place during transfer, and this is achieved by placing ice packs on the infant's chest and possibly forehead, but this carries the risk of severe hypothermia.

In the precooling era, for those with severe NE, the majority died, and almost all survivors had cerebral palsy (CP). For moderate NE, few died but roughly 20% had CP, and most had obvious cognitive deficits, and for mild NE, there were no obvious abnormalities, and they were believed to be unaffected.

BOX 16.2 CLINICAL HISTORY

Hypocarbia in a Newborn With NE

A term infant with a birth weight of 4.0 kg has a diagnosis of neonatal encephalopathy. She is 8 hours old and is being ventilated because of poor respiratory effort, as her chest X-ray is normal. She is receiving therapeutic hypothermia.

The ventilator settings are pressures 22/4, rate 30/min, FIO_2 25%. The arterial blood gas shows a pH of 7.5 (normal range 7.35–7.45), pO_2 of 9.0 kilopascals ((kPa) acceptable range 6 and 12), pCO_2 of 2.9 kPa (acceptable range 4.5–8) and bicarbonate of 25 mEq/L (normal range 20–24 mEq/L). The on-call team reduce the FIO_2 to 21% but do not alter the other settings. The next blood gases 4 hours and 8 hours later are similar, the pCO_2 values being 3.0 and 2.8 kPa, and the pH being 7.5 and 7.51, respectively.

At the consultant round, the ventilator settings were adjusted with a reduction in both the inspiratory pressure and the rate. The next gas showed a pCO_2 of 5.0, pH of 7.35 and bicarbonate of 22.0.

The infant subsequently had an abnormal brain MRI and ultimately developed dyskinetic cerebral palsy.

Clinical Pearls

Hypocarbia most commonly occurs when the infant is receiving mechanical ventilation for poor respiratory effort, and the lungs are normal.

Hypocarbia is variously defined as a pCO_2 under 3.0 to 4.0 kPa. The likelihood of its significance is increased when the pH is over 7.4 as in this case.

The clinical understanding is that when the pCO_2 is abnormally low, then vasoconstriction of the cerebral blood vessels follows. This vasoconstriction has the potential to cause cerebral ischaemia and ultimately brain injury.

When the blood gas reading shows a pCO_2 under 4.0 kPa, it is important to make appropriate ventilation adjustments in order to increase the pCO_2. The options are to decrease the ventilator pressures or decrease the ventilator rate or both. A follow-up blood gas should be undertaken 1 hour later to ensure that the pCO_2 has increased to over 4.0. If this has not been achieved, further ventilator adjustments are required.

Pitfalls to Avoid

Hypocarbia is defined as a pCO_2 under 4.0 kPa and is a potential risk whenever an infant is receiving mechanical ventilation.

It is the main reason that blood gas measurements need to be performed 4 hourly. Its significance is increased when the pH is above 7.1.

The hypocarbia is corrected by reducing the ventilator pressures and/or the ventilator rate. The ventilatory adjustments that have been made should be carefully documented in the infant's notes.

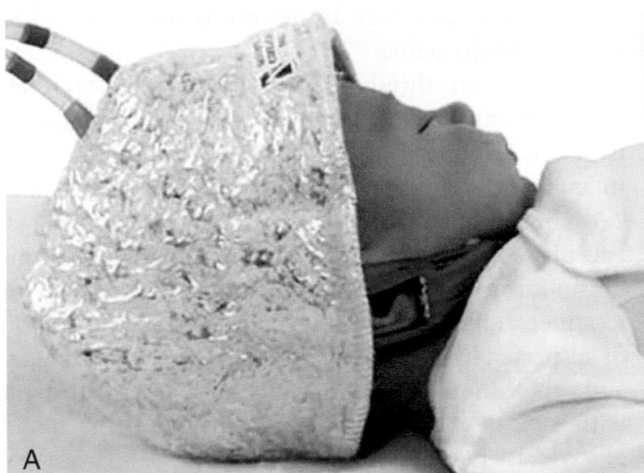

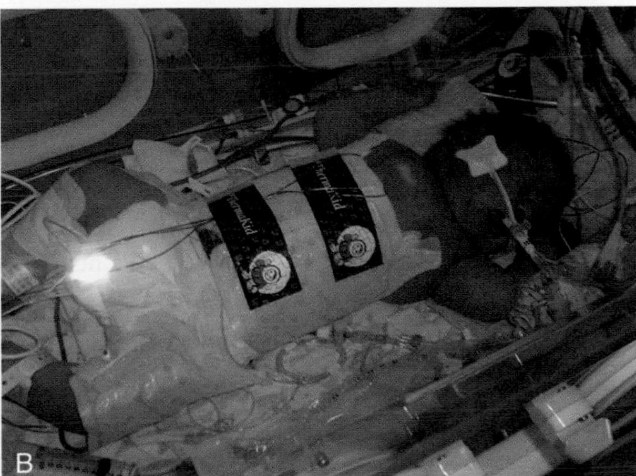

Fig. 16.3 Two approaches to hypothermia. (A) Selective head cooling with head wrap and chin straps. (B) Infant receiving whole-body therapeutic hypothermia via body wrap. (Source: Volpe JJ, et al. *Volpe's Neurology of the Newborn*. 6th edition, 2018, Elsevier Inc.)

RECOGNITION OF SEPSIS

In dealing with preterm infants in NICU, sepsis is always a possibility and intravenous antibiotics are often commenced after birth for the first 48 hours until cultures return.

The *Neonatal Early Onset Sepsis (NEOS) Calculator*[7] is a helpful clinical decision support tool in determining which infants need blood cultures and antibiotics. It uses a composite of risk factors – gestational age, maternal temperature, GBS status, duration of rupture of the membranes (ROM) and the infant's clinical examination.

Preterm infants have a greater susceptibility to infection due to being of low birth weight, having an immature immune system, the invasive procedures in NICU and overcrowding in NICU with consequent understaffing. It is quite challenging to pick up sepsis in infants who may have increased apnoeic episodes, worsening respiratory distress, increased jaundice, intolerance of feeds or who seem 'off' as these are frequent observations of residents of NICU. Sadly, investigations such as the white cell count, CRP, procalcitonin and other acute phase reactants are unhelpful. Serial repetition of some of these tests (for instance, CRP) may help if diagnostic uncertainty persists.

Suspect sepsis if an infant has a poor colour, prolonged capillary refill time (more than 2 seconds), tachycardia (over 160 per minute), a drop in BP (under 30 mmHg if preterm), apnoea or tachypnoea (over 60 breaths per minute).

> Early onset sepsis is within 48 hours of birth and may be associated with a rapid onset of fulminant multisystem disease.

Pneumonia is a prominent feature and over 75% are associated with maternal risk factors for infection. These include a prolonged rupture of the membranes, maternal pyrexia in labour, foul-smelling liquor, Group B *Streptococcus* (GBS) carriage or bacteriuria or a history of GBS in a prior delivery.

Antibiotic choice for early onset sepsis is penicillin and gentamycin intravenously with the addition of cefotaxime if meningitis is suspected or likely. Antibiotics are continued for 7 to 10 days and, if uncomplicated meningitis, for 14 to 21 days in total (Box 16.3).

Late-onset sepsis is where the onset is beyond 48 hours of age. It is usually associated with in-dwelling devices (such as a PICC line).

> *Coagulase-negative Staphylococcus* (CONS) is the predominant pathogen in late-onset sepsis, and hand hygiene is a key factor in prevention.

HYPOGLYCAEMIA

Hypoglycaemia is defined as a blood glucose less than 2.6 mmol/L and is a common reason for a newborn to be admitted to the neonatal nursery.

Clinical presentations where checking the blood glucose is warranted include hypothermia not attributable to environmental factors, suspected sepsis, seizures, excessive lethargy, severe hypotonia or reluctance to feed. There is no need to check blood glucose levels in asymptomatic appropriately grown term infants who are reluctant to feed in the first 48 hours of life. Do not rely on a hand-held glucometer for low blood glucose readings.

Current international guidelines recommend screening for hypoglycaemia in newborns who are preterm, small for dates, born to diabetic mothers or who are large for dates. Current guidelines do not recommend screening for hypoglycaemia in healthy infants born at term.[1] Symptomatic hypoglycaemia has been linked to long-term neurological sequelae, and the association between asymptomatic hypoglycaemia and adverse neurological outcomes is unclear. Most neonatal units adhere to international hypoglycaemia guidelines and advise prompt treatment if the infant is symptomatic. Hyperinsulinism is rare in newborns but may lead to severe hypoglycaemia.

Intervention thresholds for blood glucose levels include immediate intervention if the blood glucose is under 1.0 mmol/L or if under 2.0 mmol/L and the infant is at risk for hypoglycaemia.[8] Always treat under 2.5 mmol/L if abnormal clinical signs or neonatal encephalopathy and if under 3.0 mmol/L if hyperinsulinism is suspected. Use 2.0 mmol/L as the threshold for treatment unless underlying neurological dysfunction or suspected hyperinsulinism.[8]

If the blood glucose is under 1.0 mmol/L, treat with 10% dextrose bolus and infusion. If the blood glucose is 1.0 to 2.0 mmol/L, buccal dextrose gel (40%) can be used alongside intensive feeding support if the infant is asymptomatic and under 48 hours of age (Box 16.4).[8]

BOX 16.3 **CLINICAL HISTORY**

An Infant With Neonatal Meningitis

A 2-day-old term infant on the postnatal ward develops a temperature of 38.2°C. The registrar is called to review. He is told that the infant is otherwise well, and that there are no risk factors. He decides that it is environmental and advises the nurse to open the window. Two hours later, the infant's temperature is 37.9°C. It is decided that the temperature is coming down, and that no further intervention is required.

Eight hours later the nurses phone stating that the infant is now unwell with pallor, tachypnoea and grunting respirations.

He is admitted to the NICU. The vital signs on admission are tachycardia 180/min, respiratory rate raised at 75/min, capillary refill time 4 seconds and mean BP 30 mmHg. He is acidotic with a pH 7.0, HCO_3 10 mmol/L.

The clinical impression is sepsis and possible meningitis. Blood cultures are taken, and he is immediately commenced on intravenous antibiotics. He is given a bolus of saline. He is intubated and ventilated. When he is stabilised, a lumbar puncture was performed, and the CSF was turbid.

The subsequent diagnosis was Group B *Streptococcus* sepsis and meningitis.

The cranial ultrasound and MRI scans showed ischaemic changes. The baby subsequently had a significant neurological disability.

Clinical Pearls

A temperature of 38°C or higher should always be considered as clinically significant in a neonate. A warm room may cause a transient rise in temperature but not above 37.5°C. The infant's temperature remained elevated despite measures to reduce the room temperature.

Common cot side findings in early sepsis are drowsiness combined with irritability when disturbed. One simple tip is to note how many items of clothing that you can gently remove from the infant before he starts crying. Irritable infants often start crying before one has even removed one. In early sepsis the infant's tone is frequently reduced.

They have a tachycardia in excess of that expected by the rise in temperature. Infants are allowed 10 beats/min for each 1-degree rise in temperature. In this case a heart rate over 170/min suggests sepsis.

The infant's rapid deterioration is typical of neonatal sepsis. Every hour counts if a good outcome is to be achieved. The standard of care is that antibiotics must be administered within 1 hour of encountering a baby with sepsis. The mantra is 'prescribe them, get them, give them'.

Pitfalls to Avoid

A newborn with a raised temperature should always be medically reviewed. Particular note should be made of the infant's colour, heart rate and alertness. A temperature of 38°C or above is significant and should be acted on.

Environmental temperatures do not exceed 37.5°C, and they are transient. They should not be present for more than 1 hour.

A pyrexia in a newborn requires decisive, immediate action. Any delays can have a serious adverse outcome.

SEVERE HYPERBILIRUBINEMIA

We need to be aware that jaundice is more difficult to both detect and assess in infants of colour, and that the Bilimeter is a simple non-invasive way of measuring the bilirublin level. The Bhutani nomogram[9] is an excellent and recognised tool to guide doctors in terms of responding to bilirubin levels (either serum or by Bilimeter). Kernicterus is now exceedingly rare (about 1 in 100,000) and tends to be seen in term infants or preterms above 35 weeks gestation who are exclusively breastfed and where there may be a delay in presentation. There are also infants with glucose-6-phosphate dehydrogenase (G6PD) deficiency with coincident late-onset sepsis with a consequent dramatic rise in unconjugated bilirubin.

RETINOPATHY OF PREMATURITY

Regular and timely screening is required to pick up retinopathy of prematurity (ROP). ROP is a developmental vascular proliferation disorder.[10] The more severe form of ROP can lead to macular dragging, retinal detachment and blindness if not identified and treated promptly (Fig. 16.4).

Fortunately, with the advent of screening, early detection and effective therapies for ROP, blindness has become rare.

ROP affects infants under 32 weeks gestation. Infants at 28 to 31 weeks gestation usually have mild ROP. The more severe types of ROP are encountered in preterm infants under 28 weeks gestation.

BOX 16.4 CLINICAL HISTORY

A Newborn With Persistent Hypoglycaemia

An 18-hour-old term infant with a birth weight of 3.9 kg is noted to be jittery by the postnatal nursing staff. The blood sugar reading is 0.8 mmol/L. He is administered Glucogel and admitted to the NICU. On admission his repeat blood sugar is 1.0 mmol/L. He is administered 10% dextrose 2 mL/kg stat and commenced on 10% dextrose in 0.45 saline. His repeat blood sugar 2 hours later is 0.8 mmol/L. He is administered a further 2 mL/kg bolus of 10% dextrose and the infusion is increased to 12.5%. One hour later the blood sugar is 1.5 mmol/L. The infusion rate is increased to 120 mL/kg, and the glucose concentration is increased to 15%. The drip tissues. There is difficulty re-siting the line. There is an interruption to the infusion for 1 hour. The next blood sugar reading is 0.9 mmol. The consultant is called, and an umbilical venous line inserted. The glucose infusion is attached to the umbilical line. The next blood sugar is 1.6 mmol/L.

The infant subsequently had a series of seizures, each lasting approximately 90 seconds.

The endocrinology team in the tertiary paediatric centre was contacted. They advised to increase the glucose concentration to 20%, commence a glucagon infusion and to transfer the infant.

Following admission to the endocrinology centre a diagnosis of hyperinsulinism was made. The hypoglycaemia was successfully managed with diazoxide.

Clinical Pearls

The blood glucose on initial presentation was 0.8 mmol/L. The blood sugar should have been checked every 30 minutes and additional treatment given until it had normalised. A secure line either umbilical or PICC should have been sited. This would have avoided the hour that was lost when the infant was not receiving any glucose.

The glucose infusion rate (GIR) should have been calculated, the normal being 6 to 8 mg/kg/min. Values over 10 mg/kg/min are in keeping with hyperinsulism. Even at an early stage in this case the GIR was over 10 mg/kg/min.

The critical samples were not taken despite several opportunities when the infant was hypoglycaemic. The insulin measurement is the most important component of the critical sample in this particular case. When the infant is hypoglycaemic, the insulin level should be zero. The presence of insulin in this case confirms hyperinsulinism.

Pitfalls to Avoid

A blood glucose under 1.0 mmol/L is a neonatal emergency. If it is not rapidly treated and stabilised, the baby may suffer long-term neurological disability. Therefore, following the administration of an initial IV bolus of dextrose, the infant's blood glucose should be monitored every 30 minutes until normalised.

A secure central line should be obtained at an early stage so that concentrated glucose solutions as 12.5%, 15% and even 20% can be given if necessary.

The addition of a glucagon infusion can be extremely helpful during the acute phase of the hypoglycaemia, particularly when the dextrose concentration has reached 15%. It acts within 1 hour, and the median rise in blood glucose after its commencement is 2.5 mmol/L.

Always ensure that an infant being treated for hypoglycaemia has an apnoea monitor in place. The occurrence of an apnoea episode should immediately alert the nursing staff to the occurrence of a further bout of hypoglycaemia.

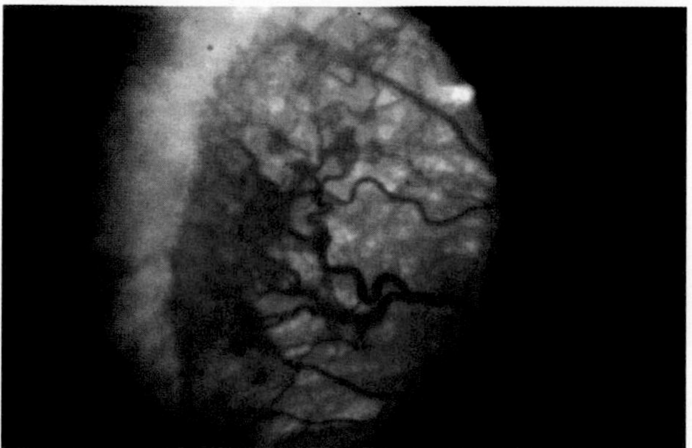

Fig. 16.4 Stage 3 retinopathy of prematurity. (Source: *Ophthalmology Secrets*. 5th ed. 2023.)

The screening for ROP is performed at 31 weeks corrected gestational age. It is a complex, skilled procedure undertaken by an ophthalmologist with a special interest in ROP. It is important to pause the procedure if there is a decrease in the infant's heart rate or oxygen saturation, as the infant may deteoriate during the procedure.

The treatment modalities for ROP are laser photocoagulation or the anti-VEGF agent bevacizumab administered by intravitreal injection.

ERB'S PALSY

Erb's palsy is where C5, C6, C7 and C8 nerve roots are affected, and the risk is increased if there is shoulder dystocia prior to delivery. Presentation is with decreased

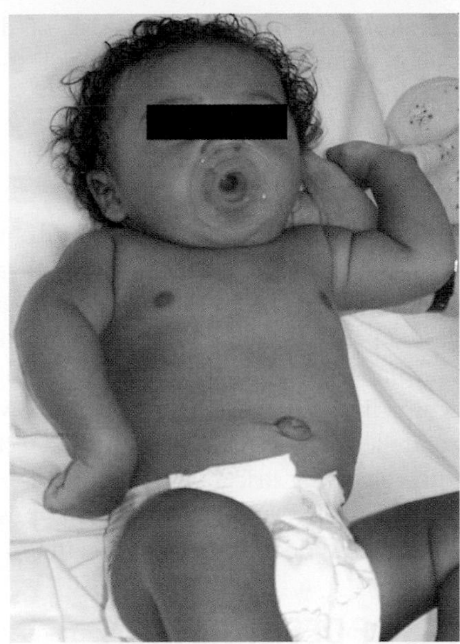

Fig. 16.5 Right-sided brachial plexus injury (Erb-Duchenne palsy) in newborn infant. The Moro reflex was absent in the right upper extremity. Recovery was complete. (Source: Chung, K., Yang, L.J., & McGillicuddy, J.E. (Eds.), (2011). *Practical Management of Pediatric and Adult Brachial Plexus Palsies*. Philadelphia: Saunders.)

movement, a 'waiter's tip' posture and an asymmetrical Moro reflex. When placed in ventral suspension, the affected arm 'hangs down' while the normal arm flexes (Fig. 16.5). The nerve roots C5 and C6 are always affected and lead to reduction in external rotation of the shoulder, elbow flexion and supination of the forearm. C7 is involved in 50% of cases leading to wrist drop and weak finger extensors. C8 and T 1 are only affected in very severe cases.

Early physiotherapy passive exercises are important in the prevention of contractures while waiting for function to return. Most recover spontaneously with only 10% having any deficit by 3 months of age. In cases of Erb's palsy with a good outcome, improvment starts within a few weeks with a return of wrist extension being an early sign. The Toronto test score is the best clinical tool in assessment with a maximum score of 10 and a score under 3.5 indicating a poor outcome for recovery.[11] It is imperative to document the severity of Erb's palsy and to re-assess at two weekly intervals. Involve a physiotherapist from the outset and refer to a specialist Erb's clinic at an early stage unless the infant has mild symptoms or is improving.

Request a chest X-ray to out rule fractures or phrenic nerve palsy, physiotherapy to aid recovery and early referral to neurosurgery (using Toronto criteria) is advised if injury fails to resolve.

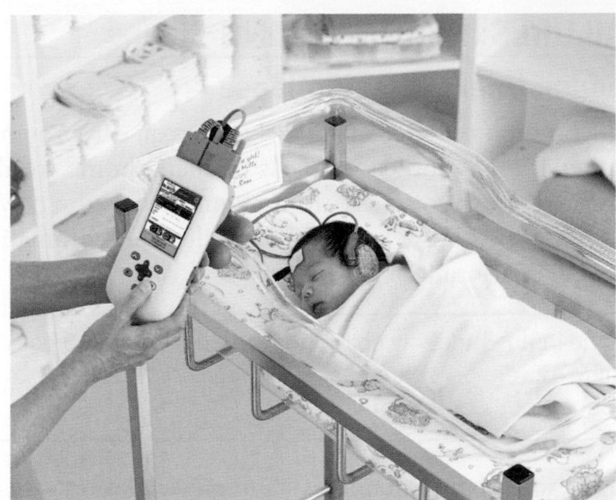

Fig. 16.6 The newborn hearing screen has an immediate pass/fail result that indicates whether the infant needs further audiological testing. The screener sends a series of soft clicking sounds to a device placed over the newborn's ears. The newborn's brain responds with a specific brain wave pattern called the auditory brainwave response (ABR). The screener automatically compares the newborn's ABR to a stored template from infants with normal hearing. Newborns with an abnormal result will be referred for follow-up evaluation. (Source: Gloria Leifer. *Introduction to Maternity and Pediatric Nursing*, Ninth Edition, 2023.)

CONGENITAL CYTOMEGALOVIRUS INFECTION

Either universal or targeted screening of asymptomatic newborns with congenital cytomegalovirus (CMV) might enable early antiviral treatment and the earlier identification of hearing loss (Fig. 16.6).

> Antiviral therapy, if started within 4 weeks of birth, will reduce the deterioration in hearing in those infants with symptomatic congenital CMV infection.

Congenital CMV is the most frequently seen non-genetic cause of sensineural hearing loss and may be progressive in up to 50% of cases whereby the initial newborn hearing screen may have been passed. Screening for congenital CMV using salivary PCR testing, would enable the earlier detection of infants with CMV-related sensineural hearing loss, but the treatment of these infants with antiviral therapy remains controversial.[12]

FAILURES IN MONITORING

Sudden Unexpected Collapse

The common practice of early skin-to-skin care, rooming in with the mother and early discharge home are all desirable but may inhibit close monitoring of the newborn infant with the potential for sudden and dramatic clinical deterioration.

> If the infant suddenly collapses after taking a first breath think of either congenital diaphragmatic hernia or a spontaneous pneumothorax.

Likewise, a preterm infant stable on ventilation with a dramatic deterioration may have a dislodged ET tube or a pneumothorax (Box 16.5). If preterm, transillumination is helpful in picking up a pneumothorax (Fig. 16.7). A neonatal stroke may be associated with a sudden collapse or onset of seizure activity.

Be aware that preterm infants of 35 to 37 weeks gestation may run into unexpected problems and are at risk of respiratory distress, becoming cold and developing hypoglycaemia. Term infants are at risk of developing persistent pulmonary hypertension of the newborn (PPHN) (Box 16.6).

LINE COMPLICATIONS

Central lines are now very popular in NICU and obviate the need for frequent changes of intravenous and intraarterial access. Always verify the position of both umbilical (UAC and UVC) and peripheral long line by imaging. Remove these central lines when nonfunctioning or no longer necessary.[1] Central line (PICC) infections are a known complication, and the risk is lessened by improved techniques with insertion including strict hygiene standards.

Ensure the line is inserted properly, well-positioned and maintained, and do not leave the line in too long.

EPISODES OF DESATURATION

In a term infant, an episode of apnoea should be considered a seizure until proven otherwise. In stark contrast, apnoea, bradycardia and desaturations are very frequent

BOX 16.5 CLINICAL HISTORY

Respiratory Distress Syndrome (RDS) in a Preterm Infant

A preterm infant of 29 weeks gestation, birth weight of 1.2 kg, is delivered by emergency caesarean section because of maternal preeclampsia (PET). There was insufficient time to give antenatal steroids. Apgar scores were 8 at 1 minute, 9 at 5 minutes. He is given nasal prong oxygen to maintain his O_2 saturation over 92%. He develops grunting respirations.

He is commenced on CPAP 5 cm with FIO_2 of 25%. Over the next 6 hours he develops increasing intercostal recession. The chest X-ray is consistent with respiratory distress syndrome (RDS).

At midnight the registrar is called to review because he is now requiring FIO_2 40% to keep the O_2 saturation above 92%. She decides to increase the FIO_2 to 45% and to continue with the present management.

Four hours later the infant had a respiratory arrest. He did not respond to bag and mask ventilation resuscitation. There are a number of attempts at intubation and the consultant was called. The infant was intubated and given surfactant. On chest transillumination, there is a large left pneumothorax which is needled and 50 mL is aspirated. The infant remains very unstable and requires artificial ventilation and insertion of a chest drain.

Clinical Pearls

This preterm infant had RDS. The natural history is for the condition to get progressively worse in the early hours after birth, as occurred in this case. The likelihood was greater in the absence of antenatal steroids.

The main warning sign, however, was when the FIO_2 progressively increased to 40%. At that point the management should have been escalated and a blood gas performed.

In this case the RDS was allowed to progress. It was not appreciated that the lungs were becoming increasingly stiff with progressive atelectasis. This ultimately led to respiratory failure and a tension pneumothorax.

Pitfalls to Avoid

Preterm infants with RDS should only be managed in neonatal units equipped with the necessary staff and equipment to provide full respiratory care.

There must be a clear set out step-by-step RDS management guideline.

An increasing FIO_2 requirement and a pH under 7.2 indicate significant lung pathology.

The neonatal team must have a low threshold for considering the development of a pneumothorax and be able to aspirate it effectively.

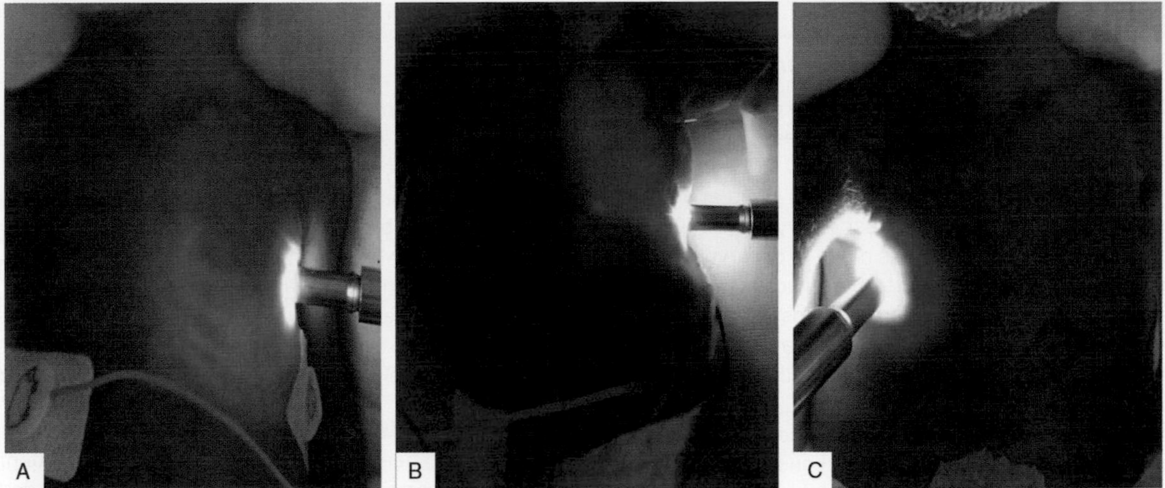

Fig. 16.7 High-intensity fibre optic light demonstrating increased transillumination on left half of chest suggestive of left-side pneumothorax (A–B) compared to normal right chest (C). (Source: Rajiv PK et al. *Essentials of Neonatal Ventilation*. 1st edition, 2018, Elsevier India.)

in preterm infants especially those under 28 weeks gestation. The caveat is, of course, that increased episodes of apnoea and desaturation in preterm infants may indicate sepsis or necrotising enterocolitis (NEC).[13] Caffeine has proved to be quite effective in limiting the number of apnoeic episodes in preterm infants.

Caffeine tends to be discontinued at around 34 weeks postconceptual age, and the infant is observed off caffeine for a number of days prior to discharge home.

NEONATAL SEIZURES

> Neonatal seizures are often quite subtle and may be challenging to pick up.

The timing of the seizures is important in determining the cause, as seizures due to neonatal encephalopathy develop shortly after birth and are associated with perinatal asphyxia and abnormal neurological behaviour.[14,15]

An important cause of seizures is neonatal stroke with typically the infant being normal at birth. The seizures develop a few hours later. The area of infarction on the MRI is usually in the distribution of the left middle cerebral artery (Fig. 16.8). They generally do well, but some develop hemiplegia or seizures in childhood. Neonatal brain malformations are another group of disorders causing seizures and are picked up on MRI.

Inborn errors of metabolism associated with seizures in newborns include maple syrup urine disease, organic acidurias (such as glutaric aciduria, propionic aciduria and methylmalonic aciduria), urea cycle disorders, nonketotic hyperglycinaemia and pyridoxine-dependent seizures.

These will require the expertise of a specialist metabolic service.

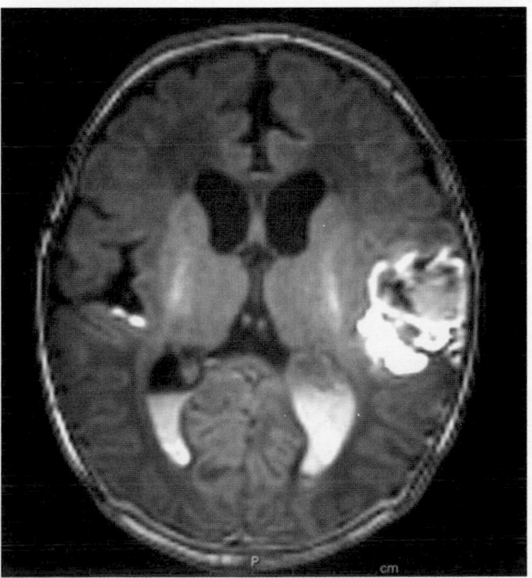

Fig. 16.8 Neonatal haemorrhagic stroke, left. (Source: *Developmental-Behavioral Pediatrics*. 5th ed. 2023.)

BOX 16.6 CLINICAL HISTORY

Persistent Pulmonary Hypertension of the Newborn (PPHN)

An infant with a birth weight of 3.8 kg was delivered by elective caesarean section at 38 weeks. The indication was a previous caesarean section.

The doctor was called to review the infant at 4 hours of age because of an elevated respiratory rate of 70 breaths per minute. The decision was made to observe and review in 2 hours. At that time the infant had a respiratory rate of 90 per minute, there were intercostal recessions, she was slightly cyanosed, and her temperature was 35.8°C.

She was immediately admitted to the NICU. On initial assessment the infant required FIO_2 50%, and the pH was 7.15. There was a 15% difference between the pre- and postductal saturations. Her condition continued to deteriorate. She required intubation and ventilation and subsequently nitric oxide. Despite these measures her oxygenation index reached 40, and she required ECMO. She responded well to ECMO treatment.

Clinical Pearls

This was a case of persistent pulmonary hypertension of the newborn (PPHN). The precipitating risk factor was the elective caesarean section at 38 weeks gestation. These infants may become progressively difficult to oxygenate. The signification difference between oxygen saturations in the upper and lower limbs encountered in this case, is indicative of right-to-left shunting. Differences greater than 10% are regarded as abnormal.

During the period on the postnatal ward the infant's respiratory problems had worsened. She became hypothermic which would have depleted her surfactant.

The correct initial management should be to admit to the NICU, place in an incubator to maintain her temperature, stop oral feeds, commence on IV fluids and commence on nasal prong O_2 if O_2 saturation is under 95%.

Pitfalls to Avoid

Infants with transient tachypnoea require careful attention and monitoring particularly the group that are borderline preterm.

If they become cold, distressed and hypoxaemic there is a risk that they will develop PPHN. Once PPHN develops it is frequently difficult to manage.

When the infant requires intubation and ventilation, the oxygenation Index (OI) should be calculated. It provides a useful indication of the severity of the PPHN. Values below 15 are indicative of mild PPHN, 16 to 25 moderate PPHN, 26 to 40 severe PPHN and over 40 signals the need for ECMO.

KEY LEARNING POINTS

Neonatology is a constantly changing speciality with new approaches to noninvasive ventilation, the use of antibiotics and postnatal steroids, new approaches to term infants with neonatal encephalopathy and a far greater awareness of pain experienced in the newborn nursery.

Neonatal transport adds a further layer of complexity and requires regional and national transport teams, close collaboration and support of smaller units, so-called retro transfers to enable growing infants to be repatriated closer to home and national resuscitation guidelines and courses.

The care provided by teams in modern neonatal intensive care is highly complex, and communication and good teamwork are essential.

Events in the first few hours after birth affect both neonatal mortality and morbidity. Skilled resuscitation, maintaining normothermia, controlling acid-base status and rapidly obtaining intravenous access to prevent hypoglycaemia are all important.

A Cochrane meta-analysis has demonstrated that therapeutic hypothermia (TH) given in the first 6 hours after birth will help to mitigate the hypoxic ischaemic encephalopathy. TH offered after 6 hours has limited or no value, so time is of the essence.

Early onset sepsis is within 48 hours of birth and may be associated with a rapid onset of fulminant multisystem disease.

Late-onset sepsis is where the onset is beyond 48 hours of age. It is usually associated with in-dwelling devices (such as a PICC line). *Coagulase-negative Staphylococcus* (CONS) is the predominant pathogen in late-onset sepsis, and hand hygiene is a key factor in prevention.

Retinopathy of prematurity (ROP) affects infants under 32 weeks gestation. With Erb's palsy, know your Toronto score, and unless the infant is mild or has shown improvement, early referral to a specialist Erb's palsy clinic is recommended.

Antiviral therapy, if started within 4 weeks of birth, reduces a deterioration in hearing in those infants with symptomatic congenital CMV infection.

Always verify the position of both umbilical (UAC and UVC) and peripheral long line by imaging.

Caffeine has proved to be quite effective in limiting the number of apnoeic episodes in preterm infants

Neonatal seizures are often quite subtle and may be challenging to detect.

REFERENCES

1. Fanaroff JM, Goldsmith JP. The most common patient safety issues resulting in legal action against neonatologists. *Semin Perinatol.* 2019;43(8):151181. doi:10.1053/j.semperi.2019.08.010.
2. Yeaney NK, Murdoch EM, Lees CC. The extremely premature neonate: anticipating and managing care. *BMJ.* 2009;338:b2325. doi:10.1136/bmj.b2325. Published 2009 Jun 22.
3. Shah PS, Rau S, Yoon EW, et al. Actuarial Survival Based on Gestational Age in Days at Birth for Infants Born at <26 Weeks of Gestation. *J Pediatr.* 2020;225:97–102.e3. doi:10.1016/j.jpeds.2020.05.047.
4. Jacobs SE, Berg M, Hunt R, Tarnow-Mordi WO, Inder TE, Davis PG. Cooling for newborns with hypoxic ischaemic encephalopathy. *Cochrane Database of Systematic Reviews.* 2013. doi:10.1002/14651858.CD003311.pub3 Issue 1. Art. No.: CD003311.
5. Abate BB, Bimerew M, Gebremichael B, et al. Effects of therapeutic hypothermia on death among asphyxiated neonates with hypoxic-ischemic encephalopathy: A systematic review and meta-analysis of randomized control trials. *PLoS One.* 2021;16(2):e0247229. doi:10.1371/journal.pone.0247229. Published 2021 Feb 25.
6. Liu W, Yang Q, Wei H, Dong W, Fan Y, Hua Z. Prognostic Value of Clinical Tests in Neonates With Hypoxic-Ischemic Encephalopathy Treated With Therapeutic Hypothermia: A Systematic Review and Meta-Analysis. *Front Neurol.* 2020;11:133. doi:10.3389/fneur.2020.00133. Published 2020 Feb 25.
7. Loughlin L, Knowles S, Twomey A, Murphy JFA. The Neonatal Early Onset Sepsis Calculator; in Clinical Practice. *Ir Med J.* 2020;113(4):57. Published 2020 Apr 3.
8. Levene I, Wilkinson D. Identification and management of neonatal hypoglycaemia in the full-term infant (British Association of Perinatal Medicine-Framework for Practice). *Arch Dis Child Educ Pract Ed.* 2019;104(1):
29–32. doi:10.1136/archdischild-2017-314050.
9. O'Reilly P, Walsh O, Allen NM, Corcoran JD. The Bhutani Nomogram Reduces Incidence of Severe Hyperbilirubinaemia in Term and Near Term Infants. *Ir Med J.* 2015;108(6):181–182.
10. Darlow BA, Gilbert C. Retinopathy of prematurity - A world update. *Semin Perinatol.* 2019;43(6):315–316. doi:10.1053/j.semperi.2019.05.001.
11. Greenhill DA, Lukavsky R, Tomlinson-Hansen S, Kozin SH, Zlotolow DA. Relationships Between 3 Classification Systems in Brachial Plexus Birth Palsy. *J Pediatr Orthop.* 2017;37(6):374–380. doi:10.1097/BPO.0000000000000699.
12. Hilditch C, Liersch B, Spurrier N, Callander EJ, Cooper C, Keir AK. Does screening for congenital cytomegalovirus at birth improve longer term hearing outcomes? *Arch Dis Child.* 2018;103(10):988–992. doi:10.1136/archdischild-2017-314404.
13. Jones IH, Hall NJ. Contemporary Outcomes for Infants with Necrotizing Enterocolitis – A Systematic Review. *J Pediatr.* 2020;220:86–92.e3. doi:10.1016/j.jpeds.2019.11.011.
14. Ramantani G, Schmitt B, Plecko B, et al. Neonatal Seizures – Are We there Yet? *Neuropediatrics.* 2019;50(5):280–293. doi:10.1055/s-0039-1693149.
15. Ziobro J, Shellhaas RA. Neonatal Seizures: Diagnosis, Etiologies, and Management. *Semin Neurol.* 2020;40(2):246–256. doi:10.1055/s-0040-1702943.

ADDITIONAL READING

Buis ML, Hogeveen M, Turner NM. The new European Resuscitation Council guidelines on newborn resuscitation and support of the transition of infants at birth: An educational article. *Paediatr Anaesth.* 2022;32(4):504–508. doi:10.1111/pan.14406.

Crowley N, Fox GF. Review of the new BAPM framework for practice (2019): Perinatal management of extreme preterm birth before 27 weeks of gestation. *Arch Dis Child Educ Pract Ed.* 2021;106(3):162–164. doi:10.1136/archdischild-2019-318719.

Dyer C. Coroner calls for new guidance on umbilical venous catheters after baby's death. *BMJ.* 2021;372:n290. doi:10.1136/bmj.n290. Published 2021 Jan 29.

Fox GF. Controversies and discussion of the BAPM Framework for the perinatal management of extreme preterm birth before 27 weeks of gestation. *Arch Dis Child Educ Pract Ed.* 2021;106(3):160–161. doi:10.1136/archdischild-2020-318836.

Gilfillan M, Bhandari A, Bhandari V. Diagnosis and management of bronchopulmonary dysplasia. *BMJ.* 2021;375:n1974. doi:10.1136/bmj.n1974. Published 2021 Oct 20.

Madar J, Roehr CC, Ainsworth S, et al. European Resuscitation Council Guidelines 2021: Newborn resuscitation and support of transition of infants at birth. *Resuscitation.* 2021;161:291–326. doi:10.1016/j.resuscitation.2021.02.014.

NICE guideline [NG124] Specialist neonatal respiratory care for babies born preterm. Published: 3 April 2019. Accessed online at- https://www.nice.org.uk/guidance/ng124/chapter/Recommendations#monitoring

Parker SJ, Kuzniewicz M, Niki H, Wu YW. Antenatal and Intrapartum Risk Factors for Hypoxic-Ischemic

Encephalopathy in a US Birth Cohort. *J Pediatr*. 2018;203:163–169. doi:10.1016/j.jpeds.2018.08.02.

Resuscitation Council UK. Newborn resuscitation and support of transition of infants at birth Guidelines. 2021. Accessed online at https://www.resus.org.uk/library/2021-resuscitation-guidelines/newborn-resuscitation-and-support-transition-infants-birth

Wassink G, Davidson JO, Dhillon SK, et al. Therapeutic Hypothermia in Neonatal Hypoxic-Ischemic Encephalopathy. *Curr Neurol Neurosci Rep*. 2019;19(2):2. doi:10.1007/s11910-019-0916-0 Published 2019 Jan 14.

17

Ordering and Interpreting Tests in Children

Kevin Dunne, Alf Nicholson, Aengus O'Marcaigh, Michael Riordan, Ellen Crushell, Niamh McGrath, Annemarie Broderick, Jonathan Hourihane, James Foley, James O'Byrne

"Technology is a useful servant but a dangerous master".
—*Christian Lous Lange*

CHAPTER OUTLINE

BACKGROUND

The history and examination are both key in making a differential diagnosis for particular symptoms, but investigations and their accurate interpretation are essential to clinch the diagnosis. Some illnesses or conditions such as a viral exanthem or rashes such as atopic dermatitis, acute tonsillitis or minor head shape abnormalities are relatively common and readily recognisable on examination. For most other diagnoses, investigations are important and do help confirm the suspected diagnosis.

AVOID UNNECESSARY TESTS

In general, with regard to children and young people, we advise that investigations should be focused and directed by the presenting symptoms and examination findings. Be aware that a general trawl of investigations is not advised and that individual investigations should be justified. We advise against performing unnecessary radiological investigations or blood tests. A full blood count, routine biochemistry, serum calcium and magnesium are not routinely indicated in young children presenting with a febrile seizure. While parents sometimes push for additional investigations, one should always be aware that there is a risk of stepping on an 'investigation train' where it is not easy to step off, and the final destination is unclear. This applies in particular to functional symptoms where exploration of the biopsychosocial model is preferred to an ever-lengthening list of tests. As an example, in this chapter, we will explore recommended conventional allergy tests and again stress the importance of the history rather than a fruitless 'fishing expedition' of unnecessary investigations.

POINT-OF-CARE TESTING

Point-of-care testing has become increasingly popular, especially in emergency departments. These investigations include urine microscopy and dipstick testing (in practice for many years), on-site chest ultrasound (looking for effusion) or abdominal ultrasound (in cases of acute abdominal pain), but these radiological investigations are generally not available in family practice. A family doctor can dipstick a urine sample obtained by ideally using a clean catch method and determine if a urinary tract infection (UTI) is likely. Obtaining urine is challenging in infants under 12 months of age, and it is important to have an accurate diagnosis of UTI in this age group who may just present with a fever and malaise. Dipstick testing in primary care is helpful in older children if a UTI is suspected, and treatment can commence while awaiting formal urine cultures.

For primary care doctors and other first responders, checking the blood for blood sugar and ketones is important in the early pick up of diabetes mellitus.

> Do not order an investigation without first seeking the result and being able to interpret the findings.

A key principle when ordering an investigation is to be able to interpret the result. Ordering an investigation and not seeking or misinterpreting the result is not advisable and can lead to adverse outcomes with medico-legal consequences.

We will focus on a number of frequent pitfalls in terms of interpretation of investigations commonly requested with illustrations based on case examples.

URINE COLLECTION AND TESTING FOR URINARY TRACT INFECTION

Prompt diagnosis of UTI is important as timely treatment reduces short-term distress, prevents renal scarring and avoids progression to more serious bacterial infection. The diagnosis poses unique challenges not least the fact that only a minority of infants and children have typical UTI symptoms. As a primary care doctor, it is not feasible or acceptable to obtain urine via suprapubic aspiration or via catheterisation. Recent studies have supported clean catch urine collection with additional bladder stimulation or cold application to accelerate urination.[1] The Quick-Wee method has recently been highlighted and employs a cold stimulus to promote urine voiding.[2] Urine is often collected within five minutes, and this results in far greater parental satisfaction and reduces delays in collection.

The contamination rate for a clean catch urine is 5% and is comparable to catheterisation. Nappy pads and bag specimens have far higher rates of contamination (over 30%) and thus are not recommended.

FULL BLOOD COUNT AND COAGULATION PROFILE

Newborn infants have relatively high circulating haemoglobin, and the haemoglobin level reaches its lowest point (usually 10 g/dL) at 2 to 3 months of age. The mean haemoglobin level rises gradually during childhood (equally for boys and girls) until puberty when the level in boys is 20% higher than in girls.[3]

> The reticulocyte count is key to categorise anaemia.

An elevated reticulocyte count is suggestive of a bone marrow response to either acute blood loss (usually clinically obvious) or increased red cell destruction or hemolysis. A low reticulocyte count in the setting of anaemia indicates bone marrow failure. In the setting of a normal haemoglobin, the absolute reticulocyte count is approximately 40 to 160 × 10^9/L.

The mean corpuscular volume (MCV) can also be used to classify anaemia, with a high MCV being indicative of macrocytosis and a low MCV suggesting microcytosis. Normal ranges of MCV are age-related.

Macrocytosis is rare in childhood and may relate to vitamin B12 or folate deficiency, Fanconi and Blackfan-Diamond anaemias and rarely severe hypothyroidism. Vitamin B12 and folate deficiencies are rarely seen in childhood. Check RBC folate to measure folate levels. B12 deficiency can be seen in children on strict vegan diets, congenital pernicious anaemia, and with terminal ileitis in Crohn disease.

Microcytosis in childhood is associated with iron deficiency, thalassemia, and rare conditions such as sideroblastic anaemia and lead poisoning.

Evaluation of the white cell count (WBC), WBC differential and platelet count are imperative in the setting of anaemia.[4] Consider bone marrow aspiration or biopsy if there is either neutropenia or thrombocytopenia in addition to anaemia.

An elevated indirect (unconjugated) bilirubin and elevated LDH can be seen in acute or chronic haemolysis. The direct Coombs test will be positive for autoimmune haemolytic anaemia.

Haemoglobin electrophoresis will identify haemoglobinopathies such as sickle cell disease or thalassemia. If there is acute haemolysis, check the red blood cell enzyme levels (for example G6PD).

The prothrombin time (PT) is prolonged either by deficiency of a clotting factor (apart from factors V11 and X111) or if an inhibitor is present. The PT measures both the extrinsic and common coagulation pathways.[5]

The partial thromboplastin time (APTT) is prolonged if there are deficiencies of factors V111, 1X and X1. Factor X11 deficiency may cause a prolonged APTT in an otherwise asymptomatic child. The APTT measures both the intrinsic and common pathways.

The bleeding time will be prolonged in platelet function abnormalities, thrombocytopenia and von Willebrand disease (Fig. 17.1) (Box 17.1).

Features seen in disseminated intravascular coagulation (DIC) include the prolongation of both PT and APTT, low fibrinogen levels, a low platelet count and elevated D-dimer levels.

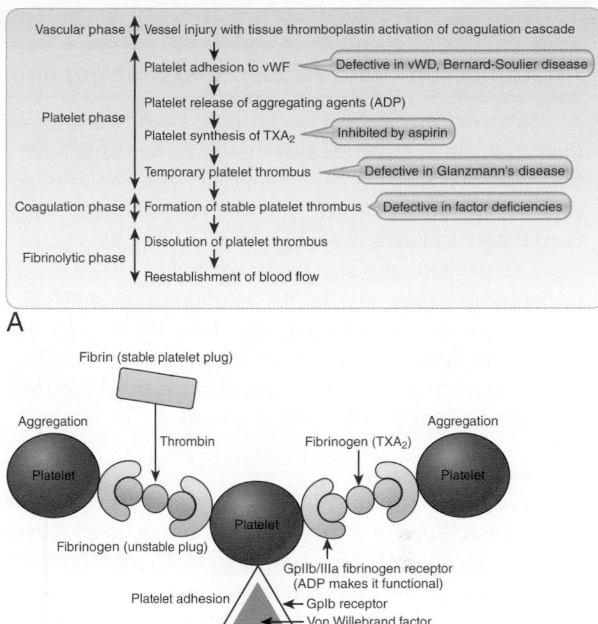

Fig. 17.1 (A) Small vessel hemostasis response to injury. A vascular phase, platelet phase, coagulation phase, and fibrinolytic phase are involved in small vessel hemostasis with formation of a platelet thrombus. (B) Platelet receptors and platelet aggregation. Disruption of the endothelial surface of small vessels exposes von Willebrand factor (vFW). This allows the GpIb receptor on the platelet to adhere to vWF on the endothelium, which is called platelet adhesion. The platelet releases preformed adenosine diphosphate (ADP) immediately after adhesion. ADP produces conformational changes in the GpIIb/IIIa fibrinogen receptor so that it is now able to bind to fibrinogen molecules. Thromboxane A2 (TXA2) is then synthesized de novo by the platelet. TXA2 enhances fibrinogen attachment to the GpIIb/IIIa receptors on adjacent platelets causing platelet aggregation and the formation of a temporary platelet thrombus. The platelet thrombus is unstable until thrombin, which is locally produced by activation of the coagulation system, converts fibrinogen to fibrin. This produces a stable platelet thrombus that stops bleeding from damaged small vessels. ADP, Adenosine diphosphate; TXA2, thromboxane A2; vWD, von Willebrand disease; vWF, von Willebrand factor. (*Rapid Review Pathology: First South Asia Edition*; 2015).

C-REACTIVE PROTEIN (CRP) AND PROCALCITONIN

C-reactive protein is, at times, helpful in the evaluation of a febrile infant or child for sepsis.[6] Along with procalcitonin[7], it is an acute phase reactant, but it does have significant limitations. Serial CRP measurements are helpful in terms of neonatal sepsis where a decline in CRP aligns with clinical recovery. While it is not recommended to perform a CRP in all febrile children, CRP should be easily accessible and may aid the decision-making process in the Emergency Department. Additional diagnostics, such as procalcitonin, repeat CRP measurement or other novel biomarkers may be helpful in infants and children who present with fever and where diagnostic uncertainty remains (Box 17.2). CRP has largely replaced ESR in

BOX 17.1 CLINICAL HISTORY

An Adolescent with Widespread Bruising and Heavy Periods

A 13-year-old girl is seen in the emergency department with multiple large bruises on her arms and legs, and a diagnosis of possible nonaccidental injury was considered. She had a coincident history of heavy menstrual losses. Blood tests including full blood count and clotting screen were requested, and she was admitted to hospital. Her investigations showed a normal prothrombin time (PT) and a prolonged partial thromboplastin time (APTT). Her von Willebrand factor activity was measured by ristocetin-induced platelet aggregation and was found to be reduced. Her factor VIII level was found to be low.

Clinical pearls

Von Willebrand disease (vWD) is associated with the delayed formation of platelet plugs and is generally inherited in an autosomal dominant fashion with desmopressin (DDAVP) being the treatment of choice.

Von Willebrand disease is relatively common with an incidence of up to 1%.

Presenting features include easy bruisability, menorrhagia, gum bleeding post tooth brushing and bleeding post-surgery. The commonest is type 1 vWD with a low level of von Willebrand factor and factor VIII.

Pitfalls to avoid

In vWD, advise against the use of aspirin or nonsteroidal antiinflammatory drugs.

Menorrhagia is a frequent symptom in vWD, and the observation that improvement occurs after starting oral contraceptives is insufficient to outrule vWD.

DDAVP is useful in those with vWD with low vWF levels but needs to be avoided in type 2B vWD where it causes thrombocytopenia.

BOX 17.2 CLINICAL HISTORY

A 10 Month Old with a High Fever

A 10-month-old female infant presents to an emergency department (ED) with a high fever and being off form. Her temperature on arrival is 40°C. She is observed for 6 hours in the ED and has a negative urinalysis and a normal CRP of 15. She is discharged home with safety netting advice to return if the parents are concerned.

36 hours later she is brought back to hospital with marked lethargy, pallor, and low-grade fever. On this occasion, she appears quite lethargic and thus has a full septic screen. Her CRP on this occasion is markedly elevated at 350, and her CSF and blood cultures grow *Streptococcus pneumoniae*. She is treated promptly and makes a full recovery.

Clinical pearls

Under 12 months of age, assessment for sepsis is indeed challenging and, early in the process, the CRP may be normal, and clinical markers for sepsis such as lethargy, meningism, tachycardia and delayed capillary refill time may be absent.

The CRP taken in isolation may be falsely reassuring if normal and should always be interpreted in terms of parental concerns and clinical indices of sepsis.

At the second presentation, this infant was clearly unwell, and the CRP had risen markedly.

Procalcitonin is superior to CRP in terms of diagnostic performance and has greater accuracy than CRP or the white cell count in detecting bacterial meningitis in children. Beyond the first few days of life, procalcitonin should be undetectable in serum in the absence of infection. In essence, procalcitonin is better at identifying infants and children who are not septic than those who are and thus should not be used as a standalone diagnostic test but rather just one component of a sepsis evaluation. Therefore, measuring procalcitonin over time can support the earlier cessation of antibiotics leading to shorter and safer courses.

Pitfalls to avoid

CRP values taken in isolation may be misleading, especially if normal. Repeating the CRP level and looking for a further rise can be helpful, especially in a child who re-presents to the hospital.

assessing the infant or child with suspected osteomyelitis or septic arthritis. CRP values must always be linked to clinical status and tend to be most useful if markedly elevated. CRP is also used in the assessment of a child with suspected acute appendicitis. CRP has been found to be helpful in the prediction of complications in community-acquired pneumonia. The biological half-life of CRP is approximately 20 hours and thus a drop in CRP levels is linked to clinical improvement and a slow decrease or new rise may herald complications.

ROUTINE BIOCHEMISTRY

This includes a high or low serum sodium and a high or low serum potassium and their interpretation[8] (Box 17.3).

BLOOD GLUCOSE

For the purposes of further investigation and achieving a diagnosis, hypoglycaemia is defined as a blood glucose under 2.6 mmol/L. The symptoms of hypoglycaemia are varied but may include sweating, anxiety, hunger, weakness, pallor, lethargy, headache, irritability, and rarely loss of consciousness. Idiopathic ketotic or so-called 'starvation' hypoglycaemia usually occurs in early childhood during an intercurrent gastroenteritis illness and the risk of hypoglycamia lessens as the child gets older. An enlarged liver may indicate Glycogen Storage Disease (GSD) which can also cause ketotic hypoglycaemia.

Persistent hypoglycaemia in infancy may be due to hyperinsulinism (either congenital hyperinsulinism or insulinoma) with characteristically very high glucose infusion rates required to prevent hypoglycaemia.[9] Hypopituitarism predisposes to fasting hypoglycaemia and may present with microphallus in males.

Fasting hypoglycaemia is also a feature of Addison's disease and hepatic glycogen storage disorders due to an inability to release glucose from glycogen.

Infants and children with medium-chain acyl-coenzyme A dehydrogenase deficiency (MCADD) have hypoketotic hypoglycaemia usually brought on by fasting stresses, typically, but not always, during intercurrent illness (Box 17.4).

BOX 17.3 CLINICAL HISTORY

A 4-Year-Old with Severe Gastroenteritis and a High Serum Sodium

A 4-year-old child is admitted with a 3-day history of vomiting and poor oral intake and very frequent loose stools. She has 8 to 10 loose stools per day and is felt to be 10% dehydrated (Fig. 17.2). Her electrolytes show a serum sodium of 158 mEq/L.

Clinical pearls

Clinical assessment by history and examination enables the correct interpretation of electrolyte measurements with a focus on taking the history of both fluid intake and fluid losses. Fluid losses may be in stool, vomit, or urine.

The focus of clinical examination should be an assessment of the child's volume status looking for the dryness of mucous membranes, pulse rate, capillary refill time and blood pressure.

Hypernatraemia (a serum sodium greater than 145 mEq/L) is usually prevented by thirst and renal concentrating mechanisms.

A water deficit is by far the most common cause of hypernatraemia and is due to inadequate water intake or excessive water loss associated with severe gastroenteritis (as in this instance). Loss of water may also occur with insensible losses in extreme heat, in diabetes insipidus with high volumes of dilute urine or in preterm infants with reduced renal concentrating power.

Excessive salt intake can cause hypernatraemia with examples including the iatrogenic administration of excess sodium, incorrect reconstitution of infant formula or deliberate salt poisoning.

Pitfalls to avoid

In managing hypernatraemia, be guided by your assessment whether the child is dehydrated or not. In the initial phase of treatment normal (0.9%) saline should be used to replace the fluid deficit slowly over 48 to 72 hours. Isotonic fluids are not recommended, as they may cause an overly rapid correction in serum sodium leading to cerebral oedema and possible central pontine demyelinosis.

Close monitoring is essential, and a rate of fall in serum sodium of no more than 1 mEq/L per hour should be the target.

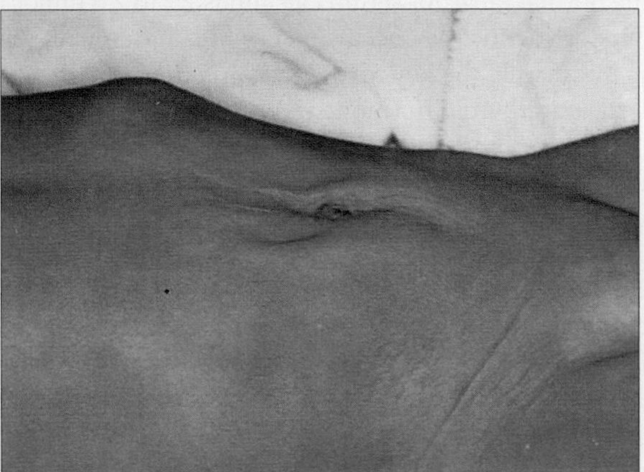

Fig. 17.2 'Standing skin folds' as a clinical sign of dehydration in a 7-year-old child with acute watery diarrhoea. (Nothdurft HD, et al. *Travel Medicine*. 2nd edition, Mosby, 2008, Elsevier Inc.)

BOX 17.4 CLINICAL HISTORY

An 8-Month-Old with Hypoglycaemia

An 8-month-old is seen in the emergency department with a one-day history of fever and increasing lethargy and unresponsiveness. A bedside glucose level is 1.1 mmol/L and a blood glucose confirms this result. Point-of-care blood ketones are 0.1 mmol/L (very low, normal being <0.6) and ketones are negative on urine testing. CK and LFT are raised. Urine organic acids and Acylcarnitine profile were abnormal and confirmed a diagnosis of Medium Chain Acyl Co-A Dehydrogenase Deficiency (MCADD).

Clinical pearls

The brain solely relies on glucose as a primary source of energy, but during periods of starvation, the brain uses ketones as an alternative source of energy.

MCADD may present with poor feeding during an intercurrent illness with associated lethargy progressing to encephalopathy and evident hypoglycaemia.

Typical features of acute MCADD include hypoketotic hypoglycaemia (they may have trace ketones), abnormal liver function, mild hyperammonaemia and dicarboxylic acids on urine organic acid testing with elevated medium-chain acylcarnitines (C8 and C10) on bloodspot acylcarnitine analysis.

Pitfalls to avoid

Always check the blood glucose in an infant or child with a seizure or impaired level of consciousness. If the blood glucose is low (under 2.6 mmol/L), check the blood or urine for ketones and take a critical sample. The absence of ketones in the urine or blood should prompt consideration of hyperinsulinism or a fatty acid oxidation disorder.

When well, children with MCADD do not have abnormal clinical or biochemical findings on routine exams or biochemical testing. Specific metabolic tests (bloodspot acylcarnitine profile and urine organic acids) however will be abnormal even when asymptomatic, and these are the tests of choice to make, or exclude the diagnosis.

Mortality in MCADD can be as high as 20% on first presentation prompting many countries to introduce neonatal screening for MCADD (through acylcarnitine analysis). Episodes of decompensation can be prevented through the avoidance of fasting and an emergency regimen of glucose polymer drinks and frequent feeds when unwell. If vomiting is present or decompensation occurs, it is best managed by admission to hospital for intravenous (IV) glucose administration.

For the emergency treatment of hypoglycaemia, give an IV bolus of 10% dextrose rapidly and thereafter a continuous infusion to maintain normoglycemia. If a child with MCADD is unwell, a supraphysiological infusion rate of dextrose is used acutely to prevent catabolism and reverse decompensation.

SERUM CALCIUM

The normal range for serum calcium is 2.2 to 2.6 mmol/L. Hypocalcaemia may occur in very ill children with sepsis but if well, the key investigation is the measurement of the parathyroid hormone (PTH).[10]

Children with mild hypocalcaemia are often asymptomatic. Paraesthesiae, muscle cramps, laryngospasm, tetany, and seizures are seen in severe hypocalcaemia. Chvostek and Trousseau's signs should be checked (Fig. 17.3). Hypocalcaemia may present with seizures which tend to be multifocal in neonates (Box 17.5) and generalised tonic-clonic in older children. Some newborns may also have stridor or apnoea.

Children with mild hypercalcaemia are often asymptomatic but if severe, they can have symptoms such as drowsiness, irritability, and a depressed level of consciousness. Other symptoms include thirst, anorexia, confusion, and depression.

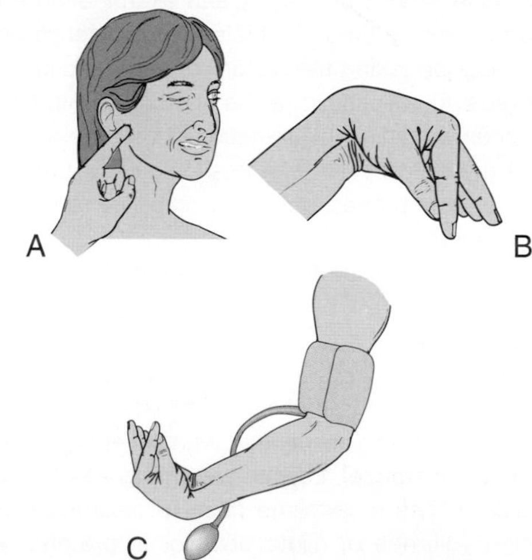

Fig. 17.3 Tests for hypocalcemia. (A) Chvostek sign is the contraction of facial muscles in response to a light tap over the facial nerve in front of the ear. (B) Trousseau sign is a carpal spasm induced by inflating a blood pressure cuff above the systolic pressure for a few minutes (C). (Harding M, et al. *Lewis's Medical-Surgical Nursing: Assessment and Management of Clinical Problems*. 11th ed. Elsevier Mosby; 2020).

BOX 17.5 **CLINICAL HISTORY**

A 7-Day-Old with Jitteriness and a Low Serum Calcium

A 7-day-old female infant is admitted with excessive tremors and jitteriness of the face, arms and legs and a possibility of seizure activity. Blood sugar is normal, and a serum calcium and magnesium are taken. Her serum calcium is 1.1 mmol/L.

Subsequently, she has significant feeding issues, and a diagnosis of a submucous cleft palate is made. She is referred to the specialist cleft palate service, and they notice a number of subtle dysmorphic features with a prominent nose, micrognathia and low-set ears (Fig. 17.4). She has a chest X-ray performed which shows an absent thymus. Subsequent echocardiography showed an interrupted aortic arch. Her renal ultrasound shows a horseshoe kidney. Her subsequent investigations (fluorescent in-situ hybridisation or FISH test) showed a microdeletion of 22q11 region confirming DiGeorge syndrome.

Clinical pearls

Within 72 hours of birth, hypocalcaemia is relatively common and is seen most often in infants of diabetic mothers, preterms and those with birth asphyxia.

Hypocalcaemia *after 72 hours* may be due to congenital hypoparathyroidism, maternal hyperparathyroidism, and vitamin D deficiency. In DiGeorge syndrome (22q11), there is hypoplasia of the parathyroid glands with associated congenital hypoparathyroidism.

Pitfalls to avoid

Hypocalcaemia after 72 hours of birth is uncommon, and the above causes need careful consideration.

Closely examine for a cleft of the soft palate, and pursue further investigations including FISH analysis if found.

All infants with suspected 22q11 microdeletion should have formal echocardiography, as over 75% have congenital heart disease.

Absent of the thymus (as in this case) is linked to defective T cell function with associated risks of giving live vaccines (including BCG vaccine) or nonirradiated blood transfusions.

Significant learning issues are frequently seen in di George syndrome with many having psychiatric issues at or prior to adolescence.

Follow-up in a multidisciplinary specialist service is indicated.

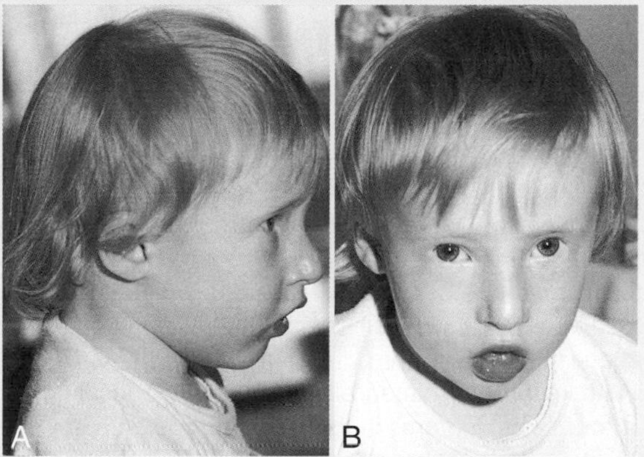

Fig. 17.4 Two-year-old with chromosome 22q11.2 deletion syndrome/DiGeorge syndrome. Facial dysmorphisms include hypertelorism, low-set ears, micrognathia, small fishlike mouth, short philtrum, malformed nose, and down-slanting palpebral fissures. The cardiac defect was truncus arteriosus. (Perloff JK, Marelli AJ. *Perloff's Clinical Recognition of Congenital Heart Disease*. 6th ed. Saunders/Elsevier; 2012:547).

LIVER FUNCTION TESTS

The key investigations are aspartate aminotransferases (AST), Alanine aminotransferases (ALT), serum total and direct bilirubin, gamma glutamyl transferase (GGT), alkaline phosphatase, serum albumin, international normalized ratio (INR) and prothrombin time. Changes can be found in many liver conditions from infectious diseases such as hepatitis A, COVID-19 (Box 17.6), autoimmune liver disease, drug-induced liver toxicity, metabolic conditions affecting the liver and many others.[11]

AST levels of 10 to 100 times normal are found in hepatitis A and the diagnosis is confirmed by hepatitis A IgM.

Both ALT and AST are useful biomarkers of the natural history of viral hepatitis where high levels fall as the child recovers. The degree of elevation of both ALT and AST is not a good marker of hepatocellular damage. The main markers of how the liver is functioning are the INR and serum albumin, as these reflect best the synthetic functions of the liver.

Liver ultrasound is a very useful investigation if transaminases are persistently raised and may show structural lesions such as benign hamartomas or

BOX 17.6 CLINICAL HISTORY

A Jaundiced Girl with a History of Recent SARS-CoV-2 Infection

A 2-year-old girl is seen in the emergency department with a three-day history of yellow discolouration of the eyes and skin (Fig. 17.5). She had no recent travel, and her other symptoms included vomiting with loose stools which were also noted to be pale. She had a confirmed SARS-CoV-2 infection diagnosed 21 days prior to this presentation but had relatively mild symptoms and received paracetamol for 24 hours in age-appropriate doses. Blood tests performed included liver function tests and a hepatitis screen. Hepatitis serology (A to E) was negative. Her INR was 2.3 at presentation, and both her total and direct bilirubin were also elevated. Tests for autoimmune liver disease and Wilson's disease were negative. She subsequently developed hepatocellular failure and was transferred to a specialist liver unit. She later required a liver transplant which went well, but she requires lifelong immunosuppression.

Clinical pearls

Children under 16 years with negative hepatitis serology may have acute hepatitis of unknown aetiology. In 2022 a significant number of such cases have been described worldwide with a small number developing fulminant hepatic failure.

With mild and isolated elevation of the transaminases without any symptoms in the child, the best strategy is to repeat several weeks later and if back to normal the child can safely be discharged.

Pitfalls to avoid

Rarely fulminant hepatitis may follow hepatitis of unknown origin but may also happen in autoimmune liver disease, Wilson's disease, and concealed paracetamol overdose. This rare condition is very likely to have a complex pathology, and the definitive cause remains elusive despite a significant international effort.

In acute liver failure, the single most important investigations are the prothrombin time (PT) and INR. If the INR is prolonged, then vitamin K should be given intravenously and then the INR repeated. If the INR remains prolonged, this suggests impaired hepatic synthesis, and urgent referral to a liver unit is required.

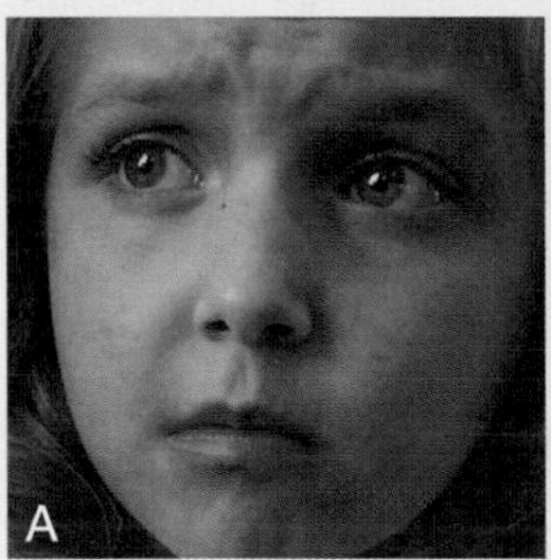

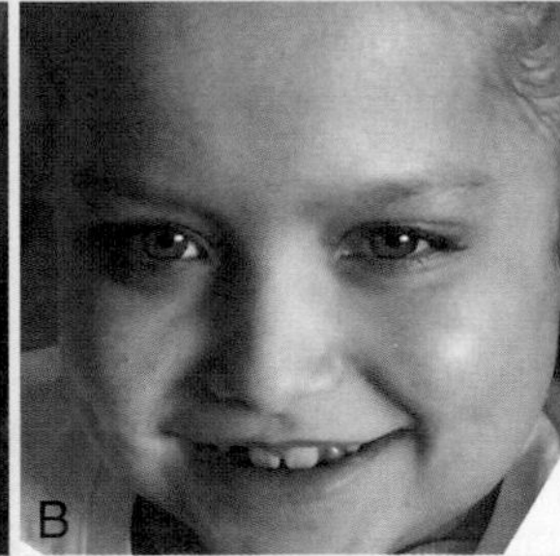

Fig. 17.5 Jaundice/icterus. (A) Note the skin discolouration (jaundice) and yellow hue of the sclerae (icterus) in this child with chronic liver disease. (B) Resolution of both jaundice and icterus just 2 weeks after liver transplantation. (*Zitelli and Davis' Atlas of Pediatric Physical Diagnosis.* 8th ed.; 2023).

hepatoblastoma, gallstone disease, choledochal cyst, liver echotexture changes such as fatty liver or changes in the blood supply to and from the liver such as portal vein thrombosis.

THYROID FUNCTION TESTS

Hypothyroidism may be congenital or acquired. The congenital form is picked up on newborn screening.

Congenital hypothyroidism is picked up by an elevated TSH level on the newborn Guthrie card test. With an elevated TSH in the newborn screen, thyroid function tests are coordinated, and a thyroid scan will pick up an absent or lingual thyroid gland (Box 17.7).

Acquired hypothyroidism in childhood is usually due to autoimmune thyroiditis. Children with Turner syndrome, Klinefelter syndrome, Down syndrome, coeliac disease, or diabetes mellitus are at increased risk of autoimmune thyroiditis. The examination may show a goitre, growth deceleration, dry hair and delayed return of ankle jerk reflexes.

In auto-immune hypothyroidism investigations show a low or low normal thyroxine (T4), a high level of thyroid stimulating hormone (TSH) and positive antithyroperoxidase and antithyroglobulin antibodies.[12]

BOX 17.7 **CLINICAL HISTORY**

A 7-Day-Old with an Abnormal Thyroid Screen

A 7-day-old infant is referred with an abnormal thyroid screen result on heel-prick testing. The infant is asymptomatic, bottle-fed and thriving. Thyroid function tests are taken.

Clinical pearls

The treatment of hypothyroidism is L-thyroxine with normalisation of the TSH level indicating adequate dosage.

Pitfalls to avoid

In hypopituitarism, an elevated TSH will not be seen on the newborn screen, and thus hypothyroidism may be missed.

Acquired central hypothyroidism (low T4 and low TSH) is due to central nervous system tumours affecting the hypothalamus (hamartoma) or anterior pituitary gland, cranial irradiation, or head trauma.

If the TSH fails to fall on L-thyroxine treatment, always consider first noncompliance with treatment, but be aware that drugs (such as rifampicin and carbamazepine), the timing of giving L-thyroxine (not during or immediately after meals) and malabsorption conditions of the small intestine (where it is absorbed) may all interfere with delivery of L-thyroxine.

CONVENTIONAL ALLERGY TESTS

The key to making the diagnosis of food allergy is the recognition of a strong temporal relationship between the exposure to a foodstuff and the onset of quite stereotyped allergic symptoms (Box 17.8).

The most common offenders in Europe are cow's milk, eggs, peanuts, tree nuts (almonds, brazil nuts, cashew nuts, hazelnuts, walnuts), fish and shellfish (prawns, mussels, crab). Exposure is usually through ingestion, and if symptoms are immediate and florid there is little difficulty in recognising the cause and effect.[13]

Skin prick tests (SPT) and specific IgE blood tests may confirm the presence of an IgE-mediated reaction to a particular food, but they do have limitations. In children seen in an allergy clinic with a history of reactions the pretest probability of a true positive is much higher.

A negative SPT is always useful. SPT performs much better with a false positive rate of just 20-25% and a true negative rate of 95%. SPT should only be done for relevant foods, not in wide-ranging fishing expeditions.

The size of the wheal and flare response relates to the age and sex of the child, the quality of the allergen extract (which may vary greatly) and whether the child is on medications such as antihistamines or topical steroids. Antihistamines must be discontinued a week before testing as they may suppress skin reactivity to skin prick tests. Topical steroids are not a problem, and if possible SPT should be delayed for about a month after oral steroid treatment

The serum-specific IgE test measures circulating allergen-specific IgE-antibody levels (which are zero in nonallergic people). IgE tests and skin prick tests usually give similar results, so negative IgE-specific tests mean food allergy is very unlikely (95%), and positive tests properly ordered – in a child with symptoms – can be interpreted with confidence. Sp IgE blood tests are not affected by antihistamine or corticosteroid use.

Food challenges are the gold standard diagnostic test but should only be performed by those with expertise. Food challenges do help confirm the parent's story of food allergy and to see if the child has grown out of it. Food challenges need to be performed in closely monitored situations, as there is always a risk of a severe anaphylactic reaction.[14] Adrenaline use can range from 1–2% to 10% in positive food challenges. Patient selection based on the likelihood of reaction means the rate of positive challenges can be as low as 5% if only challenging those who are very likely to pass, to 50%, when there is less pretest certainty about the outcome.

Food elimination and re-introduction at home is akin to a food challenge and is the only diagnostic test for cow's milk protein intolerance (CMPI) in infancy where the diagnosis cannot be based on SPT and IgE levels. A therapeutic trial of elimination of cow's milk protein leading to symptomatic improvement is only technically positive if recurrence of symptoms is seen when cow's milk protein is reintroduced. Never simply take a food out of a child's diet without a plan to consider when to reintroduce it.

Antihistamines are very effective for cutaneous, nasal and ocular symptoms of allergy but are not sufficient for evolving or established anaphylaxis involving lower airway compromise or hypotension.

Adrenaline given intramuscularly is very safe and starts to work within 5 to 10 minutes and can be repeated with supervision of senior staff. There is no contraindication to

BOX 17.8 CLINICAL HISTORY

Sudden Collapse in a 13-Year-Old Boy

A previously well 13-year-old boy with a background history of atopy and asthma presents with a sudden episode of respiratory distress while out at a restaurant. He appears extremely frightened and says that he 'cannot breathe'. He has been having issues with a number of his peers, and his mother is concerned that the episode might reflect an anxiety episode or panic attack. She takes him outside for some fresh air, but his distress continues. She calls an ambulance, and he is taken to hospital some 15 minutes later. In the hospital, he is noted to be quite distressed with stridor, difficulty in breathing and a faint rash around his mouth. He receives oxygen via face mask and nebulised salbutamol and ipratropium via nebuliser. He does not settle and therefore receives a bolus of magnesium sulphate, and the paediatric intensive care consultant is called. She arrives within 5 minutes and makes a diagnosis of acute anaphylaxis and administers intramuscular adrenaline with an almost immediate effect on his respiratory distress. He settles over the next 30 minutes. He is referred to the Allergy team for further assessment. It transpires on SPT and spIgE testing that he is allergic to shellfish.

He and his family are instructed in the use of a home adrenaline pen for emergency use.

Clinical Pearls

Anaphylaxis is a clinical diagnosis.

Anaphylaxis can be life-threatening, but in reality, the majority of reactions do not result in severe outcomes.[14] The case fatality rate is 1 in 10 million which equates to the chances of being struck by lightning! Tragically, deaths due to anaphylaxis still occur.

The most common trigger in children and young people is food with symptoms typically beginning within 15–30 min of exposure.

Anaphylaxis is likely when there is an acute onset of illness with flushing, urticaria and angioedema in tandem with the life-threatening features of lower airway or circulation compromise.

The most common food trigger for fatal anaphylaxis in children in the UK is milk, followed by peanuts and tree nuts. A severe allergic reaction (anaphylaxis) to bee stings is also potentially life-threatening (Fig. 17.6). Allergy skin prick tests and allergen-specific IgE blood tests do not predict reaction severity, and anaphylaxis can occur in patients with high, low, and even negative tests.[14]

Pitfalls to avoid

Delay in appropriate treatment almost certainly contributes to fatalities.

In older children the usual evolution of nonspecific allergic reactions into anaphylaxis makes it hard to distinguish from differential diagnoses including a vasovagal episode (which will have a slow heart rate and pallor, not raised heart rate and flushing) or a panic attack (high heart rate, pins and needles in hands and around the mouth).

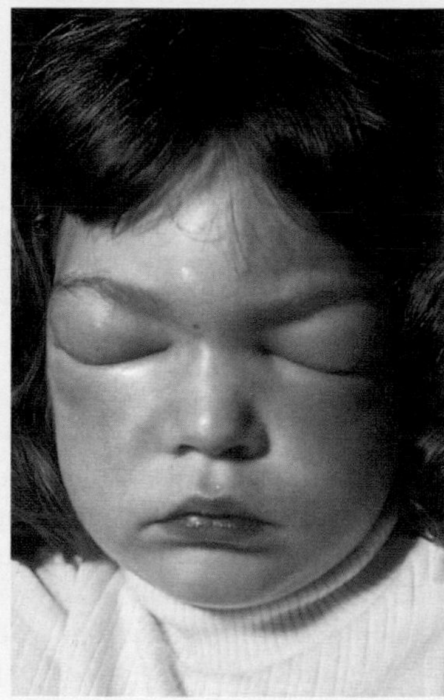

Fig. 17.6 Type I hypersensitivity reaction. Severe swelling of the eyelids in this child is the result of an allergic response to a bee sting. In some children and adults, difficulty breathing may be the first symptom of anaphylaxis. Intervention can be delayed until it is too late because there is no visible sign of narrowed airways (Fireman P. *Atlas of Allergies and Clinical Immunology*. 3rd ed. Mosby; 2006).

using adrenaline in any emergency scenario where anaphylaxis is a possible diagnosis. Delay can kill if it is anaphylaxis and adrenaline is not given. If the diagnosis turns out not to have been anaphylaxis, the pretreatment risk-benefit ratio is always in favour of 'treating, not watching'.

> Children, young people, and their families need to be told to use their autoinjector in the event of any respiratory symptoms where anaphylaxis might the cause, irrespective of severity.[14] Antihistamines are not effective in anaphylaxis.

TABLE 17.1 Key Differences in the Interpretation of Paediatric ECGs Compared to Adults
The normal heart rate is much higher with a heart rate of 110-160 per minute normal under 12 months of age.
The right ventricle can be dominant up to three years of age, and this leads to dominant R waves in Lead V1.
A superior axis on ECG in a cyanosed infant suggests tricuspid atresia and, if acyanotic, suggests an atrioventricular septal defect.
The corrected QT interval of less than 490 milliseconds (ms) is normal in newborns, and values up to 440 ms are considered normal in older infants and children.
In terms of acquired heart conditions, the P-R interval is often prolonged in acute rheumatic fever, and concave ST segment elevation is a feature of acute pericarditis.

ELECTROCARDIOGRAM (ECG) INTERPRETATION

The paediatric ECG is both a friend and foe to trainees and general paediatricians.[15,16,17] It is different from an adult ECG (Table 17.1) and requires a systematic appraisal. It is best to adopt a stepwise approach using a checklist as outlined below.

STRUCTURED APPROACH TO ECG INTERPRETATION

Rate

Firstly, calculate the rate (in essence the number of large boxes between two R waves divided into 300).

Rhythm

Calculate the rhythm which you expect to be normal sinus rhythm, but be aware that sinus arrhythmia (alterations of the heart rate with inspiration) is commonly seen in children.

QRS Axis

The QRS axis is calculated by using the net vector of ventricular depolarisation in leads 1 and a VF. The QRS axis is +110 degrees in neonates, +70 degrees from one month to three months of age and +60 degrees from 3 months to 16 years of age.[17]

Another way is to see whether the QRS net deflection is positive or negative in Lead 1 and aVF. The normal axis is positive in both 1 and aVF. Left axis deviation is positive in lead 1 and negative in aVF.

P Waves

Look for P wave abnormalities such as a broad P wave (over 80 to 100 ms) with a notch indicating left atrial enlargement and peaked P waves (over 3 mm) indicating right atrial enlargement due to pulmonary hypertension.

P-R Interval

One expects each P wave to be followed by a QRS complex, and the P-R interval should be measured. A prolonged P-R interval (over 200 ms) indicates first degree heart block, and a short P-R interval (under 80 ms) is indicative of preexcitation and is seen in Wolff Parkinson White syndrome where a slurred upstroke of the QRS or delta wave are also seen.

QRS Complex

The QRS complex represents ventricular depolarisation and is best assessed in leads V1 and V6. Right ventricular hypertrophy leads to tall R waves in Lead 1 with deep S waves in Lead V6.

In left ventricular hypertrophy, one sees a large R wave in Leads V5 and V6, abnormal Q waves in V5 and V6 and inverted T waves in Lead 1 and a VL.

Q-T Interval

Possibly the most important measurement is the Q-T interval, and this must be calculated for every ECG performed. The manual calculation is more accurate. The most commonly used formula used to calculate the QTc is Bazett's formula.

A QTc interval over 0.45 seconds (or 450 msec) warrants further attention. Congenital long QT syndromes include Romano-Ward syndrome or Jervell-Lange-Nielsen syndrome. Acquired long QT conditions relate to electrolyte disturbances (low potassium, calcium, or magnesium) myocarditis or severe head injury.

The typical arrhythmia associated with a long QT interval is the so-called Torsade de pointes which is a ventricular tachycardia and, if no pulse, should be treated with defibrillation. In Torsade de pointes, the QRS complexes are wide and appear to be twisting around the ECG baseline[17] (Fig. 17.7) (Box 17.9).

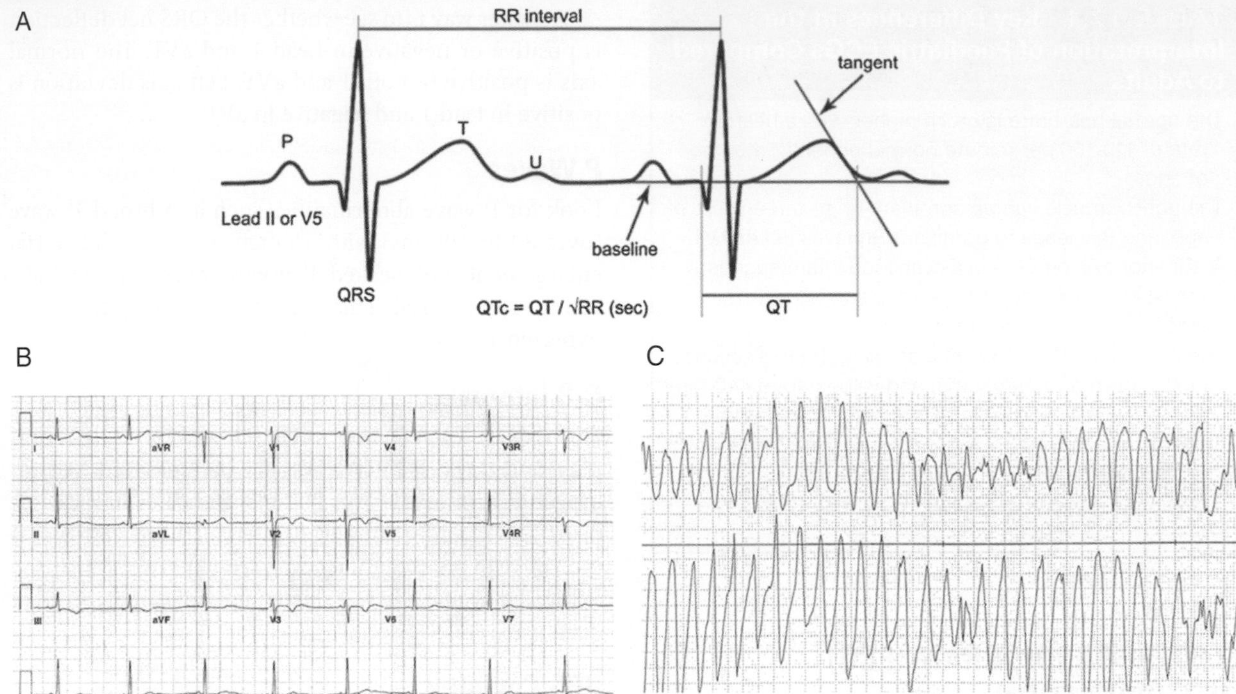

Fig. 17.7 ECG Manifestations of the Long QT Syndrome. Panel A illustrates the tangent method with Bazett's correction for assessment of the QT interval. The end of the T wave corresponds to the intersection of the tangent and baseline. Panel B is the ECG of a 14-year-old girl with long QT syndrome. Note the QTc is over 600 ms and low-amplitude bifid T waves are present. Panel C shows an example of Torsade de pointes (polymorphic VT in the presence of prolonged QT interval). (Pyeritz RE, et al. *Emery and Rimoin's Principles and Practice of Medical Genetics and Genomics.* 7th edition, 2020, Elsevier Inc.)

T Wave and ST Segment

Generally, T waves in leads V1 to V3 are upright for the first few days as a newborn and then become inverted throughout childhood. They revert to being upright in adolescence. Pathological T waves and ST segment elevation are seen in acute pericarditis.

THE ERA OF GENOMIC AND PRECISION MEDICINE

The era of genomic medicine has arrived and will play a significant role in all branches of medicine including paediatrics. In 2003, scientists from several countries working in collaboration with each other sequenced a single human genome over a period of 13 years. This has helped to unravel the complex world that underpins disease-causing alterations in our DNA. In 2017, a national genomic service was launched in the United Kingdom with the lofty aims of predicting and diagnosing inherited and acquired diseases and with a view to personalised treatment and interventions.[18]

Today such sequencing is commercially available and can deliver results within 24 hours. We are now in the era of reaping the rewards of the Human Genome Project, and developments are progressing at an impressive speed.

Since then the technology to sequence a human genome has become far more efficient, primarily due to the development of next generation sequencing (NGS), resulting in tumbling costs and increased access to genomics. This has resulted in an increased diagnostic rate of difficult and novel diagnoses and has helped to unravel the complex world that underpins disease-causing alterations in our DNA.

Some believe that by the end of this decade, a DNA profile will be part of everyone's health record, which will allow for the potential to identify at-risk individuals of developing diseases years before they manifest. This will allow for a paradigm shift to occur within health systems whereby reactive heath systems will be replaced by more proactive systems with the possibility to identify

BOX 17.9 **CLINICAL HISTORY**

A 14-Year-Old with Repeated Episodes of Collapse on Running

A 14-year-old female presents with repeated episodes of acute collapse. The episodes tend to occur when she is swimming or running and forces her to stop participation on most occasions due to concern of by-standers and her coach. The initial working diagnosis was of vasovagal syncope, and the family were reassured. She had one or two myoclonic jerks noted on one occasion and was therefore referred to a paediatric neurologist. Subsequent EEG and MRI brain scan were normal. She continued to have occasional exercise-related episodes and with ongoing parental concern, was forced to stop participation in swimming. An ECG was subsequently performed, and a diagnosis of a long QT syndrome was made (Fig. 17.7). She was commenced on beta blockers with an excellent clinical response and no further syncopal episodes.

Clinical pearls

Patients with prolonged QT syndrome are prone to ventricular arrhythmias which may present as sudden onset syncope without prodrome or, rarely, sudden death.

It is a familial condition inherited in an autosomal dominant fashion. Triggers that induce arrhythmias include medications that prolong the QT interval (including commonly prescribed antibiotics such as erythromycin and clarithromycin), swimming or exercise, auditory stimuli and emotional stress and rest or sleep.

Key pitfalls to avoid

Long QT syndromes are usually inherited in an autosomal dominant fashion, and thus there may be a family history of sudden death.

Long QT syndromes generally present with sudden onset syncope, brief seizure activity (including unexplained nocturnal incontinence) but not usually with palpitations or pre-syncope.

If undetected, ventricular tachycardia with a typical Torsades de pointes pattern may follow. ECG shows broad QRS complexes with absent P waves. If a pulse is felt then the emergency treatment of this type of arrythmia is cardioversion and, if no pulse is felt, then cardiopulmonary resuscitation and defibrillation is indicated.

individuals at risk of developing diseases allowing for screening or treatment initiation to occur before the manifestation of disease. This exciting era of genomic and precision medicine will transcend every medical speciality but will not be without significant challenges involving data storage, interpretation and privacy which will have to be thought through, incorporating high ethical and moral standards, to ensure that the full potential of this era is unlocked and applied in an appropriate manner.

There is a newfound interest in precision health with potential innovations including tiny electrodes in pillowcases enabling noninvasive monitoring of sleep patterns at home, special toilets that check urine for glucose and protein and stool for occult blood, smart refrigerators that display nutritional values for food in the fridge, smartphones that might pick up depression due to a fall off in use, sensors in cars that could detect drowsiness in the driver or blood alcohol levels on the breath of the driver, the now ubiquitous Fitbits to track exercise patterns and implantable technologies (already in place) to detect abnormal heart rhythms and blood glucose patterns. There is a downside, of course, and that is we will have information, from 18 years of age, about diseases we are likely to develop in our lifetime. That can be a two-edged sword and lead to many unforeseen effects.

COMMON GENETIC/GENOMIC TESTING TECHNOLOGIES NOW AVAILABLE IN PRACTICE

Karyotyping

Chromosomal G-banded analysis (or karyotyping) was previously considered the first-line test of a child with multiple malformations, but now the recommended first-line test is either high-resolution array CGH or Next Generation Sequencing.[19]

However, G-banded analysis remains an important test if a chromosomal disorder is suspected especially if there are signs suggestive of a known chromosome disorder such as trisomy 21 (Down syndrome), trisomy 13 (Patau's syndrome), trisomy 18 (Edward's syndrome) or if the infant has a suspected disorder of sexual development to thereby identify the chromosomal gender.

Chromosome abnormalities can broadly be classified into abnormalities of chromosome number or structure. Abnormalities of chromosome number are relatively common but may be difficult to recognise and may result in the early loss of a pregnancy. Triploidy (69 chromosomes) and tetraploidy (92 chromosomes) are both causes of early pregnancy loss. Inversions are generally balanced and tend not to produce any phenotypic effect. Translocations are either reciprocal or Robertsonian. Reciprocal translocations occur where there is an exchange of genetic material from one arm of a chromosome in return for genetic material from a different chromosome. They are usually balanced and without any clinical effects. On the other hand, those who carry a Robertsonian translocation involving chromosome 21 or 13 may be at significantly higher risk of having a child with Down or Patau's syndrome as an unbalanced product of the translocation.[19]

Chromosomal Microarray Analysis

Microarray testing is, in essence, a method of detecting the gain or loss of genetic material, ranging in size from several thousand to tens of millions of nucleotides. It is based on the measurement of the relative intensity of the patient versus the control fluorescent dye signal at each probe on the array[20] (Fig. 17.8).

Microarray testing will identify pathogenic chromosomal anomalies in up to 30% of infants with multiple malformations, and it is reported the likelihood of an abnormal array CGH increases with the number of clinical abnormalities.[19]

Microarray identifies microdeletions or microduplications known as copy number variants. These can be part of normal human variation, and this poses a significant challenge in their interpretation.

> Chromosomal microarray analysis is recommended as the first-line diagnostic test for developmental delay, autism spectrum disorder and multiple congenital anomalies.[21]

Microarray results are frequently inconclusive and reported as having variants of uncertain significance (VUS).

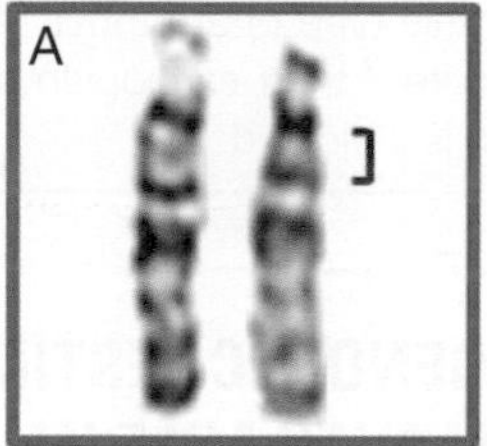

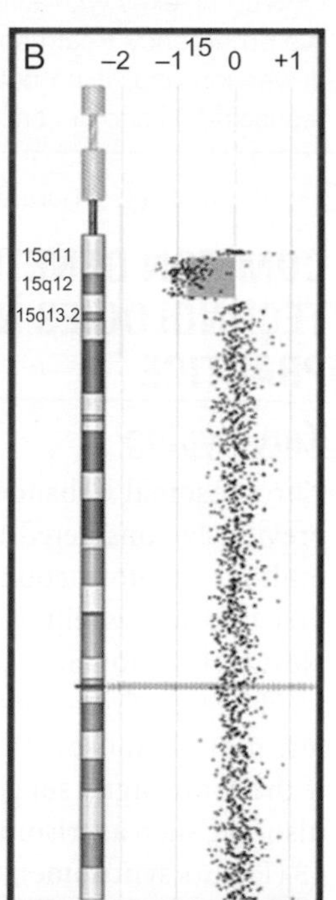

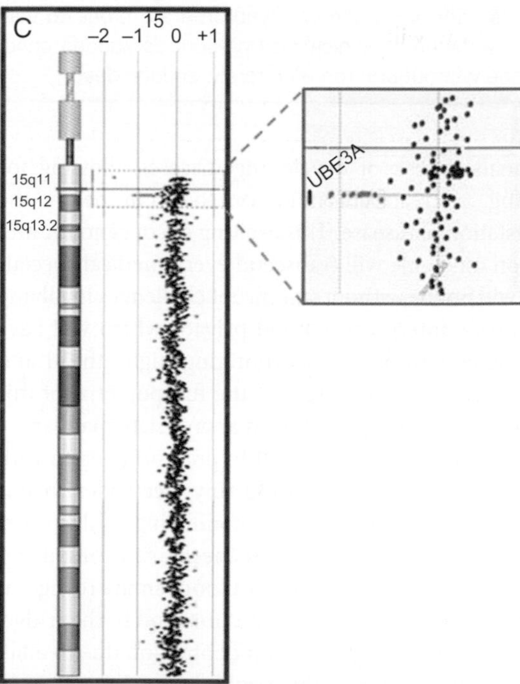

Fig. 17.8 Example of data from a microarray analysis. The upper panel shows the set of chromosomes from which chromosome 6 was chosen for examination in detail. The bands for that chromosome are shown horizontally at the bottom. In this case, the proximal long arm of chromosome 6 shows two anomalies: a duplication and a deletion. The duplication is identified by the blue box just below the chromosome panel, and the red bar denotes the smaller deletion. These are confirmed by the thick line at the top (weighted log2 ratio), series of three midweight lines in the middle (allele peaks and the single line below that (smooth signal). For the duplication, the smooth signal deflects upward, showing three copies in that region and four copies for the allele peaks. For the deletion, the smooth signal deflects downward, indicating the presence of a single copy at that locus. (These data were collected using the Affymetrix CytoScanHD System). (Source: Richard A. McPherson, Matthew R. Pincus. *Henry's Clinical Diagnosis and Management by Laboratory Methods,* 24th edition, 2022, Elsevier Inc.)

Reinterpreting prior results may increase diagnostic utility when there is additional clinical information or via a contemporary second opinion.[21] Therefore, inconclusive microarray results should be re-interpreted every two years or when a child is being considered for other genomic tests.

Whether a variant is *de novo* or inherited is a potentially powerful piece of evidence, so testing the parents is essential.[20]

For instance, if a variant is present in a parent (relatives) and they have similar symptoms, this increases the likelihood that it is significant. Likewise, if found to be *de novo* and both parents are clinically unaffected, this also supports pathogenicity.[20]

The 15q11.2 microdeletion is one variant that is relatively commonly seen in clinical practice. However, with a low penetrance and an extremely nonspecific and variable spectrum of associated features, this casts doubt whether it is a recognisable syndrome, and therefore it may not account (solely at least) for the problems of any given child.[22]

Microarray will not identify balanced chromosome rearrangements such as balanced translocations and inversions, as these do not result in any loss or gain of chromosome material. Microarray will also not detect point mutations or epigenetic abnormalities.

Reinterpretation sometime later may resolve inconclusive results especially if there is additional clinical information or a second opinion has been sought. Inconclusive microarrays should be reinterpreted every 2 years before further evaluation by other genomic tests.[21]

Fluorescent In Situ Hybridisation (FISH)

Fluorescent in situ hybridisation uses specific fluorescently labelled small DNA fragments or probes from specific regions of chromosomes which allows for targeted higher resolution analysis of specific chromosomes. One example where this technology would be commonly used is testing for Di George syndrome (22q11 deletion). FISH can also be carried out to get a rapid result for numerical chromosome anomalies such as Down syndrome or for a rapid determination of the chromosomal gender.[19]

Next Generation Sequencing (NGS) Tests

Each human genome contains about four million variants, the great majority of which are not pathogenic.

> Next generation sequencing allows for hundreds of thousands of DNA fragments to be sequenced at the same time.[18]

Whole gene sequencing sequences all the known coding regions (or exons) in the genome. It is also possible to sequence the noncoding regions or introns. NGS increases the diagnostic yield to 50% in Mendelian disorders. NGS can detect low-level mosaicism and large genomic deletions of exons or whole genes.[18]

NGS is recommended in children with a suspected monogenic condition who have global developmental delay, dysmorphic facial features and one or more major congenital anomalies. Prerequisites prior to ordering NGS include noninformative microarray results, informed consent from the parents and consultation with a clinical geneticist. Earlier diagnosis of a genetic syndrome picked up by NGS can lead to improved surveillance, changes in management and an accurate estimation of the risk of recurrence.[23]

> The use of NGS may help end the diagnostic odyssey and allow access to parent and family support groups.

NGS will not detect disorders such as myotonic dystrophy or Fragile X syndrome.

For NGS, up to 50% diagnostic yields are achieved for intellectual disability, eye diseases and in selected acutely ill children who need intensive care.[24]

These tests have become relatively inexpensive and are now considered standard for children of all ages presenting with malformations. NGS is now often suggested to be the first diagnostic test for conditions including craniosynostosis, arthrogryposis, holoprosencephaly, lissencephaly and anophthalmia and an ever-expanding list of other diagnoses.

Whole exome sequencing introduces the ability to examine the coding regions of all 23,000 genes while whole genome sequencing helps to examine both coding and noncoding regions. Both tests were made possible by the development of NGS. They also result in significant challenges such as the identification of an increased number of benign variants or variants of unknown significance (VUS). Another current significant limitation in the area is the lack of reference genomes to reflect many non-European-derived populations.

Overall next generation sequencing is the future and will play an ongoing important role.

> NGS has lots of potential benefits and is likely to become mainstream in time.

Interpreting the Results from Genetic Tests

Microarray results may be inconclusive, and VUS may be picked up requiring consultation with a clinical geneticist. Most phone calls to genetic services are from somewhat confused paediatricians looking for inspiration and asking their local specialist service to interpret the result.

> Communication between the clinicians on the ground and the laboratory is very important as is an accurate description of the phenotype of the child.

It may be difficult to establish the significance of some variants and targeted testing of other family members may be helpful. It is known that as new information is discovered and collected on gene variants the classification of some will change over time.

Precision Medicine – A 'Brave New World'

The era of Precision Health and Medicine, the natural successor to genomic medicine, has arrived, and it is estimated that about 300 new targeted therapies, many of which will be gene or genotype specific, will be available to patients by 2030. Already a number of successful treatments for genetic diseases such as spinal muscular atrophy type1,[25,26] RPE65 mutation-associated retinal dystrophy, X-linked severe combined immunodeficiency, cystic fibrosis, haemophilia[27], phenylketonuria, and Fabry disease have been successfully applied as standard of care for many patients. Genome editing technologies, such as clustered regularly interspaced short palindromic repeats (mercifully shortened to CRISPR!), are also being applied in clinical trials for many genetic conditions, an area that harbours great hope.[28] In 2015, a young 1-year-old named Layla who had leukaemia, achieved remission by means of another gene editing technology using transcription activator-like effector nucleases (TALENs)[29] to modify immune genes of donor T-cells so that they could be safely transplanted.

In general, gene therapies are considered to be more effective when given presymptomatically, and thus expanded newborn screening programmes are likely in the future. Amongst the many ethical challenges is that some gene therapies may simply transform a previously fatal condition into one with a longer life expectancy but still significant morbidity.[30] These therapies are very expensive, so cost analyses are key and necessary considerations where international health budgets are under considerable strain.

Literacy in diagnostic genetics and genomics will be a crucial and necessary skill for the next generation of clinicians and scientists to achieve for the translation of genomic and precision medicine into effective clinical practice and benefit.

REFERENCES

1. Boon HA, Lenaerts W, Van Aerde C, Verbakel JY. Outpatient urine collection methods for paediatric urinary tract infections: systematic review of diagnostic accuracy studies. *Acta Paediatr*. 2021;110(12):3170–3179. doi:10.1111/apa.16027.
2. Kaufman J, Fitzpatrick P, Tosif S, et al. Faster clean catch urine collection (Quick-Wee method) from infants: randomised controlled trial. *BMJ*. 2017;357:j1341. doi:10.1136/bmj.j1341.
3. Brandow M. Pallor and anemia. In: Kliegman RM, Lyle PS, Bordini B, Toth H, Basel D, eds. *Nelson Pediatric Symptom-Based Diagnosis*. Elsevier; 2018:661–681.
4. McNaughten B, Thompson A, Macartney C, Thompson A. How to use... a blood film. *Arch Dis Child Educ Pract Ed*. 2018;103(5):263–266. doi:10.1136/archdischild-2017-312685.
5. Kapur S, Gilmore M, Macartney C, Thompson A. How to use a coagulation screen. *Arch Dis Child Educ Pract Ed*. 2022;107(1):45–49. doi:10.1136/archdischild-2020-320925.
6. Korppi M. Serum C-reactive protein is a useful tool for prediction of complicated course in children's pneumonia. *Acta Paediatr*. 2021;110(4):1090–1091. doi:10.1111/apa.15638.
7. Downes KJ. Procalcitonin in pediatric sepsis: what is it good for? *J Pediatric Infect Dis Soc*. 2021;10(12):1108–1110. doi:10.1093/jpids/piab066.
8. Prisco A, Capalbo D, Guarino S, Miraglia Del Giudice E, Marzuillo P. How to interpret symptoms, signs and investigations of dehydration in children with gastroenteritis. *Arch Dis Child Educ Pract Ed*. 2021;106(2):114–119. doi:10.1136/archdischild-2019-317831.
9. Thornton PS, Stanley CA, De Leon DD, et al. Recommendations from the Pediatric Endocrine Society for evaluation and management of persistent hypoglycemia in neonates, infants, and children. *J Pediatr*. 2015;167(2):238–245. doi:10.1016/j.jpeds.2015.03.057.
10. Nadar R, Shaw N. Investigation and management of hypocalcaemia. *Arch Dis Child*. 2020;105(4):399–405. doi:10.1136/archdischild-2019-317482.
11. Cevik M, Rasmussen AL, Bogoch II, Kindrachuk J. Acute hepatitis of unknown origin in children. *BMJ*. 2022;377:o1197. doi:10.1136/bmj.o1197.
12. Lee YL, Yap F, Vasanwala RF. Abnormal thyroid function in paediatric practice. *Arch Dis Child*

Educ Pract Ed. 2020;105(6):361–363. doi:10.1136/archdischild-2018-316426.
13. Abrams EM, Greenhawt M, Shaker M, Alqurashi W. Separating fact from fiction in the diagnosis and management of food allergy. *J Pediatr*. 2022;241:221–228. doi:10.1016/j.jpeds.2021.10.011.
14. Anagnostou K, Turner PJ. Myths, facts and controversies in the diagnosis and management of anaphylaxis. *Arch Dis Child*. 2019;104(1):83–90. doi:10.1136/archdischild-2018-314867.
15. Evans WN, Acherman RJ, Mayman GA, Rollins RC, Kip KT. Simplified pediatric electrocardiogram interpretation. *Clin Pediatr (Phila)*. 2010;49(4):363–372. doi:10.1177/0009922809336206.
16. Harris M, Oakley C, Abumehdi MR. Making sense of the paediatric ECG. *Arch Dis Child Educ Pract Ed*. 2022;107(1):24–25. doi:10.1136/archdischild-2020-319124.
17. Lambrechts L, Fourie B. How to interpret an electrocardiogram in children. *BJA Educ*. 2020;20(8):266–277. doi:10.1016/j.bjae.2020.03.00.
18. Baralle D, Ismail V. 'Next Generation Sequencing' as a diagnostic tool in paediatrics. *Arch Dis Child*. 2021;106(1):1–2. doi:10.1136/archdischild-2020-320251.
19. Green AJ, O'Byrne JJ. Pediatric clinical genetics. In: Puri P, ed. *Pediatric Surgery: General Principles and Newborn Surgery*. Springer-Verlag; 2020:149–165.
20. Hammond CL, Willoughby JM, Parker MJ. Genomics for paediatricians: promises and pitfalls. *Arch Dis Child*. 2018;103(9):895–900. doi:10.1136/archdischild-2017-314558.
21. Shi G, Xu J, Barnes SF, et al. Chromosomal microarray reinterpretation: applications to pediatric practice. *J Pediatr*. 2022;243:219–223. doi:10.1016/j.jpeds.2021.12.036.
22. Parker MJ, Teasdale K, Parker MJ. The genetic assessment of looked after children: common reasons for referral and recent advances. *Arch Dis Child*. 2016;101(6):581–584. doi:10.1136/archdischild-2014-307215.
23. Shah M, Selvanathan A, Baynam G, et al. Paediatric genomic testing: navigating genomic reports for the general paediatrician. *J Paediatr Child Health*. 2022;58(1):8–15. doi:10.1111/jpc.15703.
24. Scott RH, Fowler TA, Caulfield M. Genomic medicine: time for health-care transformation. *Lancet*. 2019;394(10197):454–456. doi:10.1016/S0140-6736(19)31796-9.
25. Mahase E. NHS England agrees deal for gene therapy for spinal muscular atrophy. *BMJ*. 2021;372:n653. doi:10.1136/bmj.n653.
26. Gene therapy for spinal muscular atrophy. *Arch Dis Child*. 2021;106:483. doi:10.1136/archdischild-2021-322133.
27. Replacing the haemophilia gene. *Arch Dis Child*. 2018;103(3):234. doi:10.1136/archdischild-2018-314749.
28. Hirakawa MP, Krishnakumar R, Timlin JA, Carney JP, Butler KS. Gene editing and CRISPR in the clinic: current and future perspectives. *Biosci Rep*. 2020;40(4):BSR20200127. doi:10.1042/BSR20200127.
29. Sun N, Zhao H. Transcription activator-like effector nucleases (TALENs): a highly efficient and versatile tool for genome editing. *Biotechnol Bioeng*. 2013;110(7):1811–1821. doi:10.1002/bit.24890.
30. Ryan MM. Gene therapy for neuromuscular disorders: prospects and ethics. *Arch Dis Child*. 2022;107(5):421–426. doi:10.1136/archdischild-2020-320908.

ADDITIONAL READING

Contact a Family – a UK charity for families with disabled children, which offers information on specific conditions and rare disorders. Accessed at https://contact.org.uk/

Hastings R, Abhijit D. Genomic medicine for the paediatrician. *Paediatr Child Health*. 2019;29(4):185–189.

Kattamis A, Kwiatkowski JL, Aydinok Y. Thalassaemia. *Lancet*. 2022;399(10343):2310–2324. doi:10.1016/S0140-6736(22)00536-0.

Neuhaus CP, Zacharias RL. Compassionate use of gene therapies in pediatrics: an ethical analysis. *Semin Perinatol*. 2018;42(8):508–514. doi:10.1053/j.semperi.2018.09.010.

OMIM, Online Mendelian Inheritance in Man – a database of human genes and genetic disorders developed by staff at Johns Hopkins. Accessed at https://www.ncbi.nlm.nih.gov/omim

Orphanet – a database (in several languages) of genetic disorders, clinical information, clinic listings and research and diagnostic genetic testing for a wide range of disorders. Accessed at https://www.orpha.net/consor/cgi-bin/index.php

Splinter K, Adams DR, Bacino CA, et al. Effect of genetic diagnosis on patients with previously undiagnosed disease. *N Engl J Med*. 2018;379(22):2131–2139. doi:10.1056/NEJMoa1714458.

Understanding Gene testing – a website with information on basic genetic concepts, and the utility and limitations of genetic testing. Accessed at https://medlineplus.gov/genetics/understanding/testing/genetictesting/

18

Commonly Ordered Radiological Tests and Their Interpretation

Yusra Sheikh

CHAPTER OUTLINE

DIAGNOSTIC IMAGING

There have been exciting recent advances in radiology which remain central in disease diagnosis, monitoring and prognostication. There are multiple imaging modalities available to the clinician to optimise patient care with minimum radiation exposure while still ensuring the desired clinical result is achieved. For each radiological imaging referral, there must be a net benefit to the child over any potential risk associated with it. A referral general guide is provided herein, although many more of the recommended imaging indications are beyond the scope of this chapter. The referrer is advised to discuss with their local radiologist on the best radiological investigation indicated for their patient.

RADIOLOGY INVESTIGATIONS

It is essential to include appropriate clinical details in the referral letter to the radiology department to justify and optimise the radiological investigation. Imaging is performed in accordance with the principle of radiation safety ALARA (as low as reasonably achievable), to minimise radiation doses. In the postmenarchal girl, the 10-day rule should be applied and the last menstrual period (LMP) documented to avoid unnecessarily irradiating any unborn foetus.

Radiographs

X-ray machines are readily available in all radiology departments. Radiographs are the most frequently requested examinations. Although the radiation dose is quite small in comparison to computed tomography (CT), every investigation requested should be justified.

Chest Radiographs

Chest radiographs are very helpful when consolidation, pleural effusion, pneumothorax (Fig. 18.1) or inhaled foreign body (Fig. 18.2) is suspected. It is easy to misinterpret the thymic silhouette on an infant's chest radiograph due to its great variability in appearance (Fig. 18.3A,B). The normal thymus can appear quite bulky in the infant giving an impression of a widened superior mediastinum but involutes over time.

Chest radiographs are not indicated in mild to moderate bronchiolitis or for repeat acute exacerbations of asthma. Additionally, chest radiographs may not be of

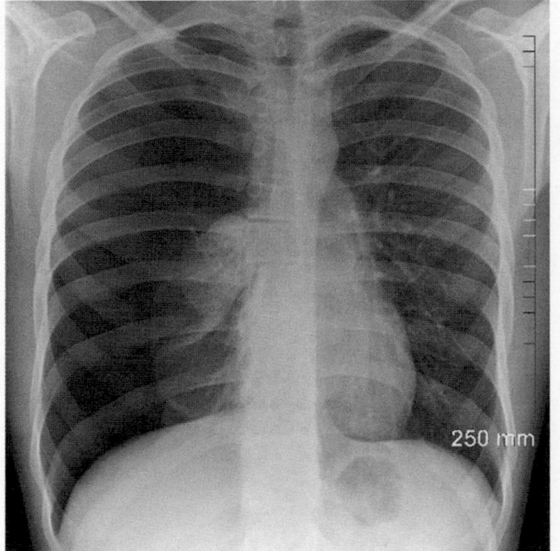

Fig. 18.1 Chest radiograph of a 14 year old who presented to ED with sharp right-sided chest pain and breathlessness. There is a large right-sided pneumothorax without any mediastinal shift (note the lack of lung markings on the right). The right lung is small and collapsed.

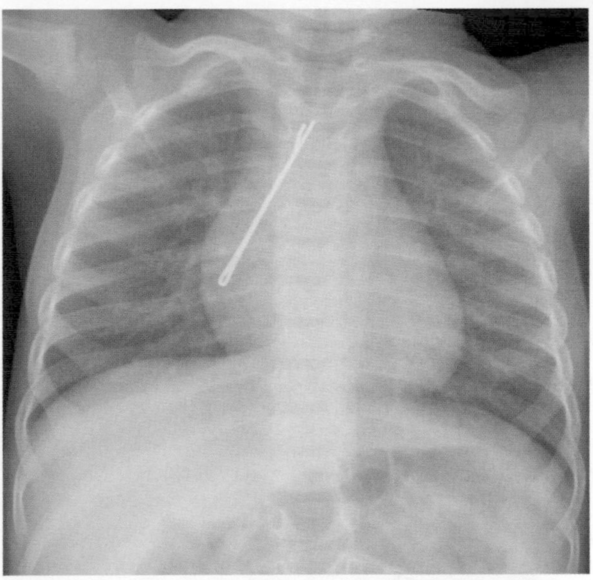

Fig. 18.2 A 1 year old presented post swallowing of a hairclip. The chest radiograph confirms an inhaled hairclip in a diagonal position, projected over the lower trachea and extending inferiorly over the bronchus intermedius.

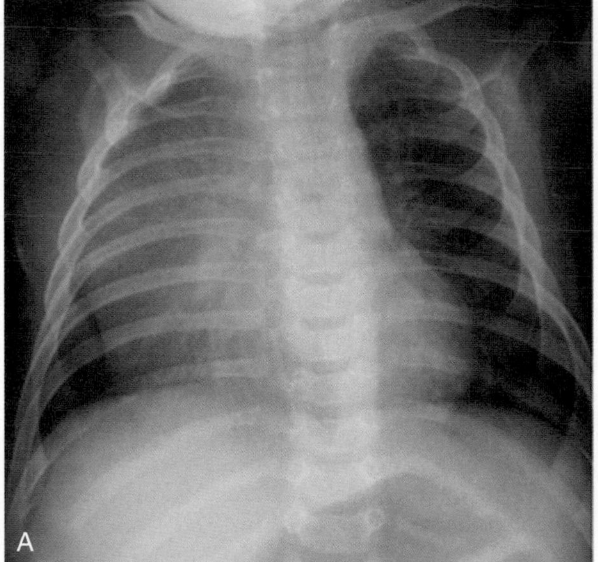

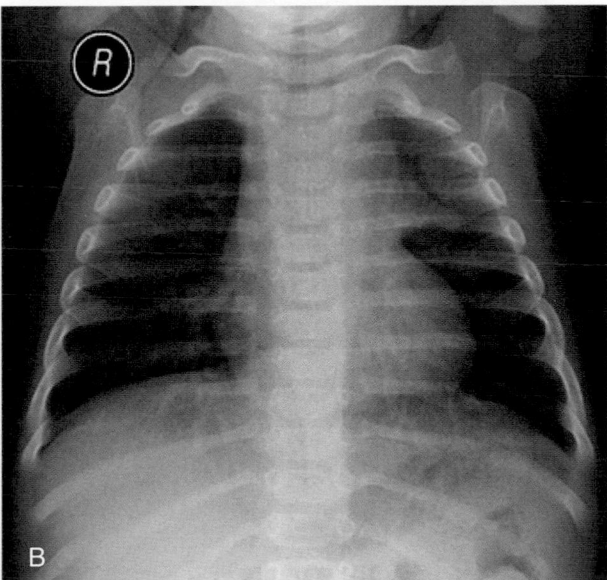

Fig. 18.3 Two different appearances of the normal thymus on chest radiograph. (A) Asymmetric right-sided opacity on chest radiograph confirmed to be the thymus on subsequent ultrasound of the chest, most suggestive of a unilobed thymus. (B) Typical sail sign of the thymus, with a sharp triangular opacity in the left superior mediastinum.

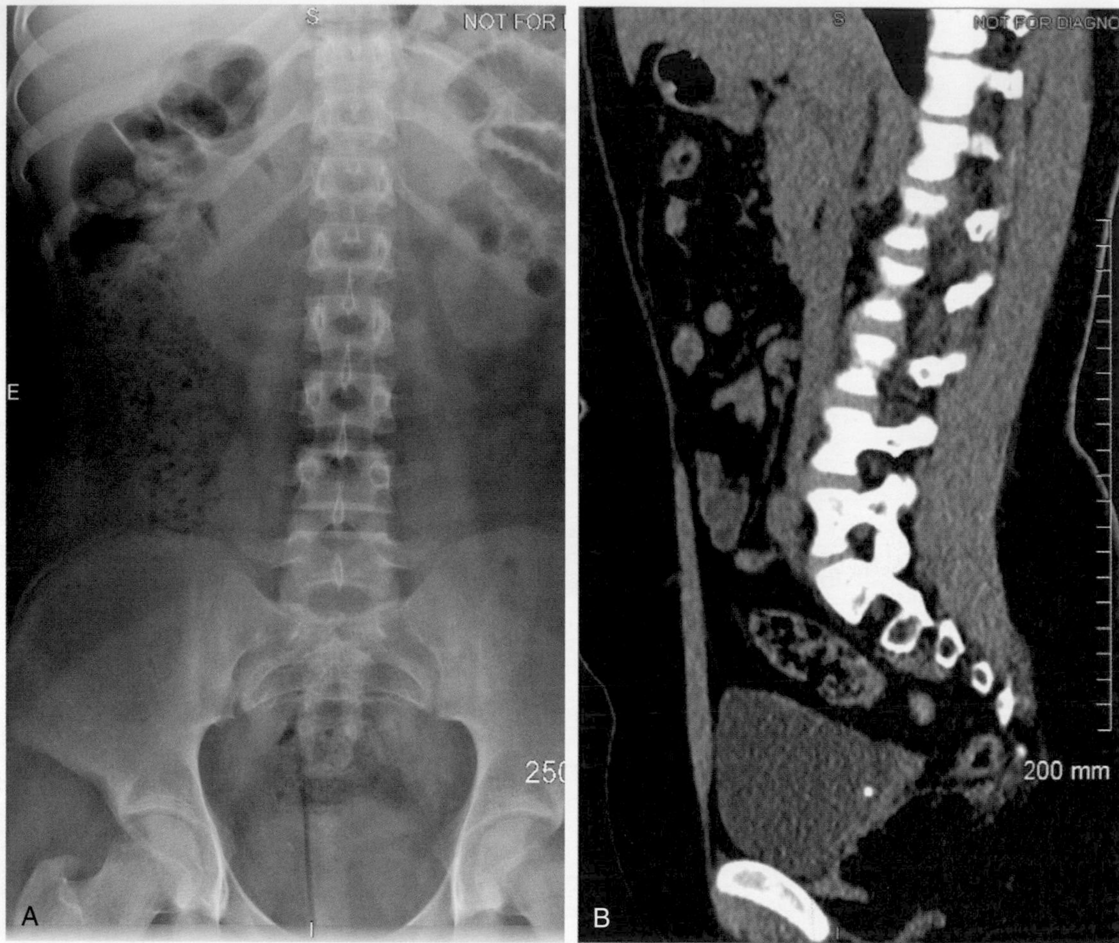

Fig. 18.4 A 15-year-old girl presented with severe right loin pain radiating to her ipsilateral groin. She also had eight episodes of vomiting in the emergency department and trace blood in her urine. (A) Plain film abdomen, demonstrated an ovoid density projected over the right hemipelvis. (B) Confirmed to be a calculus partially obstructing vesicoureteric junction on subsequent CT scan.

use in community-acquired pneumonia that is being managed in family practice, patients with prominent ribs or nonspecific chest pain.

Plain Abdominal Radiographs

A plain abdominal radiograph is helpful in the setting of an acute abdomen, haematuria to exclude radio-opaque renal stones (Fig. 18.4A,B) or ingested foreign body. It is important to recognise ingested foreign bodies such as a button battery or magnets, as these can be associated with visceral perforation (Fig. 18.5A,B). It is also useful in suspected small bowel ileus (Fig. 18.6), bowel obstruction (Fig. 18.7) or visceral perforation.

Plain abdominal radiographs are distinctly unhelpful in suspected constipation and should be avoided in such instances.

Pelvis Radiographs

Ultrasound is the ideal modality to exclude developmental dysplasia of the hips (DDH) in a young infant. There are however cases of delayed presentations (Fig. 18.8), and hip radiographs are performed in such cases. These are preferably done in infants older than 3 months of age but are not indicated for unequal groin creases or delayed walking. Additionally, hip radiographs can be performed on older children with

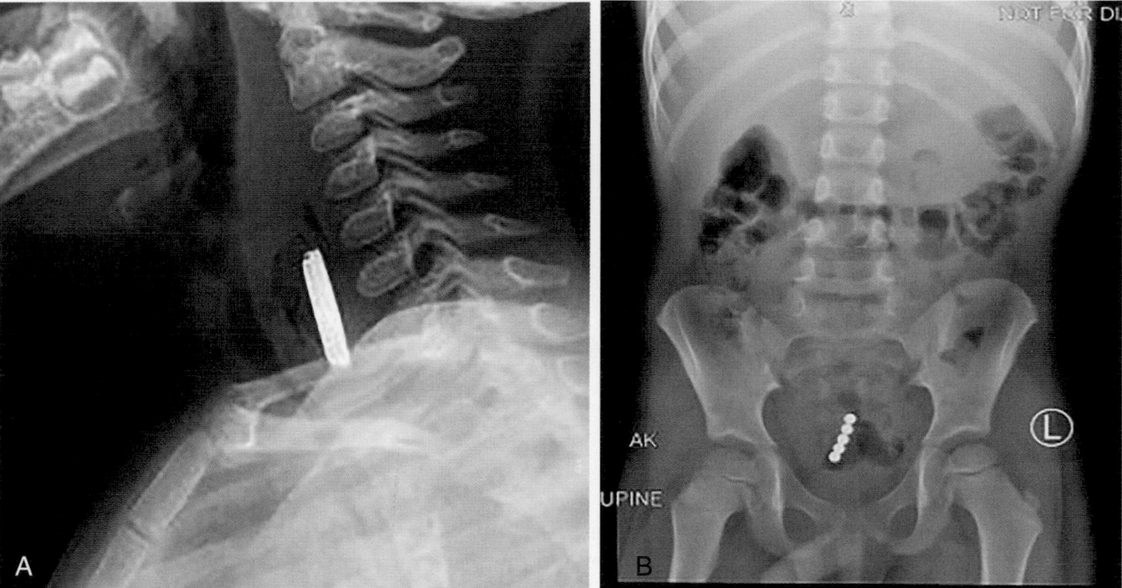

Fig. 18.5 Two different types of ingested foreign bodies to be aware of as both are associated with significant complications. (A) Impacted button battery at the level of the proximal oesophageal sphincter can cause severe corrosion with perforation and erosion into adjacent structures. (B) Five small magnets projected over the pelvis. If these are attracted together across two bowel loops, they can cause necrosis of the bowel with significant morbidity.

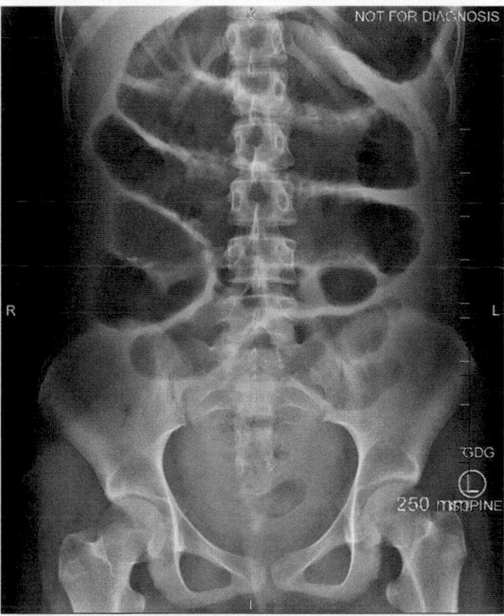

Fig. 18.6 A 15-year-old with dilated small bowel loops post appendectomy. Note air within the rectum, appearances are most suggestive of small bowel ileus rather than mechanical obstruction. Symptoms resolved on conservative management.

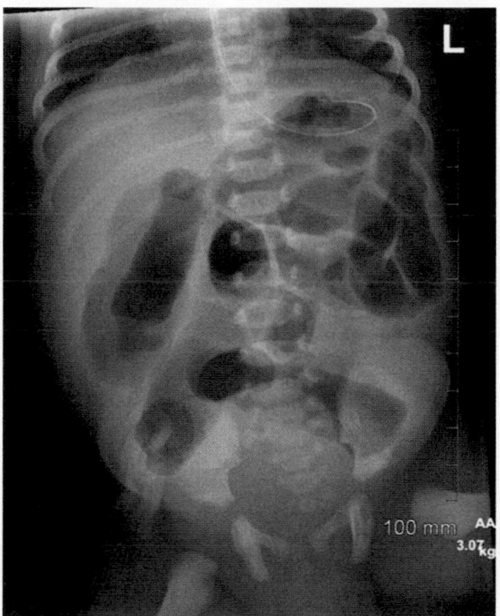

Fig. 18.7 Plain film abdomen of a term neonate on day 1 of life with a distended abdomen. A nasogastric has been placed with the tip in the stomach. There are several dilated bowel loops but no pneumoperitoneum. Note the lack of gas within the distal colon and rectum, suggestive of bowel obstruction. This was surgically confirmed to be a case of ileal atresia.

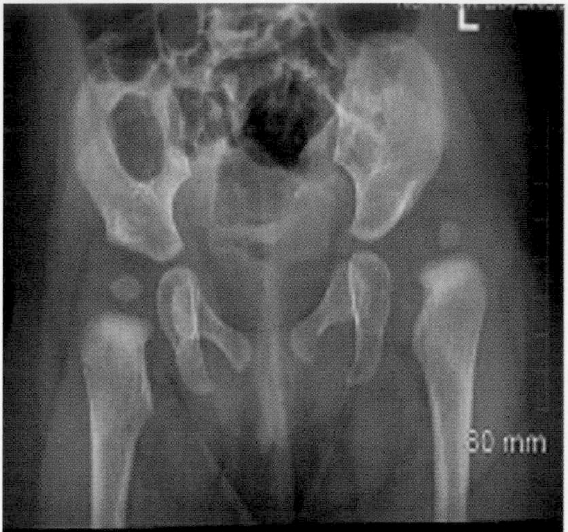

Fig. 18.8 Example of a delayed DDH presentation. X-ray of the pelvis of a 5-month-old referred by the GP with a positive left Barlow and Ortolani test. There is severe left acetabular dysplasia with superior dislocation of the left femur giving an impression of pseudoarticulation with the ipsilateral ilium. (Source: Alf Nicholson, Kevin Dunne, Sarah Taaffe, Yusra Sheikh, John Murphy. Developmental dysplasia of the hip in infants and children, BMJ 2023;383:e074507. http://dx.doi.org/10.1136/bmj-2022-074507. Published: 23 November 2023.)

traumatic or atraumatic hip pain to exclude subcapital femoral epiphysis (SCFE) slippage (Fig. 18.9A,B), avulsion fractures around the pelvis or suspected bone lesions.

Limb Radiographs

Trauma is the commonest indication for limb radiographs and the radiological investigation is tailored according to the referrer's indication on the request (Fig. 18.10A,B). The radiographs will be focused on the area of concern in accordance with the ALARA principle, therefore reducing the radiation exposure cumulative dose. Other indications for limb imaging include congenital limb anomalies, lower limb alignment such as genu vera or genu valgus, lower limb length discrepancy, a radiodense foreign body such as glass or metal and atraumatic bone pain (such as night pain for an osteoid osteoma) (Fig. 18.11).

Instances Where X-Ray Imaging Benefit Is Questionable

There are certain instances where the radiographs add minimal or no value to the suspected or concerning clinical indication. Examples are knee radiographs for Osgood Schlatter's disease, ankle radiographs for Sever's disease, skull radiographs for headaches or abnormal head shapes, sinus radiographs for suspected sinusitis and nasal bone radiographs for suspected nasal trauma. Some of these may benefit from alternative imaging, and it is best to discuss with your local radiologist for guidance.

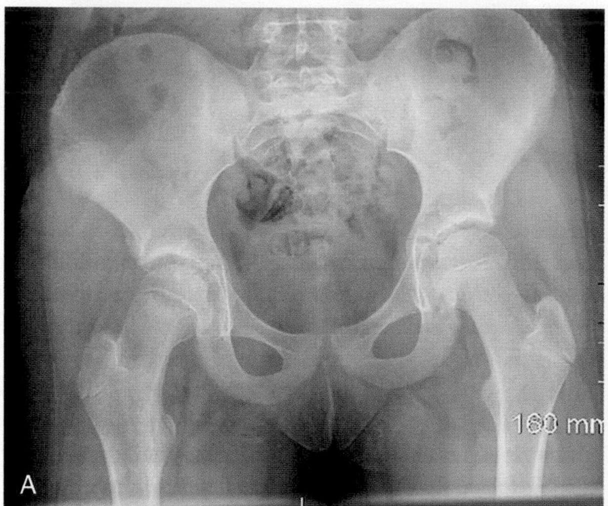

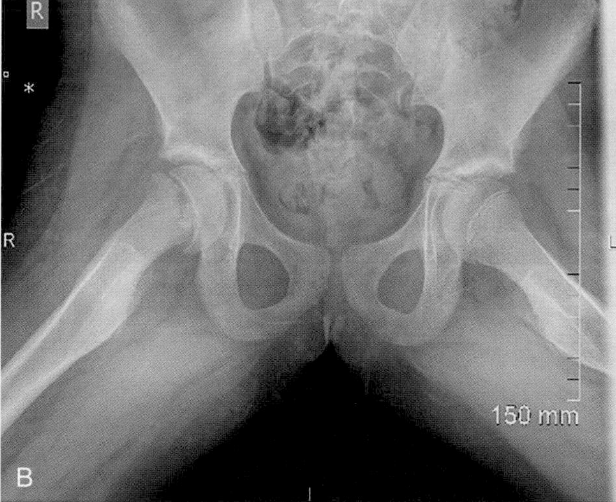

Fig. 18.9 (A) AP and (B) lateral views of the hips in a 13-year-old girl who presented with right hip pain and limp. There is right proximal femoral epiphysis posteromedial slippage with physeal widening, consistent with slipped capital femoral epiphyses (SCFE).

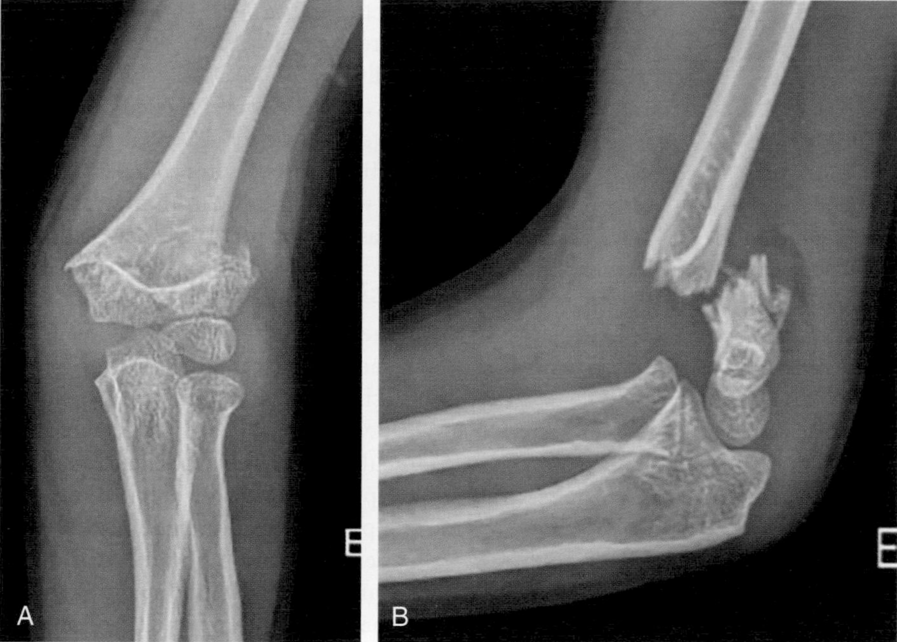

Fig. 18.10 (A) Frontal and (B) lateral left elbow radiographs of a 4 year old who fell onto his elbow (Gartland III). There is a posteriorly displaced supracondylar fracture of the left distal humerus. Radiocapitellar alignment is preserved.

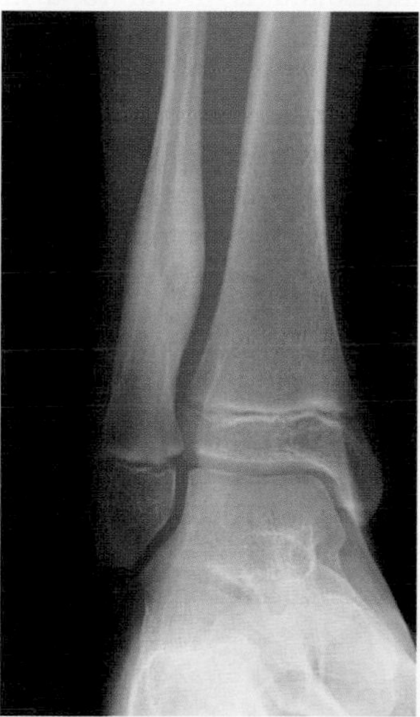

Fig. 18.11 Frontal ankle radiograph of an 11-year-old child with lateral distal leg pain, worse at night. There is thickening of the distal fibula cortex with increased sclerosis. A focal lucency and central nidus is noted medially, consistent with an osteoid osteoma. This was confirmed on CT and subsequent biopsy.

ULTRASOUND IMAGING

Ultrasound imaging is indispensable in paediatric patients due to the lack of ionising radiation, being independent of sedation in most cases and the ability of the ultrasound machine to be readily deployed to different patient locations. There are new functional ultrasound techniques that are currently in use such as contrast-enhanced ultrasound (CEUS) and elastography which further negate the need for high cost and lengthy cross-sectional imaging which may require sedation.

Abdominal Ultrasound Imaging

There are innumerable indications for abdominal ultrasound examination referrals. The commonest is a child with abdominal pain such as intussusception, hypertrophic pyloric stenosis (Fig. 18.12) or acute appendicitis. Organ-specific ultrasound can also be requested such as renal ultrasound post-UTI (please refer to your local or international guidelines) or liver ultrasound in the case of deranged liver function tests, cirrhosis or post liver transplant. Although ultrasound is impaired by bowel gas, recent technological progress and sonography experience have enabled the delineation of bowel wall

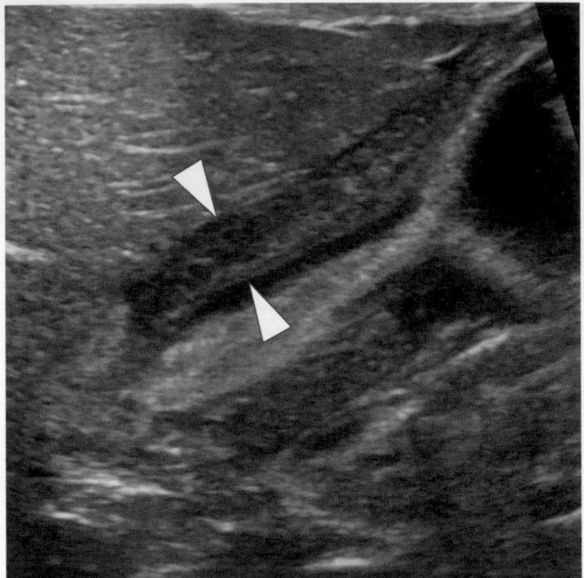

Fig. 18.12 Spot ultrasound image of a 4-week-old neonate with projectile vomiting and recent weight loss. Ultrasound confirms a long pyloric canal with thickened pyloric muscles (between the *arrowheads*), consistent with hypertrophic pyloric stenosis.

thickening, bowel dilatation, matted bowel loops and aperistaltic bowel loops.

Hip Ultrasound

Few countries use ultrasound as a universal screening tool for DDH. Many other countries recommend selective ultrasound hip screening for neonates considered high risk for DDH, (such as female, breech and family history of DDH). The hip ultrasound examination for DDH is best carried out from 6 weeks of age to 12 weeks of age (Fig. 18.13).

Hip ultrasound can also be considered if a child presents with hip pain, to look for hip joint effusion. This can be easily done in a child of any age (Fig. 18.14).

Neck Ultrasound

Some of the commonest ultrasound referrals received in radiology departments are for neck lumps. Almost all children and young adults have palpable lymph nodes. Clinical features that would warrant at least an ultrasound exam are a new, growing or painful lump; in addition, if there are associated clinical symptoms such as weight loss, fever or night sweats. Other than lymph nodes, there are other congenital/acquired cystic masses that can also present with a palpable neck lump such as a thyroglossal duct cyst (Fig. 18.15A,B), branchial cleft cyst or lymphatic malformation.

Testicular Ultrasound

Testicular ultrasound is useful to distinguish testicular torsion from epididymo-orchitis but should not delay surgical exploration. A palpable testicular lump including epididymal cyst, testicular neoplasm and scrotal hernia can easily be characterised by ultrasound.

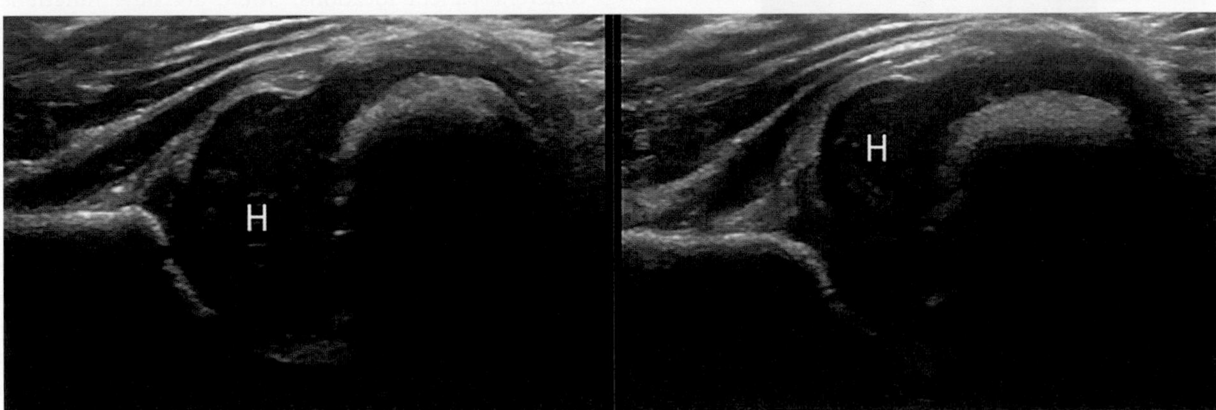

Fig. 18.13 Ultrasound hips of a 1 month old with a clinically dislocated left hip. This was confirmed on ultrasound, with the right hip enlocated and the left hip dislocated. Note the position of the cartilaginous femoral heads labelled H in relation to the acetabular. (Source: Alf Nicholson, Kevin Dunne, Sarah Taaffe, Yusra Sheikh, John Murphy. Developmental dysplasia of the hip in infants and children, BMJ 2023;383:e074507. http://dx.doi.org/10.1136/bmj-2022-074507. Published: 23 November 2023.)

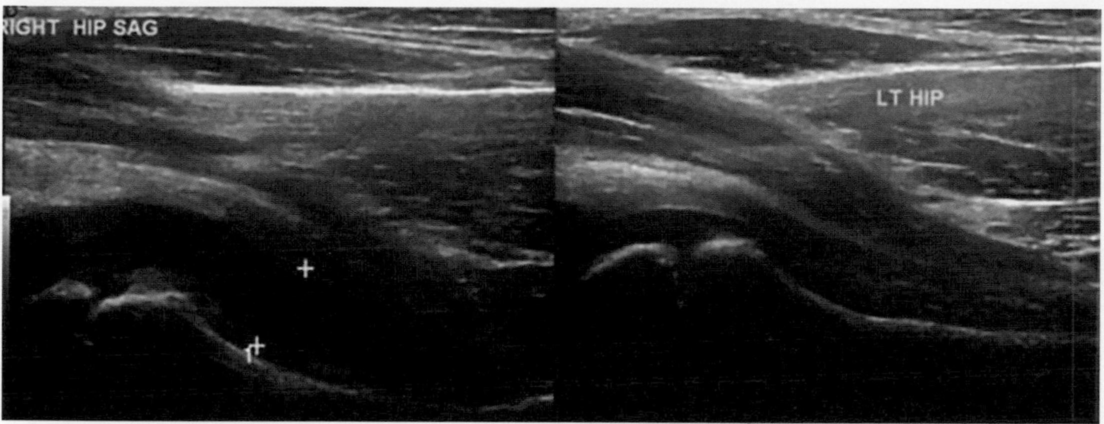

Fig. 18.14 Ultrasound of the hip joints of a 10-year-old child who presented with right-sided limp. There is a right hip joint effusion with expansion of the joint capsule (measured by the callipers). Compared to the normal left hip, no joint fluid.

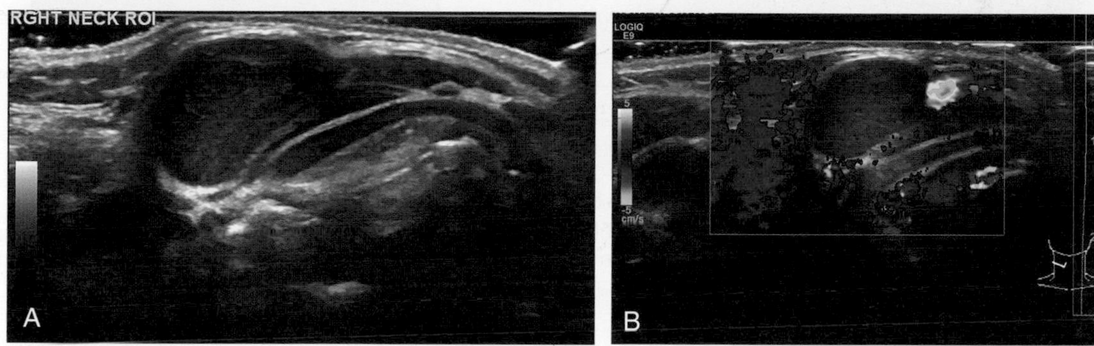

Fig. 18.15 (A) Neck ultrasound for a 2-year-old child who presented with right neck lump in the last 2 weeks. At the site of clinical concern there is a well-defined lump with no internal vascularity on (B) colour Doppler interrogation. The mass moved with tongue protrusion. Appearances are consistent with a thyroglossal duct cyst.

Soft Tissue Ultrasound

Ultrasound is useful in characterising a palpable lump by evaluating its shape, size, vascularity and local invasiveness. If the ultrasound is inconclusive, a follow-up ultrasound, further cross-sectional imaging or biopsy may be recommended. Ultrasound is also useful in evaluating musculoskeletal structures including muscles, tendons and joint spaces for joint effusions. Typically subcutaneous lumps tend to be benign whereas larger masses deep to the fascia are more likely to be malignant.

FLUOROSCOPY

GI Contrast Studies

Barium studies are now performed infrequently. Indications for a barium swallow include the exclusion of a H-type trachea-oesophageal fistula, stricture after caustic ingestion or a vascular ring, although the latter has largely been replaced by a CT angiogram. Barium contrast meal is indicated in neonates with bilious vomiting to exclude midgut volvulus (Fig. 18.16) before gastrostomy in some of the children to delineate the stomach anatomy and position or in a child with cyclical vomiting to exclude malrotation. There are instances where a barium/contrast enema may be indicated such as in a neonate with an inability to pass meconium, or in a child with chronic constipation to exclude Hirschsprung disease.

Micturating Cystourethrogram (MCUG)

The commonest indication would be part of the investigation of a child with recurrent UTI as per local guidelines to exclude vesicoureteric reflux (Fig. 18.17). Other indications may include exclusion of posterior urethral valves in a male child with bilateral hydroureteronephrosis, post major trauma in suspected bladder rupture or if there is a concern for vesicorectal/vesicovaginal fistula.

COMPUTED TOMOGRAPHY

CT is a high radiation dose examination and the study of choice in the event of major trauma, head injury (Fig. 18.18A,B) or acute neurological deterioration due to its wide availability and short scan times, which

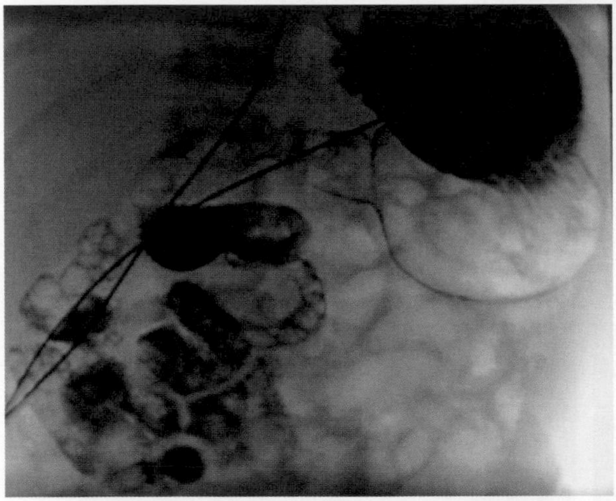

Fig. 18.16 Upper GI contrast examination in a 2 day old with bilious vomiting and abdominal distension confirms a midgut volvulus with a corkscrew configuration of the proximal jejunum.

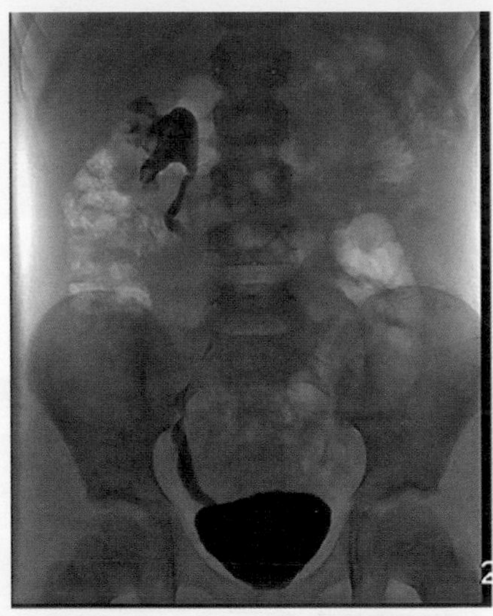

Fig. 18.17 A 5-year-old girl referred by the GP with a history of recurrent UTI. MCUG spot image demonstrates grade IV right vesicoureteric reflux.

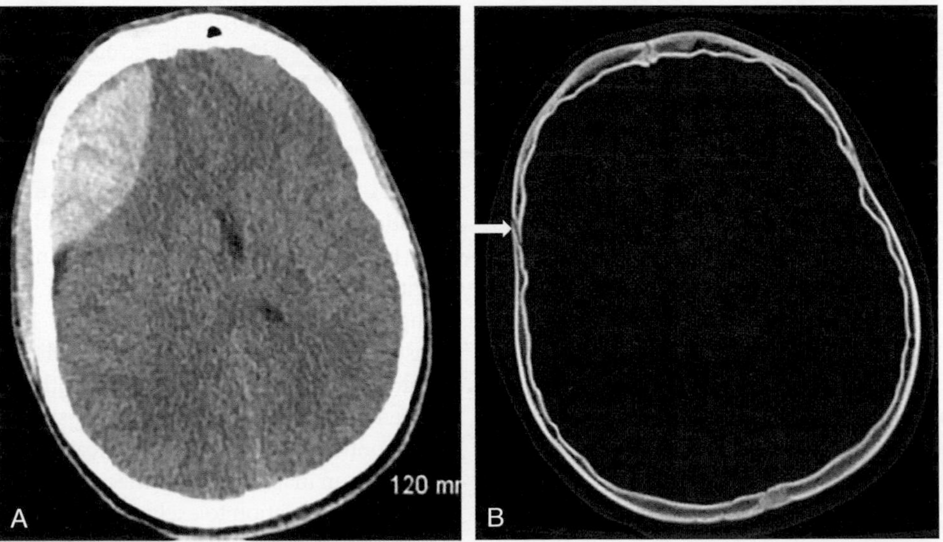

Fig. 18.18 (A) CT head of a 15-year-old boy involved in a high-impact injury with a glasgow coma scale (GCS) of 11 demonstrating a large lentiform hyperdense extraaxial hematoma overlying the right frontal lobe with associated mass effect and midline shift on the underlying brain. (B) Also, note a linear nondisplaced fracture of the left frontal bone (*white arrow*) on the bone window.

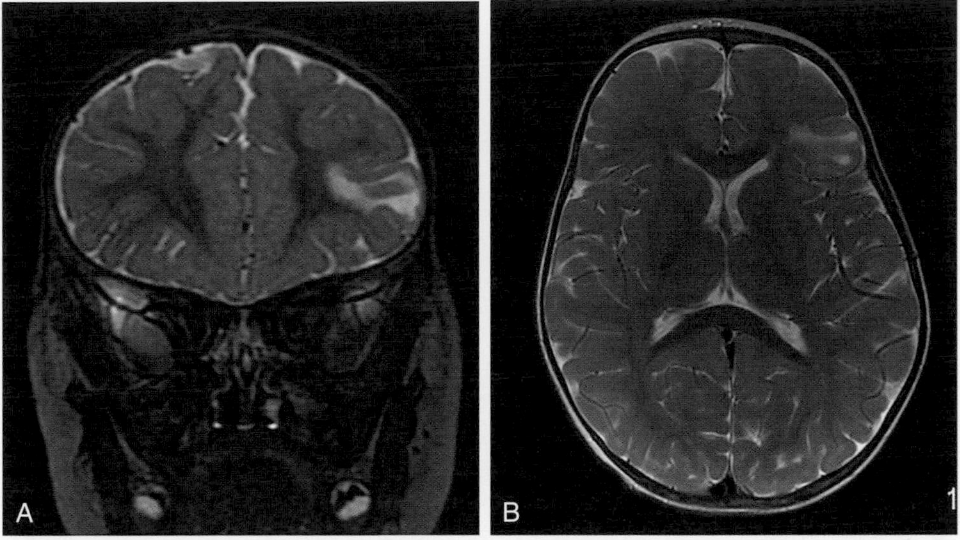

Fig. 18.19 (A) MRI brain of a 15-month-old child with generalised tonic-clonic seizures demonstrating a focal area of T2 hyperintensity within the anterior left frontal lobe cortex with (B) an associated expansion of the gyrus and poor grey-white matter differentiation. This was a pathology-proven focal cortical dysplasia.

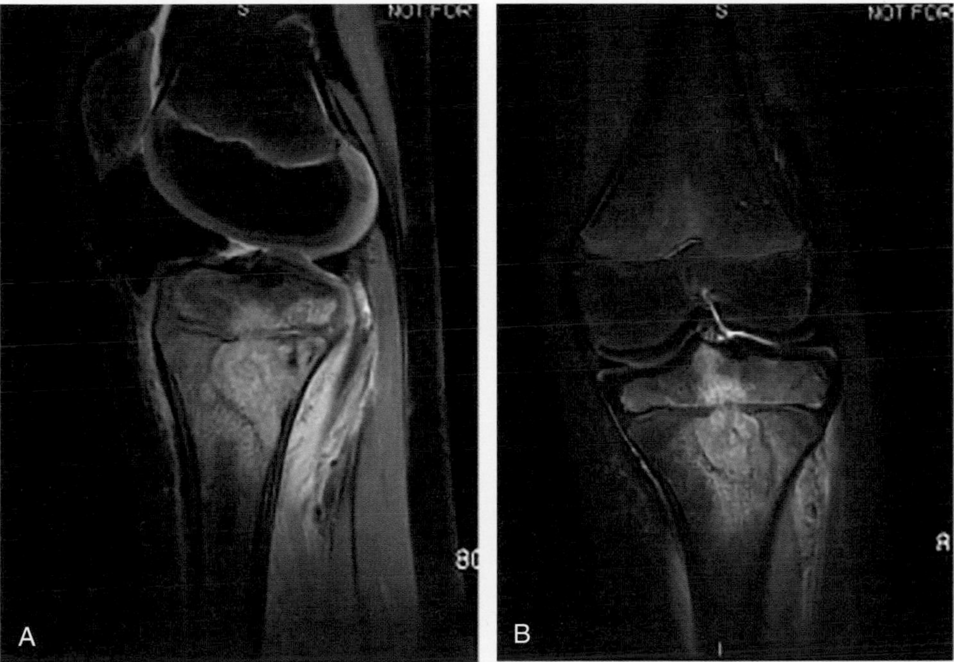

Fig. 18.20 (A) MRI of the left knee in a 9 year old referred with anterior knee pain for the last few weeks. Radiographs demonstrated a lucent lesion. (B) Subsequent MRI demonstrates an intraosseous abscess in the proximal tibia metaphysis extending to the adjacent epiphysis with some subperiosteal elevation and surrounding soft tissue oedema. Appearances are consistent with Brodie's abscess related to a focus of subacute or chronic osteomyelitis.

means children often do not have to be under sedation or general anaesthetic. Due to its tomographic and 3-D reconstruction ability, CT is extremely useful in delineating complex fractures and bone lesions, which can be used as a roadmap during interventional procedures. Children presenting with an acute abdomen, however, commonly have an ultrasound examination initially, as CT is considered a problem-solving tool in such instances.

MAGNETIC RESONANCE IMAGING

Magnetic resonance imaging (MRI) does not utilise any ionising radiation and has exquisite soft-tissue contrast. Intravenous contrast could be used to further delineate the abnormality by further enhancing the soft tissue differentiation. Patients with documented nonferromagnetic implants such as cardiac pacemakers and cochlear implants can safely have the MRI despite the strong magnetic fields. Unlike CT, MRI examinations are long, and children below 7 years may either need sedation or general anaesthetic, as motion may severely degrade the interpretation of imaging.

MRI brain imaging is indicated in infants with neonatal encephalopathy, where changes help predict the outcome. Other indications for MRI brain are in cases of suspected cerebral palsy, developmental regression with loss of skills and in intractable seizures where a focal lesion or focal cortical dysplasia (Fig. 18.19A,B) may be seen.

MRI is the imaging of choice in the diagnosis of osteomyelitis (Fig. 18.20A,B), spinal dysraphism and staging of CNS tumours.

19

Twelve Memorable Diagnoses

Alf Nicholson, Aisling Dunne, Neale Kalis, John Murphy

This chapter will highlight a number of memorable cases that are both rare and may be challenging to diagnose. A key attribute in clinical medicine (including paediatrics) is to be aware of common presentations but to be ready for a 'deeper dive' and seek further investigations if the diagnosis proves elusive and the infant or child is not improving. These memorable scenarios are somewhat subjective, but all have significant learning points.

BOX 19.1 CLINICAL HISTORY

An Infant with Profound Hypothermia

A 7-day-old male infant was brought to the local paediatric emergency department because his parents had found that he had become cold. The home temperature was a satisfactory 20°C.

His temperature on arrival was 31°C. He was very cold to touch, and his heart rate was 80 beats per minute. His respirations and BP were normal. His blood glucose was normal. He was alert. The initial measures undertaken were to place him on a heating mattress and put him in a warmed incubator. A septic screen was taken, and he was commenced on intravenous antibiotics. His temperature rose slowly to 36°C over the following 6 hours.

His background history was unremarkable. He was born at term with a birth weight of 3.8 kg. He had two older sisters, both of whom were healthy. His newborn heel prick screen had been normal.

In essence, the presentation was of a one week male infant with profound hypothermia who was otherwise medically stable.

His full septic screen was negative. Thyroid function studies and his MRI brain scan were normal. Subsequent blood tests showed reduced levels of serum copper and ceruloplasmin. The diagnosis of Menke's disease was subsequently confirmed by the presence of a mutation in the ATP7A gene. This gene affects how the body transports copper and maintains copper levels.[1]

At the time of presentation, the infant did not have the coarse kinky hair associated with the condition, as it only appears after 2 months of age.

He was treated with daily Copper Histidinate subcutaneously. This treatment increased his serum copper concentrations and helped to maintain his body temperature.

He developed seizures and a brain MRI showed the characteristic findings of cerebral atrophy and tortuosity of the cerebral blood vessels. The skeletal survey showed osteoporosis and Wormian bones. By the age of three months, he had the typical coarse, sparse, twisted hair (Fig. 19.1).

Clinical Pearls

Profound hypothermia is a very uncommon presentation in an infant. An environmental cause was

Continued

BOX 19.1 CLINICAL HISTORY—CONT'D

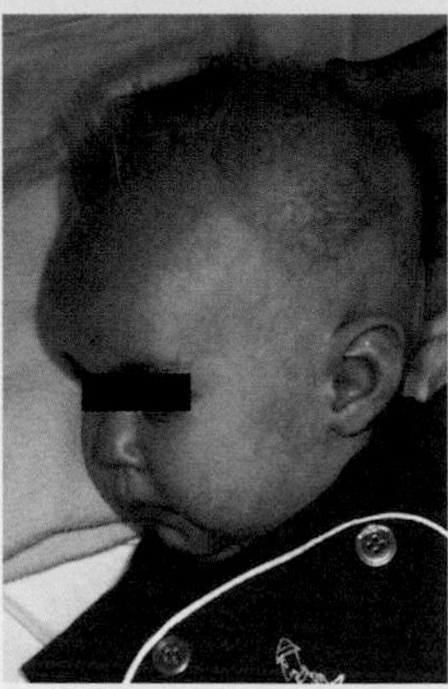

Fig. 19.1 Sparse, short, hypopigmented hair in Menkes disease. (Reproduced with permission from Schachner L, Hansen R. *Pediatric Dermatology.* Third edition, Mosby; 2003.)

excluded by the adequate home temperature. The normal Guthrie card tests effectively excluded primary hypothyroidism.

Menke's disease presents with poor weight gain, hypotonia, abnormal temperature regulation with either hypothermia (as in this case) or hyperthermia, fragile and wiry hair (later presentation) and the subsequent evolution of seizures.

Pitfalls to Avoid

Abnormal temperature regulation is an early feature of Menke's disease.

In this clinical situation Menkes disease was a valid consideration, particularly when there is no other more obvious explanation such as sepsis.

BOX 19.2 CLINICAL HISTORY

A Complication of ITP in an 8 Week Old

A male infant was born by spontaneous vertex delivery weighing 3.2 kg at birth. There were no perinatal complications, and vitamin K was administered on the first day of life. He presented at 8 weeks old with a 24-hour history of a petechial rash over the face and trunk. Family history was negative for coagulopathy. He was apyrexial, and all vital signs were normal. He was admitted for further investigation.

His examination revealed a thriving infant with a widespread petechial rash (Fig. 19.2), no hepatosplenomegaly and no evidence of mucosal bleeding.

Initial investigations showed a platelet count of 2×10^3/mcL and thus the advice of a paediatric haematologist was sought. With no active bleeding at the time, a decision was made to hold intravenous immunoglobulin (IVIG) treatment and observe with close haematology input. After 24 hours, the haemoglobin had dropped to 8.5 g% and platelets were 3. A decision to administer IVIG was made, as the blood film was consistent with immune thrombocytopenia (ITP).

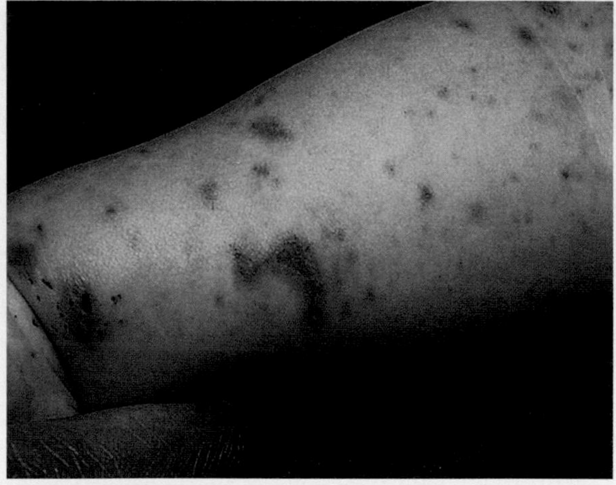

Fig. 19.2 Petechiae in lighter skin. (Singh SB. Petechial rash. In: *Pediatrics a Competency-Based Companion.* Elsevier; 2011: Case 55, Fig. 98.1).

12 hours later:

Sudden jerking of the left arm was noted on 3 occasions. An urgent CT and subsequent MRI brain were coordinated and showed a right parietal and occipital haemorrhage. The infant was intubated and transferred to pediatric intensive care unit (PICU) and given a platelet transfusion, further IVIG and Factor 7 and transexamic acid.

Subsequent progress:

Platelet count rose to 150. There were no further seizures on phenobarbitone. He spent 6 days in PICU and started an MDT rehabilitation programme.

A repeat MRI showed residual ischaemic changes and, subsequent developmental assessment showed him to be developmentally appropriate for his age. Formal neurodevelopmental review at 6 months of age showed a significant visual field defect and resolving left hemiparesis with a cystic lesion on brain MRI. The risk of epilepsy was felt to be 20%.

Clinical Pearls

The role of IVIG in the prevention of intracerebral hemorrhage (ICH) is not clear, and IVIG has potential side effects not least acute anaphylaxis and blood-borne infections.

ICH when it occurs can have very significant neurological sequelae.[2]

Pitfalls to Avoid

ICH is vanishingly rare as a complication of acute ITP in infancy and childhood.

Mucosal bleeding does *not* have to be present for ICH to occur.

The highest risk group are young infants with platelet counts under 10.

BOX 19.3 CLINICAL HISTORY

A 3-Month-Old with Apparent Sepsis

A 3-month-old male infant presented with acute vomiting and diarrhoea over 6 hours. He was noted by his family doctor to be very pale with marked lethargy and floppiness. In view of these concerns and his age, he was promptly referred to hospital with a tentative diagnosis of sepsis. On arrival he looked unwell, and his blood gases showed a metabolic acidosis. He was promptly admitted, had a full septic screen with a delayed lumbar puncture and was commenced on broad-spectrum antibiotics. All his subsequent cultures were clear, and he was discharged home after 4 days in hospital.

Some 6 weeks later, he presented with almost identical symptoms, and on this second occasion, he had a noted low temperature and was quite hypovolaemic. He received intravenous fluids and again was commenced on empirical intravenous antibiotics. Again, cultures proved negative, and the parents were quite concerned about this recurrence of unexplained symptoms. On this second occasion, some blood was noted in the stool sample passed. An ultrasound excluded intussusception. His paediatrician decided to commence a trial of exclusion of cow's milk protein. Happily, there were no further episodes, and a diagnosis of food protein-induced enterocolitis syndrome (FPIES) was made.

Clinical Pearls

FPIES is a clinical diagnosis, and there are often significant delays in making the diagnosis with up to three or more similar presentations before a healthcare professional makes the correct clinical judgement.[3]

Common trigger foods include cow's milk, fruits and vegetables, fish, and hen's eggs.[4]

Key presenting features include marked lethargy with floppiness, pallor, and diarrhoea.

Pitfalls to Avoid

Be aware of FPIES in infants who present on a number of occasions with apparent sepsis. Clinical recognition is key.

Dietary exclusion is the treatment of FPIES with subsequent challenge.

Cow's milk is the most frequently seen trigger and most tolerate later re-introduction of milk protein.

FPIES can present with symptoms of hypovolaemia and may mimic sepsis.

FPIES tends not to occur in exclusively breast-fed infants prior to the introduction of solids.

BOX 19.4 CLINICAL HISTORY

A Puzzling Case of Failure to Thrive

A 7-month-old male was admitted to hospital for assessment of faltering growth. His birth weight was 3.09 kg (9–25%) and weight on admission was 5.8 kg (under 0.4%).

He had an extended stay in hospital with dietetic and Speech and Language Therapy input and had initial significant weight gain on NG feeds, but after 7 weeks in hospital, his weight had dropped to 5.57 kg. Routine investigations including full blood count, serum electrolytes, sweat test and coeliac serology were all normal. He had a brief spell at home prior to being re-admitted 2 weeks postdischarge with further weight loss of 350 grams. He had significant cachexia due to recent weight loss.

He had further dietetic input in the hospital but continued to lose weight. At this point a further multidisciplinary and in-depth review took place.

After much deliberation, a brain MRI scan was performed, and the diagnosis was made (Fig. 19.3).

The diagnosis was diencephalic syndrome of infancy due to a pilomyxoid astrocytoma where 20% lead to diencephalic syndrome. Presenting features include profound emaciation, preserved linear growth, locomotor hyperactivity and occasional euphoria.[5,6]

Recommended management is first biopsy and then nutritional support with PEG feeds followed by chemotherapy (vincristine + carboplatin).

Clinical Pearls

Failure to thrive is a very common diagnosis and most often relates to feeding issues and psychosocial concerns.

Admission to hospital is the right strategy when weight loss is ongoing.

Many cases have social issues (often related to poverty), but infants admitted to hospital will invariably gain weight and may lose weight post discharge home again. That pattern simply did not occur here.

Pitfalls to Avoid

Always review the growth pattern, the history from the family and always entertain new and rare diagnosis if the infant is not improving or progressing along expected lines.

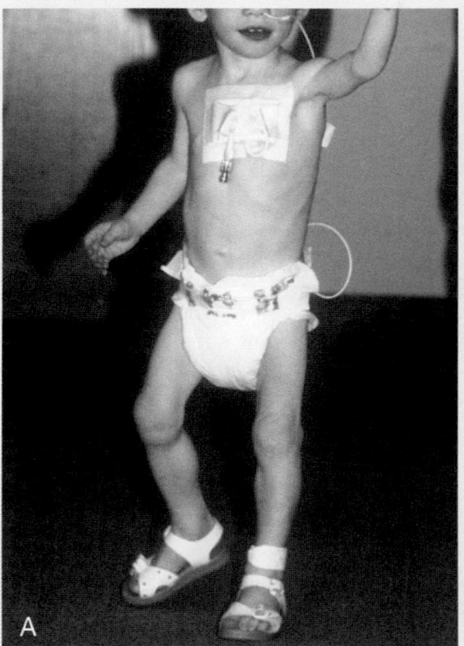

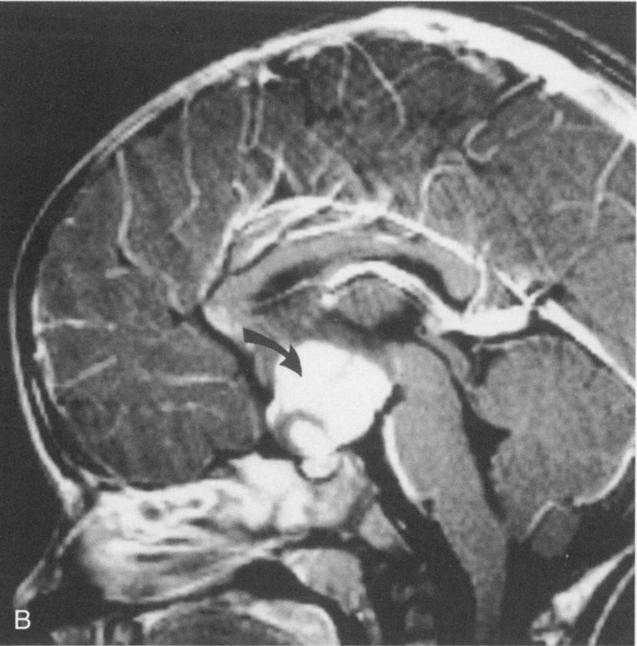

Fig. 19.3 (A) A young girl with emaciation as part of Russell's diencephalic syndrome due to a hypothalamic glioma, demonstrated in contrast-enhanced magnetic resonance imaging. (B) The arrow points to the lesion. (Source: Liu, Volpe, and Galetta's *Neuro-Ophthalmology: Diagnosis and Management,* Third Edition, 2019.)

BOX 19.5 CLINICAL HISTORY

Recurrent Hyponatremic, Hypochloremic Metabolic Alkalosis – A Surprising Diagnosis

An 8-month-old male infant presented with a history of nonprojectile vomiting not related to food intake. There was increased irritability for two days prior to admission. The infant was exclusively breast fed. Serum acid base status, electrolytes and renal function tests were requested. These showed persistent hyponatremia with a low sodium of 116 mmol/L, marked hypochloremia and metabolic alkalosis. The infant was admitted for further investigation.

The infant had two prior admissions with a similar history and metabolic profile. On both admissions the biochemical profile normalised with intravenous fluids and electrolyte supplementation. Ultrasound examinations excluded pyloric stenosis. Investigations were performed to exclude Bartter Syndrome or renal potassium wasting and happily these investigations were negative.

On examination, he was a well-nourished infant with a normal blood pressure of 100/50 mmHg. There was no clinical evidence of raised intracranial pressure or features of hypothyroidism. The remainder of the examination was normal.

On further detailed enquiry, it was found that his mother had been taking paroxetine (an SSRI for depression) during the pregnancy and postdelivery. A sample of breast milk and infant blood was sent for paroxetine levels. The presence of paroxetine in both the breast milk and the infant serum was confirmed. Breastfeeding was stopped, and the infant was discharged on no medication with a normal metabolic profile four days later. At subsequent follow up he was thriving, asymptomatic with a normal metabolic profile.

Clinical Pearls

Metabolic alkalosis with a low chloride is typically seen in hypertrophic pyloric stenosis particularly if the diagnosis is delayed. Metabolic alkalosis is also seen in newborns of mothers with bulimia. The chronic use of thiazide or loop diuretics in newborns can also lead to metabolic alkalosis. In infants with severe bronchopulmonary dysplasia with severe hypercapnia or cystic fibrosis with excessive loss of chloride via the skin, an elevated bicarbonate and reduced chloride may be seen.

Bartter syndrome and Gitelman syndrome are both rare and have an autosomal recessive mode of inheritance. In Bartter syndrome, there is a high urinary chloride, hypokalemia, metabolic alkalosis and elevated serum levels of renin and aldosterone. Infants with Bartter syndrome tend to present with poor weight gain, polyuria and tend to develop dehydration. Gitelman syndrome is milder and presents with hypokalemia, metabolic alkalosis, and a low magnesium level due to excess urinary losses of magnesium.

All the above diagnoses were entertained and excluded by history or investigations.

Paroxetine is an inhibitor of the reuptake of serotonin antidepressant included in the class of SSRI's. Hyponatremia due to the syndrome of inappropriate secretion of antidiuretic hormone (SIADH) is not infrequently seen as a side effect of SSRI's.[7] Like the other SSRI's, paroxetine is excreted in the breast milk of nursing mothers but had been considered, along with sertraline, to be safe to use while breastfeeding.

Pitfalls to Avoid

There are several drugs that are not advised if the mother is breastfeeding.

Cyclophosphamide may be linked to neutropenia in the infant and methotrexate as part of a chemotherapy regime precludes breastfeeding.

In terms of maternal anticonvulsants, ethosuximide is found in high amounts in breast milk and thus is best avoided.

In terms of illicit drugs, it is noteworthy that cocaine and marijuana are excreted in breast milk in notable concentrations and thus clearly affect the infant.

For heroin addicts on methadone programmes, methadone excretion into breast milk is minimal and thus those on methadone programmes can breast feed.

Other drugs to avoid if breastfeeding include amiodarone (which may affect thyroid function in the infant), lithium (requires close monitoring on a case-by-case basis), aspirin and opioids including codeine.

In general, avoid slow-release formulations if breastfeeding.

All breast-feeding mothers should be asked about medication intake

If the diagnosis does not fit, revisit the history and examination.

BOX19.6 CLINICAL HISTORY

Three Siblings with Central Cyanosis

Three siblings (twin boys aged four and a two-year-old girl) presented with central cyanosis (Fig. 19.4) to the paediatric emergency department. They had been put to bed with a bottle of milk at 20.00 hours and an hour later were found to have blue lips by their parents. They were rushed to hospital via emergency ambulance.

On admission, all three were cyanosed and unresponsive with respective oxygen saturations of 80%, 60%, and 50%. The two with the lower oxygen saturations required intubation and ventilation because of a deteriorating Glasgow coma scale. However, despite artificial ventilation, their oxygen saturation did not improve.

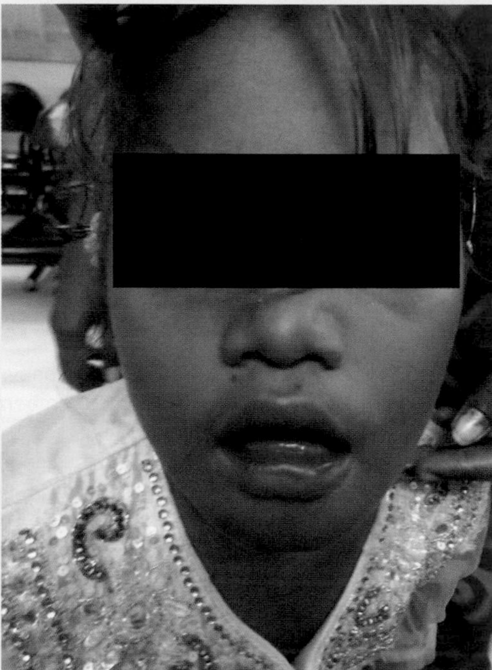

Fig. 19.4 Bluish discolouration of tongue suggestive of central cyanosis. (Source: Anupama S, Nisha R, Sai Shiva G. *Pediatrics Practical Essentials*, 1st edition, 2023, Elsevier Inc.)

The possibility of methaemoglobinaemia was considered at this point as the underlying cause of their cyanosis.[8,9] The three children were administered Methylene Blue intravenously and, almost miraculously, five minutes later all three children were pink and stable. They went on to make a complete recovery.

The subsequent methaemoglobin concentrations were between 30% and 80% with the normal methaemoglobin concentration being less than 4%.

The cause of the methaemoglobinaemia in this instance was the ingestion of sodium nitrite. Their father, who was a butcher, had brought home a small bag of sodium nitrite that he had been using to cure meat. His wife mistook it for a bag of sugar and put a teaspoonful in each child's bottle of milk when putting them to bed.

Clinical Pearls

When more than one child in a family becomes critically unwell it is important to consider whether it is something they have ingested or inhaled.

Pitfalls to Avoid

Methaemoglobinaemia is an important consideration when previously healthy children remain cyanosed despite adequate resuscitation.

Methylene Blue is safe to use, and it acts very quickly as was seen in this case.

If unexplained cyanosis in a previously well child, think about methaemoglobinaemia and have methylene blue close to hand.

BOX 19.7 CLINICAL HISTORY

A 5-Year-Old with Apparent Abdominal Pain and a Stooped Posture

Case Presentation

A 5-year-old boy presented with abdominal pain on three occasions over a six-week period to his local emergency department with the only finding of apparent constipation on plain abdominal X-ray. He received oral stool softeners, but the abdominal pain persisted.

Examination revealed a soft abdomen with no faecal masses palpable.

When he was asked to walk, it was very clear that he had a striking kyphotic posture. On palpation of the posterior spine, he was slightly tender over T 12. His repeat plain X-ray showed a compression fracture of T 12 (Fig. 19.5). An emergency spinal MRI showed compression of the spinal cord, and thus he was taken to theatre for an emergency spinal cord decompression. A biopsy confirmed a diagnosis of eosinophilic granuloma of the body of T12. This condition is benign but can be locally invasive as in this case. It accounts for up to 25% of spinal tumours in children. Happily, he made an uneventful recovery without any neurological impairment.

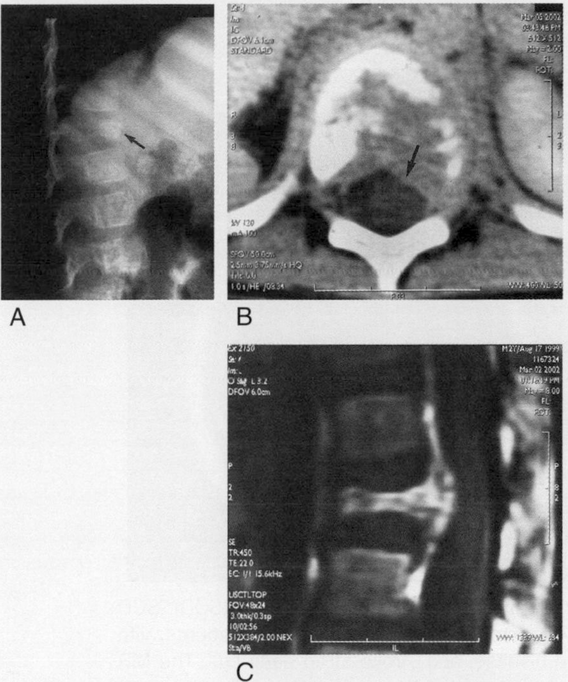

Fig. 19.5 Eosinophilic granuloma: 2-year-old boy with eosinophilic granuloma. (A) Plain lateral radiograph of the lumbar spine demonstrates at least 50% loss of height of T12 vertebral body (arrow) – 'vertebra plana' appearance. Disc spaces are preserved. Axial postcontrast CT image (B) and sagittal T1-weighted postcontrast MR image (C) show the associated soft tissue mass mildly narrowing the spinal canal (arrow in B). Enhancement of the flattened T12 vertebral body and the associated epidural soft tissue is well demonstrated on the MR image. (YSULT; 2004)

Clinical Pearls

For spinal cord tumours, symptoms that should alert the clinician include back pain (present in 2/3rds of cases), an abnormal gait (as in this instance), focal motor weakness or sphincter disturbance.[10,11,12]

Spinal cord tumours are quite rare in children, and the mean interval to diagnosis is 7.8 months.[13]

In general, a useful clinical pointer is that children with spinal cord tumours tend to resist flexion of the vertebral column due to pain and, if asked, will tend to flex their hips or knees.[14]

Other symptoms of spinal cord tumours include irritability, distressing pain and screaming at night, poor appetite with consequent weight loss, a waddling gait and fear of moving about.

Later neurological symptoms may develop including paraesthesia, a neurogenic bladder and either absence or exaggeration of lower limb deep tendon reflexes.

Painful spinal rigidity is an important clinical feature of spinal cord tumours.

Pitfalls to Avoid

In this case, his abdominal pain was referred pain from his spinal vertebral compression.

Be cautious before concluding that severe abdominal pain is due to constipation in particular where the abdominal pain is recurrent, and the child has not responded to initial stool softeners.

Observation of his gait and the examination of his spine showed significant kyphosis in this case.

Spinal tumours in children are a significant challenge to diagnose. They often present with vague symptoms.

Back pain in childhood should be considered as a sinister symptom warranting careful consideration.

BOX 19.8 CLINICAL HISTORY

A 7-Year-Old Boy with an Acute Stroke

A 7-year-old male with Sickle cell disease (SCD) was being followed up at the specialist haematology clinic. He had been fully immunised and had normal developmental milestones.

He attended the regional haematology service on a regular basis but had not attended more recently due to COVID restrictions. He thus missed his scheduled appointments for transcranial doppler screening.

He presented to a local paediatric department 100 Km from the specialist centre with an episode of collapse with a sudden loss of power in the left arm and leg. His examination revealed a depressed level of consciousness with an apparent loss of power on the left side. A diagnosis of acute stroke was made, and he was promptly referred for an urgent brain MRI (Fig. 19.6).

Clinical Pearls

Outcomes for children and adults with SCD have improved largely due to newborn screening, pneumococcal immunisation and ongoing penicillin prophylaxis and ongoing education about potential serious complications such as stroke.

Impaired immunity due to hyposplenism significantly increases the risk of life-threatening pneumonia, sepsis, and meningitis. Vaccination has helped reduce this risk, but serotypes not covered by vaccines still pose a threat.

Stroke predominantly affects children with SCD.[15]

Transcranial Doppler identifies children who are at the highest risk of developing stroke. In children with sickle cell anaemia and presentation with a rapid onset of neurological symptoms warrant investigation with both brain MRI and magnetic resonance angiography (MRA).[16]

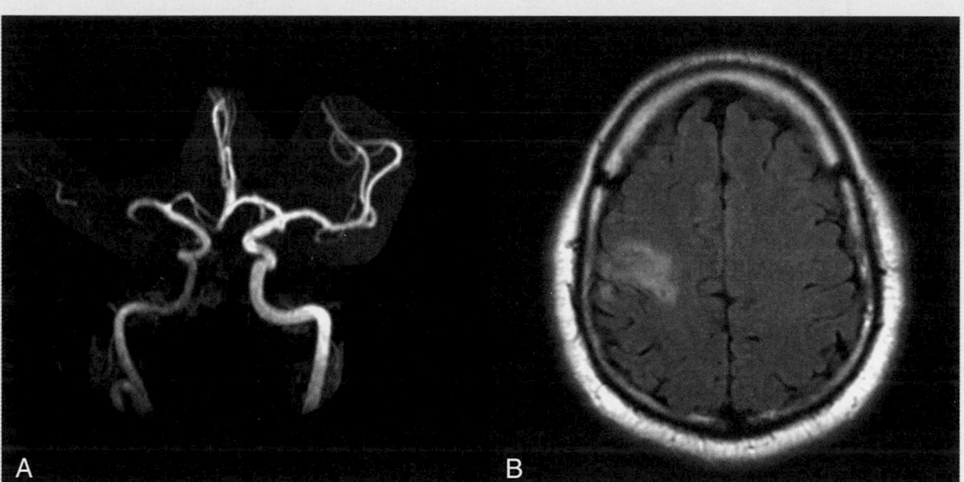

Fig. 19.6 Magnetic resonance (MR) images obtained in a patient with sickle cell disease (SCD). SCD is an autosomal recessive hemoglobinopathy caused by a mutation in the β-globin gene. Patients with SCD might develop painful crises, large artery occlusive disease, and stroke at an early age. The MR angiogram (A) shows an occlusion of the right middle cerebral artery. MR images show a hyperintense signal in fluid-attenuated inversion recovery (FLAIR) sequence (B) denoting chronic ischemic changes in the MCA territory. (Caplan LR, et al. *Primer on Cerebrovascular Diseases.* 2nd edition, Academic Press, 2017, Elsevier Inc.)

Pitfalls to Avoid

For acute stroke in SCD, the treatment is prompt exchange transfusion followed by regular transfusions to prevent stroke recurrence.[15]

Primary stroke prevention identifies children at highest risk using transcranial Doppler screening followed by a transfusion programme.

BOX 19.9 CLINICAL HISTORY

A 10-Year-Old with Apparent Psychosis

A 10-year-old boy presented to his family doctor with a history of social withdrawal, a flattened affect, general apathy, and apparent vivid hallucinations causing him great distress. The previous summer, following holidays in Spain, he had jaundice noted and was felt to have infectious hepatitis. His jaundice settled over a period of two weeks, and his liver function tests returned to normal.

His past medical history was completely normal, and his family history was negative for psychiatric illness. He had two younger siblings both of whom were well. He was referred to a consultant child and adolescent psychiatrist and had a full assessment with psychology review performed. His symptoms varied but tended to wax and wane. His neurological exam was completely normal, and both his MRI brain scan and EEG were also found to be normal. He was referred for an ophthalmology opinion where Kayser-Fleischer (KF) rings were evident (Fig. 19.7) and Wilson's disease was diagnosed.

Clinical Pearls

Disorganised thinking accompanied by delusions or hallucinations are characteristic features of psychosis.

Be aware that other mental health disorders and organic causes need to be outruled.

Typical psychotic symptoms include a flattening of affect with social withdrawal, hallucinations, delusions (fixed false beliefs) and disorganised speech and behaviour.

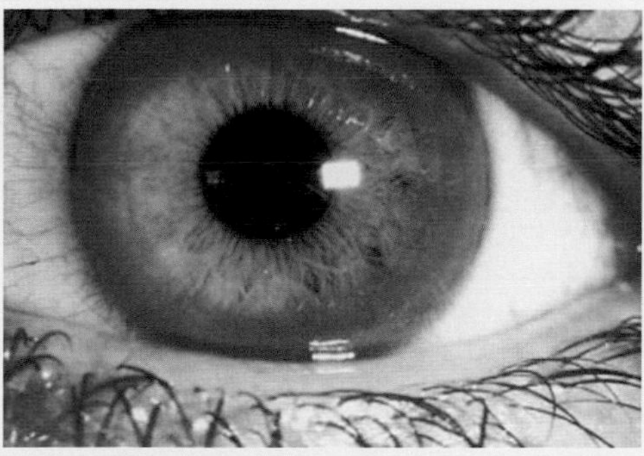

Fig. 19.7 Kayser-Fleischer rings. (Sanyal AJ, et al. *Zakim and Boyer's Hepatology*. 7th edition, 2018, Elsevier Inc.)

Key differential diagnoses in adolescence include substance abuse, delirium, and pervasive developmental disorder. Substance abuse can be picked up by history and both blood and urine toxicology.

Clinical assessment in acute psychosis requires a meticulous history.

If no organic cause is found, consider a primary psychiatric illness and refer to a child and adolescent psychiatry team.

For Wilson's disease, the average age at presentation is 13.2 years (range 5–35 years).

In Wilson disease (WD), there is a progressive copper accumulation in the liver and the brain.[17]

Treatment is chelation with penicillamine leading to a marked increase of urinary copper excretion. Rarely, liver transplantation is required usually for fulminant liver failure.

Pitfalls to Avoid

Psychosis is exceedingly rare in preadolescent children.

Always consider substance abuse or an organic diagnosis in a preadolescent with psychiatric symptoms.

Childhood presentations of Wilson disease range from asymptomatic hepatomegaly to fulminant hepatic failure.

Wilson disease may also present with movement or mood disorders or frank psychosis.

If the finding of a high bilirubin (over 300 μmol/L) is linked with modest elevation of transaminases (100–500 IU/L), GGT and ALP levels, then WD is suggested.

Kayser-Fleischer (KF) rings are gold or grey-brown opacities in the peripheral cornea that become more apparent with the progression of the disease (Fig. 19.7).

Treatment is chelation with penicillamine leading to a marked increase of urinary copper excretion.

Neuropsychiatric symptoms, common in adults with WD, are less often seen in children.

The presence of psychotic symptoms with a history of jaundice may point towards Wilson's disease.

High urinary copper excretion (over 1000 ug per 24 hours) and a low serum caeruloplasmin level are seen in Wilson disease, and the definitive diagnosis requires a liver biopsy.

Wilson disease is a treatable condition with an excellent response to agents such as penicillamine.

BOX 19.10 CLINICAL HISTORY

Chronic Constipation with an Underlying Diagnosis

A 11-year-old boy presented with an episode of collapse on to the kitchen floor. Since early childhood he had recurrent episodes of chronic constipation which led to his admission to hospital after birth and on two occasions at 7 years of age, when he received standard laxative medications to which he responded well. He was a frequent attender at the GP surgery with ongoing constipation and abdominal pains. He was admitted to hospital via ambulance, successfully resuscitated and had a diagnosis made of an enterocolitis secondary to Hirschsprung disease (HD) with associated septic shock. He made an excellent recovery and was discharged home two weeks postadmission.

Clinical Pearls

HD is an important differential in neonates with delayed passage of meconium, poor feeding or abdominal distension. HD may very rarely present in older children with chronic severe constipation or as enterocolitis (Fig. 19.8).

Always ask about the passage of meconium after birth, constipation dating from birth and unresponsive to high dose laxatives, associated failure to thrive and marked distension with the absence of overflow staining.

The gold standard for confirming the diagnosis of HD is histopathology which demonstrates the absence of the ganglion cells. A suction biopsy will confirm the diagnosis.[18]

Pitfalls to Avoid

Enterocolitis can occur even post pull-through procedure for HD and has a high morbidity and mortality.

It is sometimes easy to think that unrelenting constipation relates to noncompliance with treatment or psychosocial issues.[19]

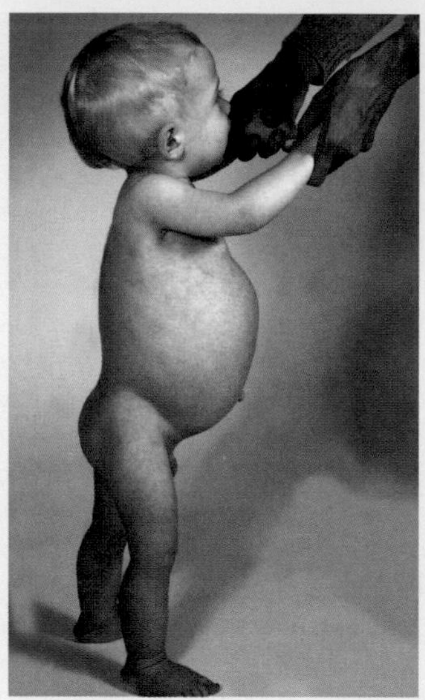

Fig. 19.8 Hirschsprung Disease. A historical photograph of a 3-year-old child with neglected Hirschsprung disease demonstrating failure to thrive, with buttock wasting and a dilated abdomen. (Quick CRG, Biers SM, Arulampalam, THA, eds. *Essential Surgery: Problems, Diagnosis and Management.* 6th edition, Elsevier.)

It is exceptionally rare for HD to present with indolent constipation.

If HD is suggested by contrast enema, then suction rectal biopsy is mandatory to confirm the diagnosis.

Constipation is incredibly common whereas HD is exceptionally rare. This is a most atypical presentation of HD.

BOX 19.11 CLINICAL HISTORY

A Rare Diagnosis Hidden Behind a Common Presentation

A 14-year-old girl presented with a three-week history of increasing respiratory distress and associated tiredness and a week long history of apparent dysphagia.

She had a background history of asthma, and the working diagnosis on admission was an acute exacerbation of asthma with coincident lower respiratory tract infection. Over the first 6 hours she deteriorated and required admission to paediatric intensive care due to repeated desaturations and increasing respiratory difficulty. Subsequently she required ventilation and had a failed extubation attempt after 3 days. She spent 8 days in intensive care and, during her stay, she was noted to be markedly anxious, and this was felt to be related to the severity of her illness and psychological support was provided. She was eventually discharged home after 2 weeks, and a respiratory clinic appointment was made.

Over the next 5 months, she developed a number of puzzling symptoms including **progressive dysphonia** (a change in voice), **dysphagia** (whereby she was unable to gag, and food gets stuck in her throat with associated regurgitation and significant weight loss), **facial and general weakness** with associated drooling of secretions, an inability to rise from the floor without assistance and a striking **personality change** with more withdrawn affect. For a while the family put these symptoms down to anxiety surrounding her six-day stay in intensive care, but after a period of months, they became progressively more concerned and therefore returned for further assessment.

On examination, she had evidence of striking weight loss and had significant neurological findings including a positive Gowers sign with proximal weakness, bilateral facial muscle weakness with bilateral ptosis (Fig. 19.9) and an absent gag reflex. A neurological consultation was swiftly sought.

Her MRI brain and spine were both normal, her EMG was diagnostic for myaesthenia gravis, and her CT thorax excluded a thymoma. Her anti-MuSK and antiacetylcholine receptor antibodies were positive.

She was commenced on pyridostigmine at increasing dosage and later oral steroids once known to be varicella immune and made an excellent clinical response to both.[20] She has regular neurology reviews.

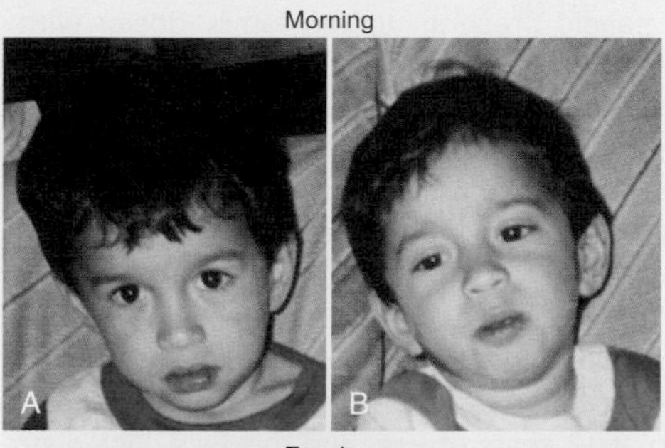

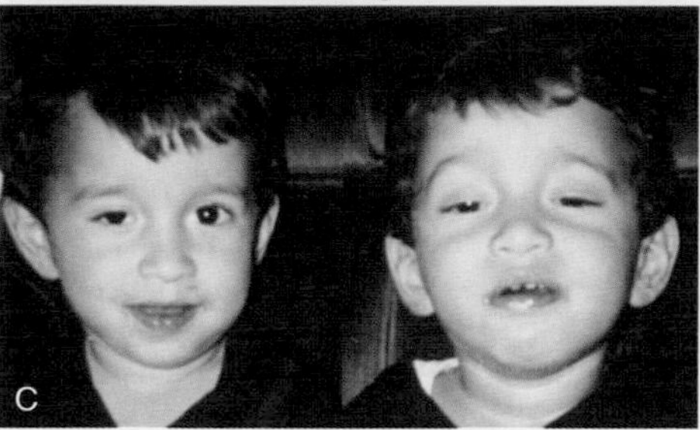

Fig. 19.9 Twins, Age 2, Both with Acetylcholine Receptor Myasthenia Gravis (A, B). In the morning, one (B) has mild bilateral lid ptosis, slightly worse on the right; ptosis is worse or has become apparent in the evening in both boys (C). (*Bradley and Daroff's Neurology in Clinical Practice*. 8th edition, 2022).

Clinical Pearls

There is a likely link between initial presentation with respiratory failure and later diagnosis of Myasthenia Gravis.

Pitfalls to Avoid

The presenting features of myaesthenic crisis are pooling of secretions, bronchospasm, paradoxical breathing and anxiety with rapid and shallow respirations, and these are the exact symptoms of her initial presentation requiring admission to intensive care.[21]

A single fibre EMG is the gold standard investigation to make the diagnosis.

Symptoms evident in this case were fatigue, anorexia, vomiting and weight loss with some very significant behavioural changes.

Rare conditions can present with relatively common symptoms, but in this case the presentation was quite atypical for acute asthma or pneumonia.

Generalised Myaesthenia Gravis can be life-threatening if presenting in myaesthenic crisis with resultant respiratory failure which affects about 1% of patients.

BOX 19.12 CLINICAL HISTORY

A 15-Year-Old Transgender Woman

A 15-year-old presents to the family doctor with panic attacks and significant anxiety. Past and perinatal history were unremarkable, and she was an excellent student excelling in all subjects. She had been subject to repeated in-person and online bullying in view of the fact that she was far more comfortable chatting with girls, had a strong interest in fashion and disliked field sports.

Her family doctor conducted a detailed review and found her to have a completely normal examination and to be in Tanners Stage 4 pubertal development. Her voice had broken at 13 years of age, and this was quite distressing to her. Following referral to a child and adolescent mental health service, she confided that she felt that she 'was a girl' and was very distressed by the changes that had occurred during her pubertal development.

She was referred by her family doctor to a specialist team in gender dysphoria, and a comprehensive review was undertaken including a full mental health assessment. After a full workup, options for treatment were discussed with both her and the family.

Her parents had great trouble coming to terms with her distress and gender identity.

Clinical Pearls

Gender dysphoria (or transgender) is an umbrella term where a person's innate and perceived sense of being differs from their assigned gender at birth. Transition or affirmation is a process whereby transgender persons can present in the gender that they identify with.

Up to 0.6% of US citizens identify themselves as being transgender. Most presentations occur during adolescence. Persons with gender dysphoria tend to experience higher rates of bullying, and they are prone to mental health issues.

The majority present in late adolescence, and the gender incongruence is persistent and evident over many years. Prior to puberty, they may present with a consistent interest in opposite-gender activities. Some find the process of pubertal development to be quite traumatic and upsetting.

Parental denial and distress in relation to gender dysphoria in their child is quite challenging. Following a history and examination several core laboratory investigations are recommended. These include LH, FSH, oestradiol and testosterone levels. Referral to a specialist clinic may be helpful.[22,23]

Transition in gender dysphoria may be reversible, partially reversible, or irreversible.

The timing of social affirmation may vary greatly.

Puberty blockers are generally used at Tanners stage 3 breast and testicular development. Halting puberty may buy time for the person and family to explore their gender roles.

Gonadotrophin release hormone (GnRH) analogues may be used later in puberty (Tanner Stage 3 to 5) and may block erectile function and the onset of menses – both very distressing to persons with gender dysphoria.

The earlier identification of gender dysphoria is important and, combined with parental support and guidance, leads to improved physical and mental health outcomes.

Irreversible transition involves surgery and is a major step.

For transgender men, giving testosterone will achieve testosterone levels in the normal range. After 3 to 6 months of testosterone therapy, an increase in facial and body hair and muscle mass, a deeper voice and the cessation of menses are expected. Testosterone therapy may lead to polycythaemia and increase the risk of endometrial cancer so hysterectomy should be considered.

For transgender women, oestrogens will lower testosterone levels, protects bone health, and will produce feminising effects. Goals include a reduction in facial hair, breast development and fat redistribution in a female pattern. Giving oestrogens after puberty will not alter either voice or height attainment.

Pitfalls to Avoid

No medical intervention is recommended prior to the onset of puberty, and the timing of social transition (in essence gender presentation in public) should be discussed with the young person and the family. Paediatricians may need extra training to support the child and family.[24]

Choices in terms of surgery should be patient-specific and should always balance the risks and benefits of surgery and a consideration of future fertility.

Surgical options for transgender women include facial feminisation, breast augmentation and genital reconstructive surgery.

Surgical options for transgender men include chest reconstruction, hysterectomy, and oophorectomy and phalloplasty.

For health professionals dealing with persons with gender dysphoria, the building of good rapport and trust with the patient is important.

Social affirmation of a different gender includes taking a new name and pronoun in the new gender as well as changes in clothing, shoes, hair and makeup.

If gender incongruence persists with pubertal onset a referral to a specialist multidisciplinary team should be made. A comprehensive assessment with skilled mental health professionals is required before medical intervention with hormonal therapy can be considered.

No medical intervention is needed prior to puberty. As puberty begins, gonadotrophin releasing hormone agonists may help to delay puberty and buy some time until a long-term treatment plan is established.

REFERENCES

1. Vairo FPE, Chwal BC, Perini S, Ferreira MAP, de Freitas Lopes AC, Saute JAM. A systematic review and evidence-based guideline for diagnosis and treatment of Menkes disease. *Mol Genet Metab*. 2019;126(1):6–13. doi:10.1016/j.ymgme.2018.12.005.
2. Elalfy MS, Eltonbary KYEM, El Ghamry IR, et al. Intracranial hemorrhage in primary immune thrombocytopenia (ITP): 20 years' experience in pediatrics. *Eur J Pediatr*. 2021;180(5):1545–1552. doi:10.1007/s00431-020-03923-x.
3. Agyemang A, Nowak-Wegrzyn A. Food protein-induced enterocolitis syndrome: a comprehensive review. *Clin Rev Allergy Immunol*. 2019;57(2):261–271. doi:10.1007/s12016-018-8722-z.
4. Stiefel G, Alviani C, Afzal NA, et al. Food protein-induced enterocolitis syndrome in the British Isles. *Arch Dis Child*. 2022;107(2):123–127. doi:10.1136/archdischild-2020-320924.
5. Curran MA, Madhavan VL, Caruso PA, Ebb DH, Williams EA. Case 31-2017. A 19-month-old girl with failure to thrive. *N Engl J Med*. 2017;377(15):1468–1477. doi:10.1056/NEJMcpc1706106.
6. Trapani S, Bortone B, Bianconi M, et al. Diencephalic syndrome in childhood, a challenging cause of failure to thrive: miniseries and literature review. *Ital J Pediatr*. 2022;48(1):147. doi:10.1186/s13052-022-01316-4.
7. Abdul Aziz A, Agab WA, Kalis NN. Severe paroxitene induced hyponatraemia in a breast fed infant. *JBMS*. 2004;16;195–198. Accessed at https://www.bhmedsoc.com/jbms/
8. Jaffé ER. Methaemoglobinaemia. *Clin Haematol*. 1981;10(1):99–122.
9. Skold A, Cosco DL, Klein R. Methemoglobinemia: pathogenesis, diagnosis, and management. *South Med J*. 2011;104(11):757–761. doi:10.1097/SMJ.0b013e318232139f.
10. Wilne S, Collier J, Kennedy C, Koller K, Grundy R, Walker D. Presentation of childhood CNS tumours: a systematic review and meta-analysis. *Lancet Oncol*. 2007;8(8):685–695. doi:10.1016/S1470-2045(07)70207-3.
11. Wilne S, Walker D. Spine and spinal cord tumours in children: a diagnostic and therapeutic challenge to healthcare systems. *Arch Dis Child Educ Pract Ed*. 2010;95(2):47–54. doi:10.1136/adc.2008.143214.
12. Merlot I, Francois J, Marchal JC, et al. Spinal cord tumors in children: a review of 21 cases treated at the same institution. *Neurochirurgie*. 2017;63(4):291–296. doi:10.1016/j.neuchi.2017.01.008.
13. Crawford JR, Zaninovic A, Santi M, et al. Primary spinal cord tumors of childhood: effects of clinical presentation, radiographic features, and pathology on survival. *J Neurooncol*. 2009;95(2):259–269. doi:10.1007/s11060-009-9925-1.
14. Fisher PG. 50 years ago in The Journal of Paediatrics. A report of 16 tumors of the spinal cord in children; the importance of spinal rigidity as an early sign of disease. *J Paediatr*. 2010;157:25. doi:10.1016/j.jpeds.2010.01.021.
15. Rees DC, Williams TN, Gladwin MT. Sickle-cell disease. *Lancet*. 2010;376(9757):2018–2031. doi:10.1016/S0140-6736(10)61029-X.
16. Hirtz D, Kirkham FJ. Sickle cell disease and stroke. *Pediatr Neurol*. 2019;95:34–41. doi:10.1016/j.pediatrneurol.2019.02.018.
17. Fernando M, van Mourik I, Wassmer E, Kelly D. Wilson disease in children and adolescents. *Arch Dis Child*. 2020;105(5):499–505. doi:10.1136/archdischild-2018-315705.
18. Thakkar H, Curry J. Hirschsprung's disease. *Paediatrics and Child Health*. 2020;30(10):341–344. doi:10.1016/j.paed.2020.07.001.
19. Bradshaw O, Foy R, Seal AK, Darling JC. Childhood constipation. *BMJ*. 2021;375:e065046. doi:10.1136/bmj-2021-065046 Published 2021 Dec 2.
20. Gilhus NE, Verschuuren JJ. Myasthenia gravis: subgroup classification and therapeutic strategies. *Lancet Neurol*. 2015;14(10):1023–1036. doi:10.1016/S1474-4422(15)00145-3.

21. Gilhus NE. Myasthenia Gravis. *N Engl J Med*. 2016;375(26):2570–2581. doi:10.1056/NEJMra1602678.
22. Pang KC, Wiggins J, Telfer MM. Gender identity services for children and young people in England. *BMJ*. 2022;377:o825. doi:10.1136/bmj.o825 Published 2022 Apr 1.
23. Safer JD, Tangpricha V. Care of transgender persons. *N Engl J Med*. 2019;381(25):2451–2460. doi:10.1056/NEJMcp1903650.
24. Ferrara P, Ruiz R, Corsello G, et al. Adequate training and multidisciplinary support may assist pediatricians in properly handling and managing gender incongruence and dysphoria. *J Pediatr*. 2022;249:121–123. doi:10.1016/j.jpeds.2022.07.009 e2.

20

Surviving and Thriving Throughout a Career in Healthcare

Sarah Taaffe, Hani Malik, Ciaran O'Boyle

'When health is absent, wisdom cannot reveal itself, art cannot manifest, strength cannot fight, wealth becomes useless and intelligence cannot be applied'.
—Herophilus 300 BC

CHAPTER OUTLINE

The above quote is as apt today as it was way back then. There is no doubt that working in healthcare is very challenging and reports of stress, burnout and ill health are now quite frequent. In this chapter we are going to explore the promotion of wellness and resilience amongst healthcare professionals. We will also explore the issue of burnout and strategies to avoid it.

Developing resilience enables doctors and nurses to adapt to challenges and discover new ways of going forward.[1] Developing personal resilience, however, is only half the answer. Many of the factors that lead to burnout are organisational, and a systems approach to well-being is also crucial. There is a need to acknowledge system-wide issues originating from workplace culture, healthcare policy and public expectations.[2]

COMPLEXITY AND CHALLENGE IN MODERN HEALTHCARE INVOLVING CHILDREN

Paediatrics, paediatric nursing and primary care can be very stimulating and fulfilling careers and the attraction of working with children and families and the great diversity of presentations are all very positive elements.[3] There is great enjoyment in the rapid recovery seen in most children, the wonders of normal development and the countless disarming moments that dealing with children brings. However, you are not just managing illness in the child but also parental fears and worries, and this adds significantly to the stress experienced by child health professionals and families.

There have been significant changes over the past number of years that have increased stress amongst primary care doctors, paediatricians and nurses. There are increasing numbers of children with highly complex needs and life-limiting conditions, and we are also seeing changed societal expectations about what can or should be done to extend life.[3] Ethical and moral dilemmas should be worked out by the clinical team and the family but are often the subject of heated debate on social media, putting added pressures on both the family and professionals.

Workforce shortages, service gaps and long waiting times all contribute to added stress and exhaustion for families and the professionals looking after them.

Most inpatient wards are no longer filled with children bouncing back to health within 48 hours but, rather, with children with medically complex conditions who have multiple healthcare needs. Families are under immense pressure, often frustrated and exhausted, and this frustration can boil over at times.

The provision of improved peer and team support structures, shared learning from high-profile events and the provision of support to families who are in a difficult and stressful situation relating to their child's illness are all helpful.

BURNOUT IN TRAINEES

For paediatric trainees, a recent Young European Academy of Paediatrics Blog (January 2022)[4] reflected responses from trainees across Europe and showed that just under 40% of trainees considered leaving the programme, and factors associated with dissatisfaction included a perceived lack of flexibility of the training programme, long working hours and 24 hours on-call shifts. Burnout was a significant issue, and the recent pandemic exacerbated the problem.

BURNOUT IN NEONATAL AND PAEDIATRIC NURSES

A recent scoping review[5] and systematic meta-analysis[6] highlighted experiences of the neonatal or paediatric nurse reflecting the unique nature of providing care to sick newborns, infants and children, the high level of empathic engagement of these nurses and the complexities of working with parents and families from varied social and ethnic backgrounds.

Burnout was most evident in those nurses working in high-intensity environments such as neonatal or paediatric intensive care or in the emergency department. Attendance and up-skilling by means of skills development courses helped to reduce burnout. Factors such as overcrowding, understaffing and poor work conditions all contributed to higher rates of burnout amongst nurses.

Coping with Stress

Low-level (termed 'healthy') stress can improve performance and is quite helpful in acute situations. When pressures exceed an individual healthcare professional's ability to cope there is a dip in performance. Resilience is the ability to cope with and bounce back from adversity and to both persevere and adapt in challenging situations. Resilience is essential for those working in healthcare.[7]

> Each of us working in healthcare should be encouraged to consider what well-being looks like through our own personal lens.

By understanding what feeds our own relaxation, we can weave some recognised recommendations as outlined below into our routine (Table 20.1).

As a pioneer in western mindfulness practice, Jon Kabat-Zinn[8] defines mindfulness as 'the awareness that emerges through paying attention, on purpose, and nonjudgmentally to the unfolding of experience moment by moment'. There are mindfulness courses that are specially geared to healthcare professionals; one such example is *Mindful Medics,*[9] a UK-based course, which supports medical doctors in managing their own stress and stresses often unique to medical practitioners and shares the latest in neuroscience and evidenced-based techniques in this evolving area.

Wellness and Health in Doctors

There is no doubt that being a doctor is both rewarding and demanding, as medicine is challenging both physically and emotionally. As a healthcare professional, there is an expectation that a certain level of stress is integral to our roles, and stress can therefore be used in a positive manner.

Reflecting on strategies that have worked in the past in times of challenge and adversity, having supportive colleagues and engaging in self-care are all likely to tilt the balance towards the development of strong coping skills, wellness and resilience.

On the other hand, unrealistic expectations, a perfectionist personality, always wishing to be the 'superhero' and an under-supportive culture at work can tilt the balance firmly towards work-related stress.

> Stress may dramatically increase following a sentinel adverse event or if litigation is being pursued by an unhappy family.

TABLE 20.1 Key Steps to Well-being

1	Professional connection	Connect with fellow professionals and form personal social networks.
2	Physical exercise	Engage in physical exercise be it in a team or individual sports, yoga, Tai-Chi or running.
3	Dedicated family time	Being present and dedicating time to your family and children, offering lots of kindness and compassion can help boost well-being.
4	Life-long learning	Engaging in lifelong learning and teaching others is very important and keeps one fresh learning other skills or spending time on hobbies (such as pottery, baking or art) can keep you stimulated and energised.
5	Practice mindfulness	With techniques such as breath work, meditation, exploration in nature, or focused activities such as the creative arts. Mindfulness is in essence 'staying in the moment', as awareness in the present reduces the tendency to ruminate over the past or worry about the future.[7]
6	Cultivate self-compassion	Cultivation of self-compassion can reduce stress levels associated with working in a healthcare environment.

Most training programmes are structured with a perceived expectation that doctors in training will sacrifice their own well-being for the sake of patients. During training, doctors should be encouraged to explore their attitudes to work, avoid being a 'super hero' and always be aware of their physical and mental health. Integrating self-care awareness and techniques into training programs will help nurture the well-being of healthcare providers as they navigate their medical careers.

Nobody wants to head down the slippery slope of compassion fatigue, burnout, depression or excessive anxiety or disruptive behaviours at work. Physician wellness, on the other hand, has been found to lead to improved system performance and indeed patient outcomes.

Developing Resilience

Resilience is defined as the ability to return to baseline after stressful events and to even grow as a result of facing challenges. Factors associated with resilience in doctors include job satisfaction (especially relating to the doctor–patient relationship) and the use of wellness strategies such as innate optimism, good work–life balance, friends outside of medicine and always taking your holidays. Factors most strongly linked to resilience were meeting recreational needs and the ability to tolerate uncertainty. Supportive professional relationships are incredibly important in promoting resilience.

Developing resilience is a key skill for a doctor, and working in a hospital or primary group setting requires attention to both institutional and individual factors.

> A strong and consistently supportive institutional culture is really important in ensuring the individual is able to practice with both security and confidence.

A compassionate approach to healthcare leadership and culture promotes an inclusive work environment that transcends organisational hierarchy, while promoting trust, intrinsic motivation and creative thinking in followers.

We cannot overemphasise the importance of a healthy, resilient and well-supported team working within a supportive medical culture, and it is this positive working environment that leads to excellent patient care. For a friendly and positive work environment, the key elements are a manageable workload, elements of choice and control for individuals, a system that places emphasis on fairness and respect and that offers support when needed.

Burnout

Burnout is an oft-discussed term and has three dimensions including emotional exhaustion (always running on a 'flat battery'), depersonalisation (lack of empathy for children and their families) and reduced work satisfaction with decreased feelings of work accomplishment.[10]

Emotional exhaustion may present as feelings of being worn out and having very low energy levels. Cynicism refers to a negative or detached response to elements of daily work and presents as irritability, lost idealism and even withdrawal.

Burnout is not an expected reaction to hard work; it is not the same as depression, but severe burnout can evolve into depression.[10]

> The chief factors linked to burnout include a high burden of responsibility, low perceived control, a discordance between individual and organisational values with an unsupportive working environment and isolation.[10]

Compassion and empathy are vital components of an effective physician's values. However, they are finite resources that can deplete when faced with unresolved and evolving work-related stressors. Both can decrease over time when a clinician is faced with unresolved stress. The resulting mismatch between stressors and coping responses can manifest in compassion fatigue or progress further into burnout.[11,12] There is a key distinction to be made between burnout and compassion fatigue. In many respects it is a continuum where unresolved stress leads to compassion fatigue and on to burnout with consequent mental health issues for the doctor. Burnout and compassion fatigue are both highly counter-productive to excellent patient care.

Preventing Burnout in Healthcare Professionals

Burnout tends to start very early during undergraduate education in health sciences and, if tackled and addressed, can be prevented during a later long career in healthcare.

Reflective practice is especially important for trainees to be able to reflect on experiences and their effect on them and understand that medicine and paediatrics are inexact sciences. As a tool for self-care, critical reflection reinforces professional resilience and helps clinicians improve behaviour and practices.[12] Recognising fallibility and that mistakes do occur are key learning elements of a successful training programme.

Mindfulness provides more clarity, calmness and emotional regulation especially when difficult situations are encountered. A mindful practice not only helps with stress reduction but may also avoid further stress arising. Enhanced communication skills enable both the child and family to feel heard and may help to dissipate potentially stressful situations.

> Engaging in mindfulness and exercise are very useful to promote wellness.

Exercise, laughter and meditation have all been shown to increase endorphin levels, and this contributes greatly to an overall sense of well-being. As a fundamental component of positive psychology, mindfulness practice has been found to increase plasma levels of oxytocin, the hormone linked to emotional and social well-being. Exercise is known to improve quality of life and tends to mitigate stress and thereby reduce burnout.

Likewise, many hospitals conduct regular Schwartz Rounds[13] where professionals (be they doctors, nurses, health and social care professionals or support staff) recount their experiences of clinical events that have made a significant impact on them, and thereafter a general discussion occurs in a supportive and confidential atmosphere. We have personally found these Schwartz Rounds or Balint groups to be very helpful.

While compassion is central to healthcare, many health professionals struggle to develop self-compassion. The work of Kristin Neff provides an excellent guide to developing self-compassion.[14]

The health and wellness of the doctor has a considerable impact on the health of children seen by that doctor, and a focus on wellness should commence in the undergraduate years in medical school.

In a systematic review and meta-analysis of interventions to reduce or prevent burnout, it has been shown that efforts directed both at the individual and at changes in the organisational culture are required.[15] Enhancing awareness of burnout is often the vital first step.

Mindfulness training can help the individual doctor identify early symptoms of burnout. Early symptoms might include headaches or muscular tension, irritability, sarcasm, or feelings of self-blame. Cognitive rigidity, difficulties with ambiguity, the setting of boundaries and forgiving oneself can all be acknowledged and addressed.

> Through mindfulness practice, there is an increase in awareness towards the importance of self-care, which in turn improves perceived emotional well-being and promotes self-compassion.

Mindful clinicians can refill the 'flat battery' and are then reinvigorated into instilling compassion into the clinical encounter.

In essence, doctors suffering from burnout have run out of compassion and empathy in their dealings with patients, and the first step to restoring this is by increasing self-compassion through mindfulness.

Dr Reena Kotecha's *Mindful Medics* mantra is[9]:

> 'Health Care starts with Selfcare' a phrase that reminds us that we cannot share our skills and care without first looking after ourselves.

Addressing burnout at an individual level will not be enough for either doctors working in hospital or in the community. Doctors need to be better at self-care or to learn how to integrate self-care into their everyday routine, as part of their undergraduate training.

BURNOUT IN PRIMARY CARE

In primary care, there is some evidence to suggest that the increased use of electronic healthcare records (EHR) is linked to increased burnout.[16]

Doctor well-being may be improved when workflow and communication deficiencies are addressed, and in the United States, scribes have been used to reduce the heavy burden associated with the completion of EHR's. EHRs direct the doctor's attention away from face-to-face interaction with the child and the family and towards data entry and clerical tasks. Voice recognition dictation may be a valuable approach when using EHRs. EHRs also make work possible around the clock and make it more challenging to separate work and home lives.[17]

MENTAL HEALTH ISSUES IN DOCTORS

Regrettably, burnout may escalate and lead to significant mental health issues. Doctors suffering from burnout may benefit from cognitive behaviour therapy (CBT). CBT is also helpful in treating anxiety disorders which are not uncommon in doctors. The key issue is to recognise the symptoms of excess anxiety or burnout and to seek professional help when it is required.

Paediatricians have high rates of reported burnout (over 50% in some studies), a higher rate in females and a higher rate in subspecialities such as critical care.[18] Empathy is reduced in those with burnout, and this significantly worsens the patient experience. Family doctors are also described as being at 'breaking point' and in need of respite.[19] This has worsened considerably during the recent pandemic.

In a UK study of 1651 doctors, 31% of participants reported high levels of burnout and compassion fatigue and often blamed themselves for the inability to adapt to increasing work pressure.[20] Emergency department doctors suffered from higher rates of burnout and stress in comparison to other specialties, while family doctors scored the lowest in compassion satisfaction.

Up to 20% of doctors plan to cut back on clinical work or leave medicine altogether. Burnout exacts a high personal toll leading to both depression and suicidal ideation. Isolation and loneliness may contribute to burnout whereas appreciation is a very effective counterbalance. Other countermeasures include building 'a manageable cockpit' which is free of information overload.[18] This in essence means reducing the complexity of using an EHR (completion may consume 50% of consultation time), unnecessary emails with the risk of missing an abnormal result and, in general, reducing the heavy burden of documentation and administration.

> Burnout is linked to higher rates of suicide, substance abuse and broken relationships.[18]

Studies have found a significant association between increased emotional exhaustion and suicidal ideation. Burnout is also linked to increased medical errors and can lead to a cycle of self-recrimination with feelings of anxiety, guilt, anger and sadness.

We all need to look after ourselves better to be able to care for others.

> The well-being of frontline primary care doctors and paediatricians is fundamental to the healthcare mission and offers the best return on investment.

KEY LEARNING POINTS

There is no doubt that medicine and nursing are both stressful careers, and reports of stress, burnout and ill health are now quite frequent.

Burnout is where meaningful and challenging work becomes unpleasant and unfulfilling, energy is replaced by exhaustion and enthusiasm by cynicism and efficacy turns into ineffectiveness.

Burnout and compassion fatigue are both highly counter-productive to excellent patient care.

Resilience is essential in those working in healthcare. It involves promoting well-being and protecting mental health in healthcare professionals.

Supportive professional relationships are incredibly important in promoting resilience.

We cannot overemphasise the importance of a healthy, resilient and well-supported team working within a supportive medical culture, and it is this positive working environment that leads to excellent patient care.

There is some evidence that the use of electronic healthcare records (both in general practice and in hospital) are linked to increased burnout.

Exercise, laughter and meditation have all been shown to increase endorphin levels, and this contributes greatly to an overall sense of well-being.

The chief factors linked to burnout include a high burden of responsibility, low perceived control, a discordance between individual and organisational values with an unsupportive working environment and isolation.

Burnout exacts a high personal toll leading to both depression and suicidal ideation. Isolation and loneliness may contribute to burnout whereas appreciation is a very effective counterbalance.

As the old proverb says, 'one cannot pour from an empty cup', a reminder that we all need to look after ourselves better to be able to care for others.

REFERENCES

1. Chakr VCBG. Stress management in medicine. *Rev Assoc Med Bras (1992)*. 2021;67(3):349–352. doi:10.1590/1806-9282.20200785.
2. *National Academies of Sciences, Engineering, and Medicine Taking Action Against Clinician Burnout: A Systems Approach to Professional Well-Being*. Washington, DC: The National Academies Press; 2019. doi:10.17226/25521.
3. Cass H, Barclay S, Gerada C, Lumsden DE, Sritharan K. Complexity and challenge in paediatrics: a roadmap for supporting clinical staff and families. *Arch Dis Child*. 2020;105(2):109–114. doi:10.1136/archdischild-2018-315818.
4. European Academy of Paediatrics: Young Eap Blog- Burnout in European Paediatric Training. Jan 2022. Accessed online at: https:// www.eapaediatrics.eu/young-eap-blog-january-2022-burnout-in-european-paediatrictraining/
5. Buckley L, Berta W, Cleverley K, Medeiros C, Widger K. What is known about paediatric nurse burnout: a scoping review. *Hum Resour Health*. 2020;18(1):9. doi:10.1186/s12960-020-0451-8. Published 2020 Feb 11.
6. Pradas-Hernández L, Ariza T, Gómez-Urquiza JL, Albendín-García L, De la Fuente EI, Cañadas-De la Fuente GA. Prevalence of burnout in paediatric nurses: A systematic review and meta-analysis. *PLoS One*. 2018;13(4):e0195039. doi:10.1371/journal.pone.0195039. Published 2018 Apr 25.
7. Suri S Consultant Paediatrician, Nash E GP Registrar. Resilience: surviving and thriving in the paediatric workplace. *Arch Dis Child Educ Pract Ed*. 2018;103(6): 291–295. doi:10.1136/archdischild-2017-313554.
8. Kabat-Zinn J. Mindfulness-Based Interventions in context: past, present, and future. *Clin Psychol*. 2003;10(2):144–156. Accessed online at: https:// doi.org/10.1093/clipsy.bpg016
9. Mindful Medics - Dr. Reena Kotecha l Corporate/Healthcare Professional Website (drreenakotecha.com)
10. The Lancet. Physician burnout: the need to rehumanise health systems. *Lancet*. 2019;394(10209):1591. doi:10.1016/S0140-6736(19)32669-8.
11. Jablow M. 'Compassion fatigue: the toll of being a care provider. *AAMCNews*; 2017. Accessed online at: https://www.aamc.org/news-insights/compassion-fatigue-toll-being-care-provider.
12. Malik H, Annabi CA. The impact of mindfulness practice on physician burnout: A scoping review. *Front Psychol*. 2022;13:956651. doi:10.3389/fpsyg.2022.956651. Published 2022 Sep 20.
13. The Schwartz Center for Compassionate Healthcare in Boston. Accessed online at: https://www.theschwartzcenter.org/
14. Neff K. *Self-Compassion*. New York, William Morrow; 2011.
15. West CP, Dyrbye LN, Erwin PJ, Shanafelt TD. Interventions to prevent and reduce physician burnout: a systematic review and meta-analysis. *Lancet*. 2016;388(10057):2272–2281. doi:10.1016/S0140-6736(16)31279-X.

16. Babbott S, Manwell LB, Brown R, et al. Electronic medical records and physician stress in primary care: results from the MEMO Study. *J Am Med Inform Assoc*. 2014;21(e1):e100–e106. doi:10.1136/amiajnl-2013-001875.
17. Olson K, Marchalik D, Farley H, et al. Organizational strategies to reduce physician burnout and improve professional fulfillment. *Curr Probl Pediatr Adolesc Health Care*. 2019;49(12):100664. doi:10.1016/j.cppeds.2019.100664.
18. Babineau T, Thomas A, Wu V. Physician Burnout and Compassion Fatigue: Individual and Institutional Response to an Emerging Crisis. *Curr Treat Options Peds*. 2019;5:1–10. doi:10.1007/s40746-019-00146-7.
19. Iacobucci G. GPs are at 'breaking point' and in need of respite, leaders warn. *BMJ*. 2021;373:n1139. doi:10.1136/bmj.n1139. Published 2021 May 4.
20. McKinley N, McCain RS, Convie L, et al. Resilience, burnout and coping mechanisms in UK doctors: a cross-sectional study. *BMJ Open*. 2020;10(1):e031765. doi:10.1136/bmjopen-2019-031765. Published 2020 Jan 27.

ADDITIONAL READING

Annabi CAA. Chapter 2 Mindfulness as a strategy to weather challenges. In: Marques J, ed. *Innovative leadership in times of compelling changes strategies, reflections, and tools*. Germany: Springer International Publishing; 2021.

Bentley PG, Kaplan SG, Mokonogho J. Relational Mindfulness for Psychiatry Residents: a Pilot Course in Empathy Development and Burnout Prevention. *Acad Psychiatry*. 2018;42(5):668–673. doi:10.1007/s40596-018-0914-6.

Berwick DM. Improving patient care. My right knee. *Ann Intern Med*. 2005;142(2):121–125. doi:10.7326/0003-4819-142-2-200501180-00011.

Callahan K, Christman G, Maltby L. Battling Burnout: Strategies for Promoting Physician Wellness. *Adv Pediatr*. 2018;65(1):1–17. doi:10.1016/j.yapd.2018.03.001.

Card AJ. Physician Burnout: Resilience Training is Only Part of the Solution. *Ann Fam Med*. 2018;16(3):267–270. doi:10.1370/afm.2223.

Celia F. *Compassion fatigue: a different kind of burnout*, 2019. [Online]. Accessed online at: https://physicians.dukehealth.org/articles/compassion-fatigue-different-kind-burnout/

Chen C, Meier ST. Burnout and depression in nurses: A systematic review and meta-analysis. *Int J Nurs Stud*. 2021;124:104099. doi:10.1016/j.ijnurstu.2021.104099.

Dunne PJ, Lynch J, Prihodova L, et al. Burnout in the emergency department: Randomized controlled trial of an attention-based training program. *J Integr Med*. 2019;17(3):173–180. doi:10.1016/j.joim.2019.03.009.

Ellen Braun S, Kinser P, Carrico CK, Dow A. Being Mindful: A Long-term Investigation of an Interdisciplinary Course in Mindfulness. *Glob Adv Health Med*. 2019;8:2164956118820064. doi:10.1177/2164956118820064. Published 2019 Jan 9.

Epstein RM, Privitera MR. Doing something about physician burnout. *Lancet*. 2016;388(10057):2216–2217. doi:10.1016/S0140-6736(16)31332-0.

Germer CK, Neff KD. Self-Compassion in Clinical Practice. *Journal of Clinical Psychology: In Session*, Vol. 69(8), 856–867 (2013) C 2013 Wiley Periodicals, Inc. Published online in Wiley Online Library (wileyonlinelibrary.com/journal/jclp). doi: 10.1002/jclp.22021

Hayes B, Prihodova L, Walsh G, Doyle F, Doherty S. What's up doc? A national cross-sectional study of psychological wellbeing of hospital doctors in Ireland. *BMJ Open*. 2017;7(10):e018023. doi:10.1136/bmjopen-2017-018023. Published 2017 Oct 16.

Ito E, Shima R, Yoshioka T. A novel role of oxytocin: Oxytocin-induced well-being in humans. *Biophys Physicobiol*. 2019;16:132–139. doi:10.2142/biophysico.16.0_132. Published 2019 Aug 24.

Jablow M. *Compassion fatigue: the toll of being a care provider*, 2019. [Online]. Available at: https://www.aamc.org/news-insights/compassion-fatigue-toll-being-care-provider/

Lheureux F, Truchot D, Borteyrou X. Suicidal tendency, physical health problems and addictive behaviours among general practitioners: their relationship with burnout. *Work and Stress*. 2016;30(2):173–192. doi:10.1080/02678373.2016.117 1806

National Health Service Leadership Academy. *Medical Leadership Competency Framework*. 3rd ed. Coventry, UK: NHS Institute for Innovation and Improvement; 2011. [ebook]. Accessed online at: https://www.leadershipacademy.nhs.uk/wp-content/uploads/2012/11/NHSLeadership-Leadership-Framework-Clinical-Leadership-Competency-Framework-CLCF.pdf.

Neff KD, Germer CK. A pilot study and randomized controlled trial of the mindful self-compassion program. *J Clin Psycholc*;69(1):28–44. doi:10.1002/jclp.21923.

Oades LG, Steger MF, Delle Fave A, Passmore J. *The Wiley Blackwell Handbook of The Psychology of Positivity and Strengths-Based Approaches to Work*. Oxford: Wiley Blackwell; 2017.

Pradas-Hernández Laura, et al. Prevalence of burnout in paediatric nurses: A systematic review and meta-analysis. *PLoS one*. 25 Apr. 2018;13(4):e0195039. doi:10.1371/journal.pone.0195039.

Stewart MT, Reed S, Reese J, Galligan MM, Mahan JD. Conceptual models for understanding physician burnout, professional fulfillment, and well-being. *Curr Probl Pediatr Adolesc Health Care*. 2019;49(11):100658. doi:10.1016/j.cppeds.2019.100658.

The Stanford Model of Professional Fulfillment™. Accessed online at: https://wellmd.stanford.edu/about/model-external.html.

West M, Eckert R, Collins B, Chowla R. *Caring to change: how compassionate leadership can stimulate innovation in health care.* 1st ed. London, UK: The King's Fund; 2017. [ebook]. Accessed online at: https://www.kingsfund.org.uk/sites/default/files/field/field_publication_file/Caring_to_change_Kings_Fund_May_2017.pdf.

West MA. *Compassionate Leadership: Sustaining Wisdom, Humanity and Presence in Health and Social Care.* UK: The Swirling Leaf Press; 2021.

Wilson H, Cunningham W. *Being a doctor: understanding medical practice.* 1st ed. New Zealand: Otago University Press; 2013.

Wuest Thomas K, et al. Clinical Faceoff: Physician Burnout-Fact, Fantasy, or the Fourth Component of the Triple Aim? *Clinical Orthopaedics and Related Research.* 2017;475(5):1309–1314. doi:10.1007/s11999-016-5193-5.

INDEX

Note: Page numbers followed by '*f*' indicate figures, '*t*' indicate tables, and '*b*' indicate boxes.

N

O

P

Q

R